Workbook for

ICD-10-CM/PCS Coding Theory and Practice

Karla R. Lovaasen, RHIA, CCS, CCS-P
Coding and Consulting Services
Abingdon, Maryland

Jennifer Schwerdtfeger, BS, RHIT, CCS, CPC, CPC-H
Partner, Auditing & Coding Experts, LLC
Crofton, Maryland

ELSEVIER
SAUNDERS

ELSEVIER
SAUNDERS

3251 Riverport Lane
St. Louis, Missouri 63043

Notices

International Standard Book Number: 978-1-4557-0796-6

Publisher: Jeanne R. Olson
Senior Developmental Editor: Jenna Johnson
Publishing Services Manager: Pat Joiner-Myers

Printed in the United States of America

Last digit is the print number: 9   8   7   6   5   4   3   2   1

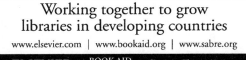

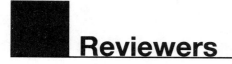

Reviewers

Betty Harr, BS, RHIA
Kirkwood Community College,
Cedar Rapids, Iowa

Dorothy M. Hendrix, MEd, RHIT
East Los Angeles College
Monterey Park, California

Karen C. Hoffman, RHIA
Health Information Technology
Southwest Mississippi Community College
Summit, Mississippi

Sandra L. Johnston, MSEd, RHIA, CPC
Clinical Assistant Professor
The University of Kansas Medical Center
Health Information Management Program
Kansas City, Kansas

Mary Juenemann, RHIA, CCS
Health Information Technology Program
Rochester Community and Technical College
Rochester, Minnesota

Brenda M. Kupecky, MS, RHIA
Ivy Tech Community College–Central Indiana
Indianapolis, Indiana

Jennifer Lamé
Medical Coding and Transcription Instructor
Southwest Wisconsin Technical College
Fennimore, Wisconsin

Judy Truempler, RHIT
North Dakota State College of Science
Whapeton, North Dakota

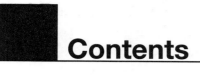

Contents

1 The Rationale for and History of Coding

ABBREVIATIONS/ACRONYMS

Without the use of reference materials, define the following abbreviations or acronyms.

1. AHIMA _____
2. CEUs _____
3. CCS _____
4. DRGs _____
5. OIG _____
6. RHIA _____
7. WHO _____

GLOSSARY DEFINITIONS

Match the glossary term to the correct definition.

1. _____ Ethics
2. _____ Procedure
3. _____ Nomenclature
4. _____ Encoder
5. _____ Credential
6. _____ Compliance
7. _____ Diagnosis
8. _____ Terminology
9. _____ Classification

A. Computer software to assist in code selection and MS-DRG assignment

B. Diagnostic or therapeutic process performed on a patient

C. System of names used as preferred terminology

D. Identification of disease by signs, symptoms, or tests

E. Adhering to accepted standards

F. Degree, certificate, or award that recognizes a course of study taken in a specific field

G. Grouping together, as with items for storage and retrieval

H. Words and phrases that apply to a particular field

I. Moral standards

MULTIPLE CHOICE

Select the correct answer for each of the following.

1. When translating a disease or a procedure to an ICD-9-CM code, one must have knowledge of
   A. Anatomy
   B. Terminology
   C. Coding rules and guidelines
   D. All of the above

2. The current coding system used in the U.S. is known as
   A. DRG
   B. ICD
   C. ICD-10
   D. ICD-9-CM

3. Coded data are not used for the following reason:
   A. Reimbursement
   B. Medical terminology
   C. Research
   D. Planning purposes

4. The purpose of a classification system is
   A. To capture health data
   B. To group like items for storage and retrieval
   C. To compare data
   D. To study patterns of disease

5. ICD-10-CM may be updated
   A. Annually
   B. Biannually
   C. Quarterly
   D. Every other year

6. Coding Certification is offered by the following professional organization:
   A. AHA
   B. NIH
   C. AHIMA
   D. CPC

7. When a compliance plan for coding is constructed, the following steps are crucial:
   A. Conduct audits
   B. Develop coding policies and procedures
   C. Cultivate a relationship with the billing department
   D. All of the above

8. Which of the following is NOT a coding credential?
   A. CCS
   B. CCA
   C. AHIMA
   D. CPC

2 The Health Record as the Foundation of Coding

ABBREVIATIONS/ACRONYMS

Without the use of reference materials, define the following abbreviations or acronyms.

1. CC _____
2. HPI _____
3. TJC _____
4. SOAP _____
5. TPR _____
6. CBC _____
7. MRI _____
8. CPT _____
9. CMS _____
10. DOB _____

GLOSSARY DEFINITIONS

Match the glossary term to the correct definition.

1. _____ Abstracting
2. _____ Symptom
3. _____ Documentation
4. _____ Comorbidity
5. _____ Integral
6. _____ Principal diagnosis
7. _____ Disposition
8. _____ Review of systems
9. _____ Consultant

A. Essential part of a disease process

B. Condition established after study to be chiefly responsible for occasioning admission of the patient to the hospital for care

C. Place a patient goes upon discharge from the hospital

D. Question and answer period between healthcare provider and patient regarding healthcare issues

E. Subjective evidence of a disease or of a patient's condition as perceived by the patient

F. Written or typed information supplied by the healthcare provider to communicate patient data and activity

G. Healthcare provider who is asked to see the patient and provide expert opinion

H. Preexisting secondary diagnosis

I. Extracting data from the health record

Select the correct answer for each of the following.

1. Which of these is NOT a purpose of the health record?
   A. Source of data
   B. Description of patient's health history
   C. Reimbursement
   D. Communication with other healthcare providers

2. A hybrid health record is
   A. A paper record
   B. An electronic record
   C. A record that requires less energy to produce
   D. A record that combines electronic and paper elements

3. According to CMS, which of the following elements apply to the general principles of medical record documentation?
   A. Legible
   B. Dated
   C. Signed
   D. All of the above

4. Which of the following is NOT a part of the UHDDS requirement for patient data that hospitals must report?
   A. DOB
   B. Race
   C. Disposition of patient
   D. Patient's employer

5. It is required by The Joint Commission that a patient's history and physical examination be completed within 12 hours of admittance.
   A. True
   B. False

6. An integrated progress note is
   A. Written by physicians only
   B. Written by any staff involved in patient care
   C. Written by physicians and nurses only
   D. Not allowed by The Joint Commission

7. A progress note written in a SOAP format does not include which of the following?
   A. History taken by the physician
   B. Statement from the patient about what the problem is
   C. A plan for care
   D. The patient's next of kin

8. A coder should commit to memory which of the following?
   A. UHDDS reportable data elements
   B. The definition of principal diagnosis
   C. The list of MS-DRGs
   D. Requirements of The Joint Commission

9. The definition of a principal diagnosis includes which of the following?
   A. Condition determined by study occasioning the admit
   B. Chief complaint
   C. Disposition of the patient
   D. Comorbidities of the patient

10. Which of the following would not meet the requirements for coding an additional diagnosis?
    A. Condition for which a patient is currently receiving treatment
    B. Condition listed by the physician in the discharge diagnosis
    C. Condition that extends the length of stay
    D. Condition that increases the requirement for nursing care or monitoring

11. To code a condition as chronic, the patient must be receiving medication.
    A. True
    B. False

12. Which of the following would NOT be considered integral to the diagnosis of pneumonia?
    A. Cough
    B. Fever
    C. Positive blood culture
    D. Infiltrates on chest x-ray

13. A coder can take the site of a fracture from the x-ray report.
    A. True
    B. False

14. The purpose of physician queries is to improve reimbursement.
    A. True
    B. False

15. It is a good practice to code from abnormal findings in lab reports.
    A. True
    B. False

16. It is acceptable to query using yes or no answers when querying for POA.
    A. True
    B. False

3 | ICD-10-CM Format and Conventions

ABBREVIATIONS/ACRONYMS

Without the use of reference materials, define the following abbreviations or acronyms.

1. NEC _____

2. MS-DRG _____

3. CPT _____

4. ICD-10-CM _____

5. WHO _____

6. NOS _____

GLOSSARY DEFINITIONS

Match the glossary term to the correct definition.

1. _____ Manifestation

2. _____ Neoplasm

3. _____ Etiology

4. _____ Nonessential modifier

5. _____ Essential modifier

6. _____ NOS

7. _____ Conventions

8. _____ NEC

A. Describes the cause or origin of a disease or condition

B. Abbreviation for "not elsewhere classifiable" that means "other specified"

C. Abnormal growth

D. Symptom or condition that is the result of a disease

E. General rules for use of the ICD-9-CM classification that must be followed for accurate coding

F. Terms enclosed in parentheses that, whether present or absent, do not affect code assignment

G. Abbreviation for "not otherwise specified" that means "unspecified"

H. Subterms used in the Alphabetic Index that affect code assignment

MULTIPLE CHOICE

Select the correct answer for each of the following.

1. A cross-reference in the code book that instructs the coder to review another main term in the Index if all required information cannot be found under this particular main term is
   A. *See also*
   B. *See*
   C. *See category*
   D. *See condition*

2. A cross-reference that instructs the coder to look under another term to locate a particular condition is
   A. *See also*
   B. *See*
   C. *See category*
   D. *See condition*

3. The word "with" should be interpreted to mean
   A. Associated with
   B. Due to
   C. All of the above
   D. None of the above

4. An instruction that directs the coder to code the causal condition if it is known is
   A. Code also
   B. *See condition*
   C. *See category*
   D. Code, if applicable, any causal condition

5. The term "and" in a category title should be interpreted as
   A. Including
   B. And/or
   C. Also
   D. With

SHORT ANSWER

Underline the main terms to be located in the Alphabetic Index in the following diagnostic statements.

1. Bee sting

2. Chronic steatorrhea

3. Acute pancreatitis

4. Acute and chronic tonsillitis

5. Adynamic ileus

Using ICD-10-CM Alphabetic Index, locate the following main terms and identify whether the bolded subterm is an essential or nonessential modifier.

6. Otitis **externa** _____

7. **Acute** otitis externa _____

8. **Streptococcal** nasopharyngitis _____

9. **Suppurative** mastitis _____

10. **Congenital** spondylolisthesis _____

Using the Tabular List, answer the following questions.

11. Is acquired clubfoot assigned code Q66.8? _____

     If not, what code is assigned? _____

12. Is passive pneumonia assigned code J18.2? _____

13. Is Crohn's disease of the small and large intestine included in category K50.1?

     If not, what code category is assigned? _____

Using the Alphabetic Index, answer the following questions.

14. Locate the main term "itch" in the Index. Is there another term for "itch" that may be located in the Index? If so, what is the term?

     _____

15. Locate the main term "polyadenitis" in the Index. Is there another term for "polyadenitis" that may be located in the Index? If so, what is the term?

     _____

16. Locate the main term "polypoid" in the Index. What cross-reference is given?

     _____

Using the Tabular List and instructional notes, assign and sequence the following code(s).

17. See code N40.1. Assign code(s) for a patient with benign prostatic hypertrophy with urinary retention.

     _____

18. See code M14.8. Assign code(s) for a patient with arthropathy of the left wrist due to erythema multiforme.

     _____

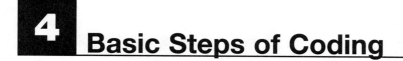

4 Basic Steps of Coding

ABBREVIATIONS/ACRONYMS

Without the use of reference materials, define the following abbreviations or acronyms.

1. CC _____

2. ER _____

3. DS _____

4. OR _____

GLOSSARY DEFINITIONS

Match the glossary term to the correct definition.

1. _____ Eponym

2. _____ Main term

3. _____ Nonessential modifier

4. _____ Discharge summary

5. _____ Subterm

6. _____ Specificity

7. _____ Alphabetic Index

A. Brief report written by a healthcare provider that summarizes a patient's hospital stay

B. Index of disease conditions listed in alphabetical order

C. Diagnosis or procedure named for a person

D. Modifier of a main term

E. Coding to the highest level of detail

F. Term used to identify a disease condition or injury

G. Words that do not affect a code that may be present or absent

CODING

Using the code book, code the following.

1. Sacral pressure ulcer, stage I _____

2. Chronic renal failure _____

3. Acute prostatitis _____

4. Hematemesis _____

5. Sialodocholithiasis _____

6. Black lung disease _____

7. Transient ischemic attack _____

8. Wolff-Parkinson-White disorder _____

9. Aortic valve insufficiency _____

10. Amaurosis _____

11. Seizure disorder, recurrent _____

12. Tic douloureux _____

13. Herpetic felon _____

14. Leiomyoma, uterus _____

15. COPD _____

MULTIPLE CHOICE

Select the correct answer for each of the following.

1. The main term for deep vein thrombosis of the femoral artery is
   A. Artery
   B. Deep
   C. Vein
   D. Thrombosis

2. The main term for abdominal aortic aneurysm is
   A. Abdominal
   B. Aneurysm
   C. Aortic
   D. All of the above

3. The procedure for a small-bowel obstruction treated with a left hemicolectomy is
   A. Obstruction
   B. Hemicolectomy
   C. Bowel
   D. Small

4. The subterm for newborn conjunctival hemorrhage is
   A. Newborn
   B. Conjunctival
   C. Hemorrhage
   D. A and B

5. Identify the nonessential modifier for pneumonia.
   A. Aspiration
   B. Fulminant
   C. Chlamydia
   D. Allergic

6. It is appropriate to code from the Alphabetic Index in ICD-10-CM.
   A. True
   B. False

7. What is a principal procedure?
   A. The condition found after study to be chiefly responsible for the admit
   B. The first procedure performed on a patient
   C. A procedure performed for diagnostic purposes
   D. The procedure that is most related to the principal diagnosis

5 General Coding Guidelines for Diagnosis

ABBREVIATIONS/ACRONYMS

Without the use of reference materials, define the following abbreviations or acronyms.

1. AHA _____
2. GPO _____
3. HIPAA _____
4. DHHS _____
5. CMS _____
6. AHIMA _____
7. NCHS _____

GLOSSARY DEFINITIONS

Match the glossary term to the correct definition.

1. _____ Acute
2. _____ Symptom
3. _____ Asymptomatic
4. _____ Conventions
5. _____ Etiology
6. _____ Sign
7. _____ Manifestation
8. _____ Combination code
9. _____ Sequelae
10. _____ Subacute
11. _____ Chronic

A. A single code used to classify two diagnoses; or a diagnosis with an associated secondary process (manifestation); or a diagnosis with an associated complication

B. Cause or origin of a disease or condition

C. Symptom or condition that is the result of a disease

D. Persistent over a long period

E. Residual condition or effect; time when the acute phase of an illness or injury has passed, but a residual condition or health problem remains

F. Subjective evidence of a disease or of a patient's condition as perceived by the patient

G. A short and relatively severe course

H. Somewhat acute; between chronic and acute

I. Objective evidence of a disease or of a patient's condition as perceived by the patient's examining physician

J. General rules for use in classification that must be followed for accurate coding

K. Without any symptoms

CODING

Assign codes to the following conditions using your code book.

1. Chronic conjunctivitis, left eye

   Code from Alphabetic Index   _____

   Code following verification in Tabular List   _____

2. Pain, right hip joint

   Code from Alphabetic Index   _____

   Code following verification in Tabular List   _____

Assign and sequence codes to the following conditions using your ICD-10-CM code book.

3. Acute and chronic cholecystitis with cholelithiasis   _____

4. Acute and chronic salpingitis   _____

5. Acute on chronic pelvic inflammatory disease   _____

6. Enteritis due to *Clostridium difficile*   _____

7. Herpes labialis   _____

8. Legionnaires' pneumonia   _____

9. Hemiplegia due to previous nontraumatic subarachnoid hemorrhage affecting right dominant side   _____

10. Subacute appendicitis   _____

6 General Coding Guidelines for Medical and Surgical Procedures

ABBREVIATIONS/ACRONYMS

Without the use of reference materials, define the following abbreviations or acronyms.

1. CAS _____
2. CMS _____
3. MCE _____
4. NPI _____
5. GEMS _____
6. CPT _____
7. PTCA _____
8. BMI _____

GLOSSARY DEFINITIONS

Match the surgical procedure to the correct root operation.

1. _____ Destruction
2. _____ Fusion
3. _____ Release
4. _____ Control
5. _____ Change
6. _____ Repair
7. _____ Bypass
8. _____ Map
9. _____ Division
10. _____ Creation
11. _____ Alteration
12. _____ Extraction
13. _____ Fragmentation
14. _____ Reattachment
15. _____ Dilation
16. _____ Resection
17. _____ Detachment
18. _____ Excision

A. Cautery of nosebleed
B. Below elbow amputation
C. Biopsy, left kidney
D. Bone marrow biopsy
E. Total lobectomy of lung
F. Thoracentesis
G. Left common carotid endarterectomy
H. Transurethral cystoscopy with fragmentation of bladder calculus
I. Neurotomy
J. Carpal tunnel release
K. Reattachment of severed left ear
L. Reduction of right radial fracture
M. Transfer radial to median nerve
N. Liver transplant
O. Femoral-popliteal artery bypass
P. ERCP with balloon dilation of common bile duct
Q. Percutaneous ligation of esophageal vein

Continued

19. _____ Occlusion		R.	Cervical cerclage using Shirodkar technique
20. _____ Insertion		S.	Change of gastrostomy tube
21. _____ Reposition		T.	Insertion of cochlear implant, right ear
22. _____ Inspection		U.	Total hip replacement
23. _____ Transfer		V.	Cystoscopy with retrieval of right ureteral stent
24. _____ Restriction		W.	Adjustment of pacemaker lead in left ventricle
25. _____ Supplement		X.	Mitral valve annuloplasty using ring, open
26. _____ Revision		Y.	Diagnostic colonoscopy
27. _____ Removal		Z.	Intraoperative whole brain mapping
28. _____ Replacement		AA.	Control of post-operative peritoneal bleeding
29. _____ Transplantation		BB.	Suture of left biceps tendon laceration
30. _____ Drainage		CC.	Abdominoplasty for cosmetic reasons
31. _____ Extirpation		DD.	Creation of penis in female for sex change
		EE.	Arthrodesis of left ankle

MULTIPLE CHOICE/SHORT ANSWER

Select the correct answer or fill in the blank for each of the following.

1. When a patient is admitted for a surgical procedure and the procedure is canceled because of an equipment problem, which cancelation Z code is used?
   A. Z53.09 Canceled due to contraindication
   B. Z53.20 Canceled due to patient's decision
   C. Z53.8 Canceled due to other reasons
   D. None of the above

2. In the acute setting, a procedure that is performed for definitive treatment rather than for diagnostic or exploratory purposes, or one necessary to take care of a complication, is the
   A. Principal diagnosis
   B. Principal procedure
   C. Secondary diagnosis
   D. Secondary procedure

3. An example of a limited coverage procedure is
   A. Cholecystectomy
   B. Appendectomy
   C. Bilateral lung transplantation
   D. Vasectomy

4. When a procedure is canceled because of a medical condition of the patient, the principal diagnosis is the reason for which the patient was to have the procedure.
   A. True
   B. False

5. To be coded as a procedure, a procedure must be performed in a designated Operating Room.
   A. True
   B. False

6. If a Z code is assigned that describes the nature of the procedure, such as admission for sterilization, it is not necessary to assign a procedure code.
   A. True
   B. False

7. When a surgical procedure has been started and for whatever reason cannot be completed, a code is assigned to identify the extent of the procedure that was done.
   A. True
   B. False

8. Ligatures, sutures and clips are not considered to be devices.
   A. True
   B. False

9. Physical eradication of all or a portion of a body part by the direct use of energy, force, or a destructive agent is extraction.
   A. True
   B. False

10. Putting back in or on all or a portion of a separated body part to its normal location or other suitable location is reattachment.
    A. True
    B. False

11. Altering the route of passage of the contents of a tubular body part is bypass.
    A. True
    B. False

12. The type of instrumentation is a component in determining the approach.
    A. True
    B. False

13. The root operation extraction always involves a device.
    A. True
    B. False

14. The term "and" when used in a code description means "and/or."
    A. True
    B. False

15. If the intended procedure is discontinued, code to the root operation that was achieved.
    A. True
    B. False

16. Exploration or inspection of a body part(s) that is integral to the performance of the procedure is coded separately.
    A. True
    B. False

17. Division is the root operation in which the sole objective is separating a nontubular body part.
    A. True
    B. False

18. Procedures that are performed using an open approach with percutaneous endoscopic assistance are coded to laparoscopic approach.
    A. True
    B. False

19. Bypass is the root operation when a body part is freed and no tissue is being manipulated or cut to free the body part.
   A. True
   B. False

20. A procedure performed using an open approach with percutaneous endoscopic assistance is coded to the percutaneous endoscopic approach.
   A. True
   B. False

Assign and sequence the following procedures using your code book.

1. Total left nephrectomy with removal of adrenal gland   _____

2. Transurethral cystoscopy with closed biopsy bladder   _____

3. Cystoplasty with biological graft (nonautologous), laparoscopic   _____

4. Percutaneous jejunostomy   _____

5. Bone marrow biopsy, percutaneous, iliac   _____

6. Total lobectomy of right upper lobe lung   _____

7. Paracentesis of peritoneal cavity, percutaneous   _____

8. Closed reduction of left humeral shaft fracture   _____

9. Left kidney transplant, cadaver donor   _____

10. Diagnostic arthroscopy, right shoulder   _____

11. CABG of LAD using left internal mammary artery, open (off-pump)   _____

12. PTCA of left anterior descending and left circumflex   _____

13. Total knee replacement with prosthesis, left   _____

14. Removal of drainage device from right pleural cavity   _____

15. Dilation of anal sphincter   _____

16. Resurfacing of right hip, acetabular surface   _____

17. Percutaneous needle biopsy of the liver   _____

18. Laparoscopic sigmoidectomy converted to open sigmoidectomy   _____

19. Fiberoptic bronchoscopy with diagnostic lavage of right main bronchus _____

20. Open reduction of right radial fracture with internal fixation device _____

21. Percutaneous aspiration of right renal cyst   _____

22. Removal of nevus left lower arm   _____

23. Vaginal hysterectomy   _____

24. Removal of foreign body from right external auditory canal   _____

General Coding Guidelines for Other Medical- and Surgical-Related Procedures and Ancillary Procedures

7

ABBREVIATIONS/ACRONYMS

Without the use of reference materials, define the following abbreviations or acronyms.

1. PET _____

2. CT _____

3. MRI _____

4. ECT _____

5. ECMO _____

GLOSSARY DEFINITIONS

Match the Other Medical- and Surgical-Related Procedures and Ancillaries to the correct root operation/type.

1. _____ Monitoring
2. _____ Performance
3. _____ Removal
4. _____ Delivery
5. _____ Restoration
6. _____ Pheresis
7. _____ Abortion
8. _____ Speech Assessment
9. _____ Assistance
10. _____ Transfusion

A. Abortion by dilatation and evacuation
B. Manually assisted vaginal delivery
C. Removal of splint, left wrist
D. Transfusion of platelets via central line
E. Holter monitoring
F. Cardiac defibrillation with successful conversion
G. Intermittent mechanical ventilation, 20 hours
H. ECMO, continuous
I. Plasmapheresis, single treatment
J. Bedside swallow assessment

MULTIPLE CHOICE/SHORT ANSWER

1. The root operation for putting pressure on a body region is
   A. Packing
   B. Dressing
   C. Immoblization
   D. Compression

2. When equipment is used outside of the body for a therapeutic purpose that does not involve the assistance or performance of a physiological function.
   A. Extracorporeal therapy
   B. Restoration
   C. Measurement
   D. Monitoring

19

3. The approach for a chiropractic manipulation is always
   A. Indirect
   B. Internal
   C. External
   D. Direct

4. Originating from the recipient, rather than from a donor, or transferred from the same individual's body.
   A. Autologous
   B. Non-autologous
   C. Extracorporeal
   D. Restoration

5. Taking over a portion of a physiological function by extracorporeal means is:
   A. Performance
   B. Assistance
   C. Restoration
   D. Measurement

6. Completely taking over a physiological function by extracorporeal means is:
   A. Performance
   B. Assistance
   C. Restoration
   D. Measurement

7. Putting in or on a therapeutic, diagnostic, nutritional, physiological, or prophylactic substance except for blood or blood products is:
   A. Transfusion
   B. Irrigation
   C. Administration
   D. Introduction

8. Compression is limiting or preventing motion of a body region.
   A. True
   B. False

9. Pheresis procedure is a type of extracorporeal therapy.
   A. True
   B. False

10. The approach for chiropractic manipulation is always internal.
    A. True
    B. False

11. The term products of conception refers to all physical components of a pregnancy, including the fetus, amnion, umbilical cord, and placenta.
    A. True
    B. False

12. Measurement is defined as determining the level of physiological or physical function repetitively over a period of time.
    A. True
    B. False

13. Fluoroscopy procedures are located in the imaging section.
    A. True
    B. False

14. Radionuclide is root type in the nuclear medicine section.
   A. True
   B. False

15. Detoxification services are a procedure that can be coded in the substance abuse treatment section.
   A. True
   B. False

CODING

Assign and sequence the following procedures using your code book.

1. Mechanical ventilation over 96 hours   _____

2. Hemodialysis, multiple sessions   _____

3. In utero repair of cardiovascular system, percutaneous approach   _____

4. Removal of packing from right nare   _____

5. Transfusion of nonautologous platelets, percutaneous via
   peripheral vein   _____

6. EEG monitoring, external   _____

7. CPAP, 48 hours   _____

8. Fascial release of the cervical region, osteopathic treatment   _____

9. Removal of sutures from abdominal wall   _____

10. Abortion induced with Laminaria   _____

11. Upper GI series, fluoroscopic imaging using barium   _____

12. Ultrasound of right breast   _____

13. PET scan of heart   _____

14. Stereotactic radiosurgery to spinal cord using gamma beam   _____

15. Medication management for mental health issues   _____

16. Educational counseling   _____

17. IQ testing   _____

18. Methadone treatment for drug dependence   _____

19. Swallowing assessment   _____

20. Hearing treatment with cerumen management   _____

Symptoms, Signs, and Abnormal Clinical and Laboratory Findings Not Elsewhere Classified, and Z Codes (ICD-10-CM Chapters 18 and 21, Codes R00-R99, Z00-Z99)

8

ABBREVIATIONS/ACRONYMS

Without the use of reference materials, define the following abbreviations or acronyms.

1. UTI _____

2. BMI _____

3. HIV _____

4. PSA _____

5. ASCUS _____

6. HGSIL _____

7. SIDS _____

8. FUO _____

9. COPD _____

10. CVA _____

GLOSSARY DEFINITIONS

Match the glossary term to the correct definition.

1. _____ Screening examination

2. _____ Symptom

3. _____ Prophylactic

4. _____ Sign

A. Objective evidence of a disease or of a patient's condition as perceived by the patient's examining physician

B. Examination that occurs in the absence of any sign or symptoms

C. Medication or treatment used to prevent a disease from occurring

D. Subjective evidence of a disease or of a patient's condition as perceived by the patient

CODING

Using the code book, code the following.

1. Near syncope _____

2. Abdominal cramps _____

3. Hoarseness _____

4. Family history of sudden cardiac death _____

5. Hypothermia (not due to environmental temperature) _____

6. Crying baby _____

7. Weight loss _____

8. Swollen glands _____

9. Vertigo _____

10. Abnormal EKG _____

11. Prediabetes _____

12. Allergy to penicillin _____

13. Exposure to rabies _____

14. Family history of hypertension _____

15. Physical examination to participate in sports _____

16. Anonymous egg donor younger than age 35 _____

17. Turn off AICD prior to surgery _____

18. Family problems with marital conflict _____

19. Genetic counseling for carrier of cystic fibrosis gene _____

20. Status post porcine heart valve replacement _____

21. Observation after motor vehicle accident _____

MULTIPLE CHOICE

Using the Z code guideline for Principal/First Listed diagnosis, select the correct answer.

1. Z99.2 Renal dialysis status
   A. First diagnosis only
   B. First or additional diagnosis
   C. Additional diagnosis only
   D. Nonspecific diagnosis

2. Z51.11 Encounter for antineoplastic chemotherapy
   A. First diagnosis only
   B. First or additional diagnosis
   C. Additional diagnosis only
   D. Nonspecific diagnosis

3. Z51.5 Encounter for palliative care
   A. First diagnosis only
   B. First or additional diagnosis
   C. Additional diagnosis only
   D. Nonspecific diagnosis

4. Z87.798 Personal history of other congenital malformations
   A. First diagnosis only
   B. First or additional diagnosis
   C. Additional diagnosis only
   D. Nonspecific diagnosis

5. Z91.81 History of fall
   A. First diagnosis only
   B. First or additional diagnosis
   C. Additional diagnosis only
   D. Nonspecific diagnosis

CASE SCENARIOS

Using the code book, code the following cases.

1. The patient fell off a bicycle, sustaining a bruise to her right elbow, an abrasion to her right leg, and she hit her head on the street. No LOC was reported. Because of suspected concussion, the patient was admitted for overnight observation. The concussion was ruled out, and the patient was discharged.
   Final Diagnosis: Concussion ruled out.

   _____

   _____

2. The patient was admitted for a takedown of colostomy. The patient underwent a colostomy 3 months ago after colon resection was performed for perforated diverticulitis. The patient was taken to the OR for colostomy reversal with end-to-end anastomosis. The patient still has a few diverticula and should follow a diverticulosis diet.
   Final Diagnosis: Perforated diverticulitis.
   Procedure: Colostomy takedown.

   _____

   _____

3. The patient was admitted for removal of his Lorenz pectus bar by open approach. The Nuss technique was used to correct his pectus excavatum. The bar has been in place for 3 years with no complications. The patient uses an inhaler for control of his asthma. The patient's pectus excavatum has resolved.
   Final Diagnosis: Removal of hardware.

   _____

   _____

4. The patient was admitted with abdominal pain in the right upper quadrant. Workup included an EGD that showed some mild erosive gastritis, and abdominal ultrasound was positive for gallstones.
   Final Diagnosis: Abdominal pain due to gastritis versus cholelithiasis.
   Procedure: Esophagogastroduodenoscopy with biopsy of the esophagus. Abdominal ultrasound.

   _____

   _____

5. The patient was admitted to the hospital for monitoring of seizure-like spells. Video electroencephalogram monitoring of these episodes was performed over three days and did not reveal any epileptic activity.
   Final Diagnosis: Transient alteration of awareness. Seizure disorder ruled out.

   _____

   _____

6. The patient was admitted for prophylactic breast removal. The patient has a strong family history of breast cancer, and severe fibrocystic disease, bilaterally. Her past medical history is negative except for Crohn's disease with recurrent flares of ileitis. The patient was taken to the OR, and a bilateral simple mastectomy was performed. The patient recovered with no problems. The pathology report showed no evidence of malignancy.
Final Diagnosis: Family history of breast cancer; severe fibrocystic disease.
Procedure: Bilateral simple mastectomy.

_____

_____

7. A 2-year-old child was admitted for investigative workup for failure to thrive. The patient was tested for evaluation of any metabolic disorders, infections, intolerance of milk protein, and other gastrointestinal conditions. The workup was entirely negative. The patient will continue to be followed by a primary care provider.
Final Diagnosis: Failure to thrive.

_____

_____

8. The patient was admitted from her primary care physician office for palpitations. The patient has never had an episode like this. The patient does have a family history of coronary artery disease and a personal history of recurrent urinary tract infections and takes prophylactic antibiotic to prevent UTIs. The patient was monitored by telemetry, but no specific cardiac arrhythmias were identified. The patient was instructed to return for follow-up if palpitations recurred.
Final Diagnosis: Palpitations; cardiac arrhythmia ruled out; family history of coronary artery disease.

_____

_____

9. The patient was admitted for biopsy of an enlarged lymph node in the area of the left axilla. The patient has a past medical history of breast cancer with a mastectomy of the left breast 1 year ago. The patient is no longer receiving any therapy for her cancer. A needle biopsy was done. The pathology report showed normal lymphatic tissue with no evidence of metastatic spread.
Final Diagnosis: Lymphadenopathy left axilla; metastasis ruled out.
Procedure: Needle biopsy axillary lymph node.

_____

_____

10. A 6-month-old infant was admitted with a febrile seizure. The patient had a temperature of 103 and had been started on antibiotics the day before for an acute bilateral otitis media. The patient was discharged to the care of the parents on the following day.
Final Diagnosis: Febrile seizure; fever due to acute bilateral otitis media.

_____

_____

Using the code book, code and answer questions about the following case studies.

8-1. CASE STUDY

History and Physical

CC: Ileostomy reversal.

HPI: Patient has finished treatment for her rectal cancer and wishes to have her ileostomy reversed. Preoperative workup is negative, and no contraindication to this procedure is present. The patient will also have her MediPort removed.

Past medical history: Rectal cancer, hypertension, diabetes, and history of renal calculi.

Social history: No tobacco, alcohol, or illicits. Married.

Allergies: NKDA.

Medications: No medications.

ROS: Constitutional: No change in weight; no fatigue or fevers. Neuro: No headache or dizziness.

HEENT: No vision problems or lymphadenopathy.

CV: No chest pain, palpitations, or PND.

Respiratory: No cough, SOB, or hemoptysis.

GI: No abdominal pain, N/V, diarrhea, or dysphagia.

GU: No dysuria or frequency.

Skin: No rashes or myalgias.

Psych: No mood changes.

PHYSICAL EXAMINATION:

Vitals: Stable.

General: No acute distress; normal affect.

HEENT: PERRLA, EOMI, oropharynx clear, no nystagmus; neck has no masses; trachea is midline.

Chest: CTA.

Breasts: Normal breast examination with no masses.

Heart: RRR, no M/R/G.

Abd: Soft, obese; ileostomy present.

Joints: No acute changes.

Skin: No rashes.

Neuro: Alert, oriented, and answers questions appropriately. CN II through XII intact.

A/P: Rectal cancer, status post neoadjuvant therapy and a coloanal anastomosis to have a takedown of her stoma.

Introduction: This 60-year-old female patient presents for an elective outpatient sigmoidoscopy. The indication for the procedure is S/P low anterior resection for rectal cancer for evaluation prior to stoma takedown.

Consent: Benefits, risks, and alternatives to the procedure are discussed, and informed consent is obtained.

Preparation: EKG, pulse, pulse oximetry, and blood pressure monitored.

Medications: No medications.

Procedure: Rectal examination: Normal. The endoscope is passed without difficulty into the rectum. The quality of the preparation is good.

Findings: Normal-appearing anastomosis and pouch with no evidence of leak.

Complications: No complications are associated with this procedure.

Impression: Normal-appearing anastomosis and pouch with no evidence of leak.

Recommendation: Radiologic studies ordered: Barium enema.

Discharge Summary

DIAGNOSES/PROBLEMS:

1. Rectal cancer. Status post resection/ileostomy/postoperative chemotherapy.

2. Diabetes mellitus, type I.

PROCEDURES:

1. Ileostomy takedown and reanastomosis.

2. Port-a-Cath removal.

HISTORY, MAJOR FINDINGS, AND HOSPITAL COURSE:

This 60-year-old female patient with the medical history described previously who completed her postoperative chemotherapy desires to have her stoma reversed. She presents on the day of admission for ileostomy takedown and reanastomosis and removal of her MediPort, both of which are performed without complications (please see the operative note for details). Postoperatively, she does quite well and on the day of discharge is tolerating a regular diet and has stable vital signs and a bowel movement. Her dressings are taken down and reveal only minimal erythema around the abdominal incision with no induration or expressible fluid. Her JP is removed after minimal output is noted.

DISCHARGE MEDICATIONS:

1. Resume home meds.

2. Oxycodone 5-10 mg PO q4-6 prn pain.

3. Colace 100 mg PO bid.

DISCHARGE INSTRUCTIONS:

Call for fevers, chills, pain not controlled by medications, drainage from wound sites, increasing wound erythema, opening up of wounds, inability to tolerate a diet, or any other concern. May shower; do not soak or bathe. Maintain good diabetic control.

Follow up with surgeon in 2 to 3 weeks; call for an appointment.

Operative Report

Title of Operation: Removal of MediPort and ileostomy takedown.

Indications for Surgery: This 60-year-old female patient completed her postoperative chemotherapy and desires to have her stoma reversed. She comes in after undergoing an endoscopic evaluation of her colonic J pouch and a Gastrografin enema, which reveals no leak. She is taken to the OR for the above procedure.

Preoperative Diagnosis: Rectal cancer status post neoadjuvant therapy and a coloanal anastomosis here for takedown of her stoma.

Postoperative Diagnosis: Rectal cancer status post neoadjuvant therapy and a coloanal anastomosis here for takedown of her stoma.

Surgeon's Narrative

The patient is taken to the OR and is placed in the supine position; general endotracheal anesthesia is administered. She is prepped and draped in the right chest wall and into the right lower abdomen. We start with the upper, taking out the Port-a-Cath first. The patient is injected with about 3 mL of 1% lidocaine. Her old incision is used to open up the skin. Once we have done this, we carefully dissect down to the Port-a-Cath itself, dissecting along the edges of the Port-a-Cath, and retrieve it. It was not stitched in. The Port-a-Cath is removed. The patient has a little oozing from the Port-a-Cath site, and this is oversewn with 3-0 Vicryl. We irrigate the Port-a-Cath site and close it with two layers of 3-0 Vicryl followed by 4-0 Biosyn and Indermil, and a dry dressing is applied. We then turn our attention toward the stoma. We carefully come around the stoma and use the Bovie cautery to make a circumferential incision. The edges of the stoma are carefully freed up until the bowel is separated from the muscle and fascial layers. Once this has been done, the edges of the bowel are reapproximated. Effusions within the intraloop are taken down. Excess skin and the mucocutaneous conjunction are removed, and the bowel was closed with interrupted 3-0 Vicryl followed by interrupted 3-0 silk, second layer Lambert stitches. Anastomosis was nice and patent when it was completed. The bowel is placed back in the abdomen. The patient is irrigated. We change gloves and close the fascia with interrupted Maxon sutures, place a drain into the subcutaneous tissue, make sure hemostasis was appropriately accomplished, and close the subcutaneous tissue with interrupted 3-0 Vicryl followed by a 4-0 Biosyn. The drain is stitched with 3-0 nylon and is placed to bulb suction; then, a dry sterile dressing is applied. The patient tolerates the procedure well. She awakes from anesthesia and is transferred to the recovery room in stable condition.

Progress Note: OP Note

Preop: Rectal Ca S/P resection/ileostomy.

Proc: Ileostomy takedown with reanastomosis. Port-a-Cath removal.

Postop: Same.

GETA: Extubated to PACU.

Specimen: None.

Complication: None.

EBL: Minimal.

Drain: JP, subcutaneous.

for addressograph plate

Date	Time	
		Op NOTE
12/27		Pre Op.: Rectal Ca s/p resection / ileostomy.
	10 15	Proc: ileostomy take down reanastomosis
		port a cath removal.
		Post Op. Dx: same.
		Surgeon: Dr Smith
		GETA → extubated to PACU
		Specimen: none
		Complication: none
		EBL minimal Cryst 2000 UO N/A.
		Drain: JP, subcutaneous
12/5	2000	Prog Note
		60 y.o. ♀ s/p ileostomy take down w/reanastomosis,
		portacath removal.
		- pt. states she feels well, mild pain @ surgical
		site
		- denies SOB, chest pain, lightheadedness, dizziness.
		- PE: pt. lying in bed in no acute distress.
		VS: T 36.1, HR 34, BP 109/52, 92-26% @ RA
		chest: CTA b/lat
		CV: HS dual, ejection systolic murmur 3/6, @ Oxygen shared bed
		AB: soft, mild tender to palp. (−) flatus.
		Dressing c/d/i, JP serosanguinous.
		#. doing well

PROGRESS NOTES

for addressograph plate

Date	Time	
12/25	0500	
		T: 76.7/76.1 HR 80-100 BP $\frac{90-110}{50's}$ 96% on baci 108-086
		76. IV: 1.2 u/o 700 BP: scant
		S: ∅ acute complaints, ⊖ current pain
		O: abd dress, soft, JPE serosang.
		drainage.
		A: S/P Ileostomy takedown POD#1
		- KVO
		- Clear Liquid diet
		- MIC HS, CITH?
12/28	10³⁰ᵃ	Ostomy Note: Ms. M. had a takedown of ileostomy -
		given various perianal ointments to use to prevent irritation.
		discussed cleaning the area and dietary issues
		Ostomy nurse

31

Chapter **8**   **Symptoms, Signs, and Abnormal Clinical Findings**

PROGRESS NOTES

for addressograph plate

Date	Time	
12/25 7:00a		36¹/36¹ 80s-90s MOS/60s 96% RA Daus 12-290
		IV 1.8 Ro F⊗ 1.7 ⊃P 2.6/1.2 NG 5/- JT 5/5
		NGT ⊝ 75cc
		S: Pt. up in chair ⊕flatus ⊕BM
		O: abd obese
		A: S/P colostomy takedown
		— HL IV
		— Reg diet
		— D/C PCA
		— alert nurse/team c̄ next BM)

CASE STUDY QUESTIONS

8-1a. Admit diagnosis: _____

8-1b. Discharge disposition: _____

8-1c. Principal diagnosis: _____

8-1d. Secondary diagnoses (indicate POA status for secondary diagnoses):

_____

_____

_____

_____

_____

_____

8-1e. Principal procedure: _____

8-1f. Secondary procedures: _____

_____

8-1g. Assign MS-DRG: _____

8-1h. Relative weight of MS-DRG: _____

8-1i. Can this MS-DRG be optimized with the addition of a CC? Yes or No

Can this MS-DRG be optimized with the addition of an MCC? Yes or No

8-1j. Is there a particular main guideline that is pertinent to selection of the principal diagnosis in this case study?

_____

_____

8-1k. Is there another diagnosis that meets the definition for principal diagnosis? Yes or No

8-1l. If yes, what is the other diagnosis? _____

8-1m. Is there any opportunity for physician query?

_____

_____

8-1n. What is the drug Colace used to treat? _____

CC: Chest pain.

HPI: The patient is a 70-year-old male with a history of coronary artery disease, hypertension, hypercholesterolemia, and prostatectomy who presents to the emergency department with a complaint of new-onset chest pain. The patient reports that he was in his usual state of health until the evening of presentation when, while eating a piece of turkey, he experienced some mild chest discomfort that lasted approximately 4 minutes and was not associated with any nausea, vomiting, shortness of breath, or jaw or left arm pain. The patient reports that he had three similar episodes over the prior 3 days, and they were all associated with eating a turkey sandwich. The patient denies any history of dysphagia or odynophagia but notes that sipping water seems to make the pain go away. He also states that he felt he had an item of food in his throat while he was having the pain. The patient notes no history of shortness of breath at rest or dyspnea upon exertion. He states that he can climb several flights of stairs without difficulty. He denies any pleuritic chest pain, any sensation of palpitations, or any other complaints. He reports that he did undergo cardiac catheterization at an outside hospital, and no interventions were performed. He states that he was found to have one lesion, which was not in need of stent placement. The patient does not know the percent occlusion of this lesion, but he states that he was told that it "had good collateralization." The patient also reports that he had a stress test a few years ago that was reportedly negative.

Past medical history:
1. CAD.

2. Hypercholesterolemia.

3. Left inguinal hernia.

4. Hypertension.

5. Prostate cancer.

Past surgical history:
1. Prostatectomy.

2. Repair left inguinal hernia.

Allergies: NKDA.

Social history: No tobacco and denies alcohol use.

Review of systems: The patient denies any fevers, chills, or night sweats and reports no weight loss or weight gain. He reports that he had a good appetite. He had no headache, seizures, lightheadedness, or dizziness and no history of syncope. The patient had no vision changes, diplopia, or hearing loss. Chest pain was as described previously. He had no palpitations, orthopnea, PND, or edema. He also had no claudication with activities. The patient reports that he had no shortness of breath, pleuritic pain, cough, wheezing, sputum production, or hemoptysis. He reports a history of occasional reflux, no abdominal pain, and no nausea, vomiting, diarrhea, or constipation. He reports no dysuria and no rashes.

PHYSICAL EXAMINATION:

General: NAD but appears anxious.

HEENT: PERRLA. EOMI. Moist membranes. No thrush. Neck is supple.

Chest: Clear to auscultation bilaterally.

Heart: S1 and S2 normal.

Abd: Normal bowel sounds. No tenderness or organomegaly.

Ext: No cyanosis, clubbing, or edema.

GU/Rectal: Deferred.

34

Neuro: Alert and oriented ×3. CN II to XII grossly intact. Coordination is normal.

Assessment and Plan: Patient with intermittent chest pain is admitted for 12-hour ruleout. Continue daily ASA. Add Protonix 40 mg.

HTN: Continue medication and monitor blood pressure.

Hypercholesterolemia: Continue Lipitor.

Anxiety: Ativan prn.

Discharge Summary

DIAGNOSES/PROBLEMS:

1. Chest pain—noncardiac.
2. History of coronary artery disease.
3. Status post prostatectomy for prostate cancer.
4. Hypercholesterolemia.
5. History of left hernia.
6. Hypertension.

PROCEDURES:

Chest x-ray: Normal except for minimal tortuosity of thoracic aorta.

HISTORY, MAJOR FINDINGS, AND HOSPITAL COURSE:

The patient is a 70-year-old male with a history of coronary artery disease, hypertension, hypercholesterolemia, and prostatectomy who presents to the emergency department with a complaint of new-onset chest pain. The patient reports that he was in his usual state of health until the evening of presentation when, while eating a piece of turkey, he experienced some mild chest discomfort that lasted approximately 4 minutes and was not associated with any nausea, vomiting, shortness of breath, or jaw or left arm pain. The patient reports that he had three similar episodes during the prior 3 days, and they were all associated with eating a turkey sandwich. The patient denies any dysphagia or odynophagia history but notes that sipping water seems to make the pain go away. He also states that he felt he had an item of food in his throat while he was having the pain. The patient notes no history of shortness of breath at rest or dyspnea upon exertion. He states that he can climb several flights of stairs without difficulty. He denies any pleuritic chest pain, any sensation of palpitations, or any other complaints. He reports that he did undergo cardiac catheterization at an outside hospital, and no interventions were performed. He states that he was found to have one lesion, which was not in need of stent placement. The patient does not know the percent occlusion of this lesion, but he states that he was told it "had good collateralization." The patient also reports that he had a stress test a few years ago that was reportedly negative.

On review of systems, the patient denies any fevers, chills, or night sweats and reports no weight loss or weight gain. He states that he had a good appetite. He had no headache, seizures, lightheadedness, or dizziness and no history of syncope. He had no vision changes, diplopia, or hearing loss. Chest pain is as described previously. He had no palpitations, orthopnea, PND, or edema and no claudication with activities. The patient reports that he had no shortness of breath, pleuritic pain, cough, wheezing, sputum production, or hemoptysis. He reports a history of occasional reflux, no abdominal pain, and no nausea, vomiting, diarrhea, or constipation. The patient reports no dysuria and no rashes.

In the emergency department, the patient is found to have a temperature of 98.6 degrees, pulse 84, respiratory rate 20, blood pressure 166/92, and saturation 98% on room air. He receives 325 mg of aspirin and 50 mg of metoprolol.

Past medical history: Please see above.

Allergies: The patient reports no drug allergies.

Medications: Lipitor 20 mg every night and atenolol 50 mg daily.

Social history: The patient denies any history of tobacco or illicit usage and does not drink alcohol.

Family history: The patient reports no history of illness for his parents.

Physical examination: On admission to the floor, the patient's temperature is 98.6 degrees, heart rate 66, blood pressure 176/107, respiratory rate 18, and saturation 98% on room air. In general, he is a well-developed male in no apparent distress who appears slightly anxious. Head examination is unremarkable; pupils are equally round and reactive to light. Extraocular movements are intact, sclerae anicteric. Mucous membranes are moist. Oropharynx is clear. Neck examination shows a JVP at approximately 6 to 7 cm; the neck is otherwise supple. Chest is clear to auscultation bilaterally. Cardiac examination reveals a regular rate and rhythm with no murmurs, rubs, or gallops. The patient has no extra heart sounds. Abdominal examination is benign. Extremity examination shows no cyanosis, clubbing, or edema and good capillary refill. Neurologic examination is also unremarkable; cranial nerves II through XII are grossly intact, and the patient ambulates without difficulty.

Laboratory data: On admission, the patient's laboratory work was remarkable for a white count of 4.4, hematocrit 48.8, and platelets 131. His complete metabolic panel was within normal limits, except for a bicarb of 29. Urine toxicology screen was negative. Urinalysis was unremarkable. No bacteria were seen. The patient's cholesterol panel was remarkable for an LDL of 86, total cholesterol of 156, and triglycerides of 72. The patient had 3 sets of cardiac enzymes, all of which were within normal limits.

EKG: The patient's EKG showed a normal sinus rhythm with inferior T-wave inversions and borderline left ventricular hypertrophy. No other EKGs were available for comparison.

HOSPITAL COURSE BY SYSTEMS:

Chest pain: The patient presented with approximately 4 months' history of chest pain. This occurred while eating a turkey sandwich and was similar to 3 or 4 prior episodes that also occurred while he was eating a sandwich. At that time, the patient stated that he felt he had something perhaps caught in the throat, and this was relieved upon drinking a sip of water. Upon arrival, the patient was chest pain free, and EKG showed inferior T-wave inversions with no prior EKG for comparison; this was not a matter of concern. No evidence of ST elevation or acute infarction was seen. The patient additionally had three sets of cardiac enzymes sent, all of which were negative. The patient underwent repeat EKG when he was admitted; no additional changes were noted.

Hypertension: The patient was continued on atenolol while in the hospital. Upon admission, his blood pressure was elevated at 170; however, systolic pressure did fall to below 140 on his home regimen.

Hypercholesterolemia: The patient was continued on Lipitor as an inpatient. His lipid panel showed an LDL of 86, total cholesterol of 156, and triglycerides of 72. Given the patient's history of coronary disease, an argument could be made that his goal LDL would be less than 70. The patient is currently on Lipitor 20 mg nightly; this could be increased now that he is an outpatient.

Disposition: The patient was discharged after a series of cardiac enzymes were completed over a 12-hour period. It was not thought that he was having a myocardial infarction. The patient was discharged on the same medications with which he arrived at the hospital, in addition to a proton pump inhibitor. The patient was to follow up with his outpatient physician. The patient states that he was feeling well at the time of discharge. The patient was discharged home in good condition.

DISCHARGE MEDICATIONS:

Pantoprazole 40 mg by mouth daily.

Aspirin 81 mg by mouth daily.

Atenolol 50 mg by mouth daily.

Atorvastatin 20 mg by mouth at bedtime.

FOLLOW-UP CARE:

The patient reported that he has a primary care physician who is managing his hypercholesterolemia, coronary artery disease, and hypertension. The patient stated that he would call on the morning after discharge to make an appointment to see this physician.

Progress Notes

DAY 1

Patient was admitted with chest pain. Received ASA, metoprolol, and Ativan in the emergency department. EKG and cardiac enzymes suggest low risk. Patient has known CAD. Will maintain current regimen and check third set of enzymes. UA is normal. Chest x-ray is normal with no infiltrate.

DAY 2

Cardiac enzymes ×3—negative. MI ruled out.

No chest pain.

Patient should take 81 mg ASA/day.

Patient encouraged to visit emergency department, or to call if recurrent chest pain.

CASE STUDY QUESTIONS

8-2a. Admit diagnosis: _____

8-2b. Discharge disposition: _____

8-2c. Principal diagnosis: _____

8-2d. Secondary diagnoses (indicate POA status for secondary diagnoses):

_____

_____

_____

_____

_____

_____

8-2e. Principal procedure: _____

8-2f. Secondary procedures: _____

_____

8-2g. Assign MS-DRG: _____

8-2h. Relative weight of MS-DRG: _____

8-2i. Can this MS-DRG be optimized with the addition of a CC? Yes or No

     Can this MS-DRG be optimized with the addition of an MCC? Yes or No

8-2j. Is there a main guideline pertinent to selection of the principal diagnosis in this case study?

_____

_____

8-2k. Is there another diagnosis that meets the definition for principal diagnosis? Yes or No

8-2l. If yes, what is the other diagnosis? _____

8-2m. Is there any opportunity for physician query?

_____

_____

8-2n. What is the drug Protonix used to treat? _____

8-3. CASE STUDY

History and Physical

CC: Dizzy.

HPI: Patient is taking BP meds only when feels dizzy. She has been dizzy for the past month.

No LOC. Positive for vertigo—lasts for 10 to 15 minutes. Vision comes and goes. Tinnitus ×2 months. Hearing is stable. Headache daily for 1 year. No fevers/chills. Has lost 45 pounds in 2.5 years because of poor appetite. She is sleeping well but is fatigued. No suicidal ideation. Has arthritis pain.

Past medical history: Hypertension, arthritis, history of breast cancer.

Social history: No tobacco, alcohol, or illicits. Retired and lives alone.

Allergies: NKDA.

Medications: Diazide 37.5/25 mg daily and Percocet prn.

ROS: Negative except for HPI.

PHYSICAL EXAMINATION:

Vitals: T 98.5, HR 125, RR 18, BP 146/91, Sao_2 97% on RA.

General: No acute distress. Normal affect.

HEENT: PERRL. EOMI. Oropharynx clear, no nystagmus. Neck is soft, nontender, and nondistended.

Chest: CTA.

Breast: Normal breast examination, no masses.

Heart: RRR, no M/R/G.

Abd: Soft. Mild diffuse tenderness, nondistended, no HSM.

Joints: No acute changes.

Skin: No rashes.

Neuro: Alert, oriented, and answers questions appropriately. CN II to XII intact.

A/P: Vertigo and dizziness in a patient with hypertension and headache. Obtain CT of head.

Discharge Summary

DIAGNOSES/PROBLEMS:

1. Vertigo.
2. Hypertension.
3. Depression.
4. Chronic renal insufficiency.

PROCEDURES:

1. Head CT.

HISTORY, MAJOR FINDINGS, AND HOSPITAL COURSE:

This is a 75-year-old patient who was taking blood pressure medications only when she feels dizzy, coming in because of dizziness for the past month with no loss of consciousness. The patient is complaining of vertigo. Apparently, the patient's hearing is stable. The patient has had daily headaches for the past year or longer. The patient denies any fevers or chills. The patient lost 45 pounds over the past 2½ years because she has a poor appetite. The patient lost her daughter, and she has not gotten over that loss.

Past medical history: Significant for hypertension, arthritis, history of breast cancer, hand surgery, face surgery, left mastectomy, and abdominal surgery.

Social history: No alcohol or drug or tobacco abuse. Lives alone.

Allergies: No known drug allergies.

Medications: Dyazide 37.5/25 mg daily. The patient is taking it only as needed; she also takes Percocet as needed.

Physical examination: The patient is not orthostatic.

Vital signs: Stable.

Chest: Clear to auscultation and percussion.

Heart: S1 and S2. Regular rate and rhythm.

Abdomen: Soft, nontender, and nondistended.

Extremities: No edema, cyanosis, or clubbing.

Laboratory workup showed a white count of 6.8, hemoglobin 14.1, BUN 15, and creatinine 1.5.

Hospital course: The patient was hospitalized and was monitored. Head CT was negative. On the second day of her admission, the patient felt significantly better. She was able to manage her daily activities on the floor, and she was discharged.

Condition on discharge: Improved.

DISCHARGE MEDICATIONS:

Aspirin 81 mg a day.

Hydrochlorothiazide 25 mg a day.

Metoprolol 25 mg twice a day.

Nifedipine XL 60 mg daily.

Motrin 600 mg 3 times a day.

Protonix 40 mg a day.

FOLLOW-UP CARE:

Follow-up appointment is scheduled with her physician next week. The patient is to talk to her doctor about colonoscopy and possible abdominal CAT scan.

Brain Without IV Contrast, CT

History: Dizziness.

Technique: Axial CT scan images were performed from the foramen magnum to the vertex without administration of intravenous contrast.

Findings: These images show no evidence of mass lesions in the brain. Ventricles and sulci are normal in size and position. No evidence of shift of midline structures is apparent. Hemorrhage in the brain is also not evident. Small areas of periventricular white matter hypodensity are most compatible, in this age group, with small vessel ischemic disease. Visualized portions of bones are unremarkable. Visualized portions of orbits, paranasal sinuses, and mastoid cells are unremarkable.

Impression: No acute intracranial abnormality.

Progress Notes

DAY 1

Patient still has some vertigo. CT of head this morning. Report still pending.

HTN: Resume patient medication.

Weight loss: Could be related to depression, but patient should have some cancer screening such as colonoscopy, possibly EGD, and so forth. This can be done on an outpatient basis.

CRI: Patient's renal insufficiency is at baseline.

Obtain PT evaluation, nutrition consult.

DAY 2

Patient is feeling better. CT of head is negative. Ready for discharge.

CASE STUDY QUESTIONS

8-3a. Admit diagnosis: _____

8-3b. Discharge disposition: _____

8-3c. Principal diagnosis: _____

8-3d. Secondary diagnoses (indicate POA status for secondary diagnoses):

_____

_____

_____

_____

_____

_____

8-3e. Principal procedure: _____

8-3f. Secondary procedures: _____

_____

8-3g. Assign MS-DRG: _____

8-3h. Relative weight of MS-DRG: _____

8-3i. Can this MS-DRG be optimized with the addition of a CC? Yes or No

Can this MS-DRG be optimized with the addition of an MCC? Yes or No

8-3j. Is there a main guideline pertinent to selection of the principal diagnosis in this case study?

_____

_____

8-3k. Is there another diagnosis that meets the definition for principal diagnosis? Yes or No

8-3l. If yes, what is the other diagnosis? _____

8-3m. Is there any opportunity for physician query?

_____

_____

8-3n. What is the drug Nifedipine XL used to treat? _____

Certain Infectious and Parasitic Diseases (ICD-10-CM Chapter 1, Codes A00-B99)

9

ABBREVIATIONS/ACRONYMS

Without the use of reference materials, define the following abbreviations or acronyms.

1. HIV _____
2. SIRS _____
3. CDC _____
4. HAART _____
5. UTI _____
6. MRSA _____
7. *C. diff* _____
8. TB _____
9. HSV _____
10. PCP _____

GLOSSARY DEFINITIONS

Match the glossary term to the correct definition.

1. _____ Parasite
2. _____ Chancre
3. _____ Nosocomial
4. _____ Communicable
5. _____ Mycoses
6. _____ Condyloma

A. Wart-type growth usually found in genital or anal area

B. Easily spread from one person to another

C. Hospital-acquired infection

D. Ulcer that forms during the first stage of syphylis

E. Fungal infection

F. Organism that lives on or takes nourishment from another organism

CODING

Using the code book, code the following.

1. Mononucleosis _____
2. Streptococcal pericarditis _____
3. Fifth disease _____
4. Lyme disease _____
5. Thrush, oral _____
6. Cold sore _____
7. Charcot joint disease _____

43

8. Viral gastroenteritis _____

9. Chronic hepatitis B _____

10. Septic shock due to *Staphylococcus aureus* _____
    septicemia

11. Monkey malaria _____

12. Urethral chancre _____

13. PCP pneumonia in immunocompromised patient _____

14. Condyloma acuminatum _____

Assign codes for the following organisms using your code book.

15. *Bacteroides fragilis* _____

16. *Enterococcus faecium* _____

17. *Stenotrophomonas maltophilia* _____

18. *Citrobacter freundii* _____

19. *Staphylococcus epidermidis* _____

20. *Viridans* streptococci _____

21. Listeriosis _____

22. *Corynebacterium diphtheriae* _____

23. Actinomycotic mycetoma _____

24. *Serratia* _____

CASE SCENARIOS

Using the code book, code the following cases.

1. A patient was admitted to the hospital with change in mental status. Upon discharge, the physician documents change in mental status due to AIDS encephalopathy.

    _____

    _____

2. A patient was admitted to the hospital with fever, cough, and low blood pressure. CXR shows infiltrates, and sputum culture is positive for MRSA. The discharge summary indicates that the patient was admitted and was given IV antibiotics for MRSA pneumonia.

    _____

    _____

3. A patient was admitted with a diagnosis of urosepsis. Urine and blood cultures are performed on admittance. Blood and urine cultures come back positive for *E. coli*. Discharge summary documents sepsis due to *E. coli*.

    _____

    _____

4. A patient was admitted to the hospital with severe diarrhea. Upon examination, the patient is found to be severely dehydrated. She is given IV fluids to correct the hydration. In the assessment, the physician suspects gastroenteritis. After stool cultures, it is determined that the patient has *C. diff* colitis.

_____

_____

5. A patient known to be positive for HIV is admitted to the hospital with high fever, malaise, and cough. PCP pneumonia is suspected. Tests reveal that the patient has mononucleosis.

_____

_____

6. A 5-month-old infant presents to the emergency department with cough, fever, and wheezing. A URI is suspected, but during the course of the examination, the patient becomes hypoxic and is therefore admitted. After testing, it is determined that the child has RSV.

_____

_____

7. An AIDS patient is hospitalized for PCP. During hospitalization, it is discovered that the patient also has thrush.

_____

_____

8. A patient with AIDS is admitted to the hospital after a car accident in which he suffered a fractured shaft of the left humerus that required an ORIF.

_____

_____

9. A patient is admitted with cellulitis of the leg. The physician orders blood cultures to be done on admission. The day after admit, the infectious disease physician documents SIRS caused by *Enterococcus*.

_____

_____

10. A college student presents to the emergency department with a severe headache and fever. He was admitted to rule out meningitis. A diagnostic lumbar puncture was performed. It was determined that the patient had aseptic meningitis. He was treated with fluids and rest.

_____

_____

Using the code book, code and answer questions about the following case studies.

9-1. CASE STUDY

History and Physical

CC: Fever, vomiting, bloody diarrhea.

HPI: This is a 3-year-old female who presented to urgent care a few days PTA. The patient was given a diagnosis of gastroenteritis and was rehydrated and sent home. Because of persistent fever, vomiting, and now bloody diarrhea, Mom returns with the child today.

Past medical history: Full-term vaginal delivery with no complications. No prior hospitalizations. Developmentally appropriate. UTD on immunizations according to Mom.

Past surgical history: No surgeries.

Social history: Lives with Mom and two older siblings. No tobacco exposure. Has pet turtle. Goes to daycare full time.

Family history: Maternal side with DM and HTN.

Allergies: NKDA.

Review of systems: Decreased appetite, vomiting, bloody diarrhea, and fever (range, 102-104 axillary). No known sick contacts, no travel, no new/unusual foods.

PHYSICAL EXAMINATION:

Vitals: T 36.2, HR 108, R 28, BP 121/64, Wt 14.6 kg.

General: Lying in mother's arms, NAD, looks tired.

HEENT: NCAT, slightly dry MM, PERRLA, EOMI. TMs clear bilaterally, clear oropharynx. Neck is supple. No lymphadenopathy.

Chest: CTA bilaterally.

CV: RRR. No murmur.

Abd: Soft, tender to deep palpation, especially in epigastric and lower abd + BS.

Ext: WNL.

GU/Rectal: Normal female.

ASSESSMENT/PLAN:

Workup for cause of gastroenteritis. Stool studies done. The patient was playing with a pet turtle and is at a peak age range for *Salmonella* diarrhea. Will give Tylenol prn for fever. Will continue IV fluids. Monitor I/Os. Clear liquid diet.

Discharge Summary

DIAGNOSES/PROBLEMS:

1. *Salmonella* gastroenteritis.
2. Dehydration.

This 3-year-old female presents with a 4-day history of fever, vomiting, and a 2-day history of diarrhea that is blood streaked. She was brought to urgent care a few days prior to admission and is sent home with recommendations for rehydration and a diagnosis of gastroenteritis. Fevers are intermittent. Bloody diarrhea persists. The patient is admitted after she presents to the emergency department. Of note is that she does have a pet turtle at home. Signs of dehydration such as decreased urine output are evident, and the patient requires normal saline bolus in the emergency department. She is maintained on intravenous fluids and gradually begins to take orals. Stool cultures are pending at the time of discharge. Stool ova and parasite examination ×1 is negative. Electrolyte panel was originally notable for a CO_2 of 19, BUN 13, sodium 133, and chloride 94. Urine culture was sent and is negative at 48 hours at the time of discharge. The patient is stable and is discharged to home.

Discharge Medications:

None.

Follow-up Care:

Return if bloody diarrhea persists, or if the child has a significant increase in abdominal pain. Follow-up is provided by the primary medical doctor.

Social Work Screening

The patient is screened; no social work services are needed at this time. If new concerns arise, please contact Social Work at that time.

Progress Notes

Day 1

The patient was admitted with a 4-day history of fever with vomiting and bloody diarrhea. She had one watery stool early this morning. Cultures are still pending. The patient has a pet turtle that she has been playing with. Therefore, the likely cause of her gastroenteritis is *Salmonella*. The patient is better hydrated with moist mucous membranes. She is hemodynamically stable.

Day 2

The patient was admitted with gastroenteritis and dehydration. She had one large, loose stool overnight. She is currently afebrile. No emesis reported since admission. May advance diet. No cardiovascular or pulmonary issues. Hep lock IV if tolerating diet.

Day 3

The patient's PO intake has improved. Urine and blood cultures are negative. Stool is negative for ova and parasites. Moist MM. Chest is clear. Abdomen is soft and nontender. The patient is ready for discharge home with mother.

CASE STUDY QUESTIONS

9-1a. Admit diagnosis: _____

9-1b. Discharge disposition: _____

9-1c. Principal diagnosis: _____

9-1d. Secondary diagnoses (indicate POA status for secondary diagnoses):

_____

_____

_____

_____

_____

9-1e. Principal procedure: _____

9-1f. Secondary procedures: _____

_____

9-1g. Assign MS-DRG: _____

9-1h. Relative weight of MS-DRG: _____

9-1i. Can this MS-DRG be optimized with the addition of a CC? Yes or No

Can this MS-DRG be optimized with the addition of an MCC? Yes or No

9-1j. Is there a main guideline pertinent to selection of the principal diagnosis in this case study?

_____

_____

9-1k. Is there another diagnosis that meets the definition for principal diagnosis? Yes or No

9-1l. If yes, what is the other diagnosis? _____

9-1m. Is there any opportunity for physician query?

_____

_____

9-2. CASE STUDY

History and Physical

CC: SOB, RLQ pain.

HPI: The patient is a 43-year-old gentleman with a history of HIV and hypertension who presents to the emergency department with 1 week of right lower quadrant tenderness, nausea, and diarrhea, as well as 3 to 4 weeks of dyspnea on exertion, night sweats, and nonproductive cough. A lapse has occurred in the patient's HIV care. He was incarcerated over the past 4 months. While in jail, he had night sweats, progressive dyspnea on exertion, and nonproductive cough. He denies fever, chills, chest pain, and orthopnea. He also admits to intermittent sharp right lower quadrant tenderness accompanied by diarrhea and nausea that were worse upon eating. The patient reports negative PPD in prison.

Past medical history: The patient was given a diagnosis of HIV 15 years ago. He does not have a record of his last CD4 count. He has only had thrush. He has a history of hypertension.

Past surgical history: Hernia repair.

Social history: The patient has smoked 1 pack per day for the past 25 years. No alcohol, no illicits. Currently unemployed.

Family history: Significant for prostate cancer and diabetes.

Medications: He is currently on none. Previously on Bactrim and Procardia XL.

Allergies: NKDA.

Review of systems: The patient denies vomiting, bright red blood per rectum, urinary complaints, and jaundice. Denies weight changes. Admits to night sweats and fatigue. Admits to a headache. Denies seizures, syncope or lightheadedness, vertigo, weakness, numbness, and tingling. Denies vision changes, cataract, hearing loss, tinnitus, and lymphadenopathy. Admits to diplopia and glaucoma. Denies chest pain, palpitations, orthopnea, and PND. Admits to exercise intolerance. Denies bowel changes, bladder changes, or rashes.

PHYSICAL EXAMINATION:

Vitals: T 37.0, HR 105–115, BP 160/94, RR 20, Sao_2 96% on 2 L.

General: NAD.

HEENT: NC/AT, dry MM, no oral thrush, EOMI, PERRLA.

Neck: No nuchal rigidity, no neck stiffness, no LAD.

Chest: Bibasilar crackles.

CV: RRR, S1 and S2, no m/r/g. JVP not elevated.

Abd: Soft, nondistended, mild RLQ tenderness, +BS.

Ext: No edema.

GU/Rectal: Deferred.

Skin/Musculoskeletal: WNL.

Neuro: Alert and oriented ×3. Cranial nerves intact.

Chest x-ray: Possible subtle interstitial infiltrate right lower lobe.

ASSESSMENT/PLAN:

This is a 43-year-old patient with HIV with a chest CT that suggests the need for concern regarding diffuse infiltrate with elevated LDH consistent with PCP.

Discharge Summary

DIAGNOSES/PROBLEMS:

1. PCP pneumonia.
2. HIV.
3. Chest pain.
4. Acute renal failure.
5. Hypertension.

PROCEDURES:

1. Bronchoscopy.

HISTORY, MAJOR FINDINGS, AND HOSPITAL COURSE:

The patient is a 43-year-old gentleman with a history of HIV and hypertension who presents to the emergency department with 1 week of right lower quadrant tenderness, nausea, and diarrhea, as well as 3 to 4 weeks of dyspnea on exertion, night sweats, and nonproductive cough. A lapse in the patient's HIV care has occurred. He was incarcerated over the past 4 months. While in jail, he had night sweats, progressive dyspnea on exertion, and nonproductive cough. The patient denies fever, chills, chest pain, and orthopnea. He also admits to intermittent sharp right lower quadrant tenderness accompanied by diarrhea and nausea that were worse upon eating. Past medical history includes HIV, which was diagnosed 15 years ago. The patient does not have a record of his last CD4 count. He has had only thrush and has a history of hypertension and a hernia repair.

Social history: He has smoked 1 pack per day for the past 25 years. No alcohol, no illicits. Currently unemployed.

Family history is significant for prostate cancer and diabetes.

Review of systems: The patient denies vomiting, bright red blood per rectum, urinary complaints, and jaundice. Denies weight changes. Admits to night sweats and fatigue. Admits to a headache. Denies seizures, syncope or lightheadedness, vertigo, weakness, numbness, and tingling. Denies vision changes, cataract, hearing loss, tinnitus, and lymphadenopathy. Admits to diplopia and glaucoma. Denies chest pain, palpitations, orthopnea, and PND. Admits to exercise intolerance. Denies bowel changes, bladder changes, or rashes.

Medications: He is currently on none. He has no known drug allergies.

On physical examination, his temperature is 37 degrees, heart rate in the 110s, blood pressure 160/94, and oxygen saturation 96% on 2 liters. His O_2 saturation had dropped down to the mid 80s on room air in the emergency department.

General: He is in no acute distress, well appearing.

HEENT: Dry mucous membranes. Normal pupils. Normal extraocular motions. No thrush.

Neck examination: No nuchal rigidity. No lymphadenopathy.

Lungs: Scattered rhonchi and rales.

Heart examination: Regular rate and rhythm. No murmurs, gallops, or rubs.

Abdominal examination: Bowel sounds, soft, nontender, except in the right lower quadrant, nondistended.

Extremities: No edema. Neurologically, normal mental status, cranial nerves, motor, sensory, and coordination.

White blood cell count is 12.3000, hematocrit 35.1, and platelet count 249. Serum sodium is 136, potassium 4.3, chloride 104, bicarbonate 18, BUN and creatinine 29 and 2.2, and glucose 103. LFTs are normal. Neutrophil count is 62%. LDH is 634, amylase and lipase 151 and 34. ABG 7.46, 24, 53, and 17 on room air. UA shows 0 white cells. Phenol is calculated at 1.27%. Urinary anion gap is positive 60. Blood cultures, mycobacterial culture, and fungal culture were sent.

EKG is sinus tachycardia at 120. Right atrial enlargement. T-wave inversion in II and III, V4 through V6, not changed since 8/06. Chest x-ray shows possible subtle interstitial infiltrate in the right lower lobe. Chest CT shows diffuse ground-glass infiltrate in the lungs and more dense infiltrates in the superior lower lobes bilaterally. No pleural effusion. Axillary adenopathy, multiple mediastinal lymph nodes, and retroperitoneal iliac and inguinal lymph nodes.

This is a 43-year-old gentleman with a history of HIV who presents with several weeks of subacute shortness of breath, nonproductive cough, and night sweats. He has a recent incarceration history and diffuse infiltrates with an elevated LDH; the causes of these are presumed to be *Pneumocystis carinii* pneumonia, bacterial pneumonia, and viral pneumonia. Tuberculosis is unlikely. He is initially started on Bactrim and is given corticosteroids for hypoxia. He is also treated for a community-acquired pneumonia, initially on ceftriaxone and azithromycin, but within 24 hours, moxifloxacin. For renal failure, he is hydrated. A renal ultrasound is checked.

HOSPITAL COURSE/PLAN:

1. PCP pneumonia: The patient was continued on Bactrim and prednisone and was placed on moxifloxacin for possible community-acquired pneumonia. Although his induced sputum was negative, a bronchoscopy revealed PCP. The patient was placed on airborne precautions until the AFB from his bronchoscopy came back negative. Moxifloxacin was discontinued. He was briefly on clindamycin/primaquine instead of Bactrim because of concern for renal failure. However, after discussion with our pharmacist, in the absence of definitive evidence of Bactrim-associated renal failure (urine eosinophils negative), we thought it safe to give the more effective anti-PCP therapy.
2. HIV: Because of our uncertainty about his follow-up, we did not institute HAART. We did place the patient on azithromycin prophylaxis.
3. Chest pain: Because of chest pain that radiated down his left shoulder and minor ECG changes, MI was ruled out and the patient was placed on IV heparin, aspirin, a beta blocker, and sublingual nitrates. After MI was ruled out, these treatments were stopped, and a TTE was performed; findings were negative.
4. Acute renal failure: With hydration, the patient's creatinine came down to 1.7 (baseline). He was started on Bicitra for a bicarbonate of 13.

DISCHARGE MEDICATIONS:

Nifedipine XL Enteral 60 mg PO daily, azithromycin enteral 1200 mg PO q7 days, aspirin enteral 81 mg PO daily. Prednisone 20 mg: take 2 pills by mouth (40 mg) daily for the next 3 days, then 1 pill by mouth (20 mg) for 11 days. Bactrim DS: take 2 pills by mouth 3 times daily for 14 days (you will need to take only 2 pills on the evening of discharge, then start 2 pills 3 times a day thereafter); Bactrim SS: take 1 pill by mouth daily (to start once you've finished the Bactrim DS). Sodium bicarbonate 1300 mg by mouth 3 times daily.

DISCHARGE INSTRUCTIONS:

Discharge to—Home.

Discharge diet—Regular.

Discharge activity—Resume normal activity.

Discharge restrictions (e.g., lifting, walking, stairs)—None.

FOLLOW-UP CARE:

Call your doctor if you have any of the following problems: chest pain, shortness of breath, or any other issues that concern you.

Indication for study: Myocardial infarction.

Interpretation summary: A 2-dimensional transthoracic echocardiogram with M-mode was performed. The study was technically adequate. The left ventricle is normal in size. Concentric left ventricular hypertrophy is mild. EF is estimated at 60% to 65%. Left ventricular wall motion is normal.

Heart rate: 71 bpm.

Left ventricle: The left ventricle is normal in size. Concentric left ventricular hypertrophy is mild. Left ventricular systolic function is normal. EF is estimated at 60% to 65%. Left ventricular wall motion is normal. No regional wall motion abnormalities are noted.

Right ventricle: The right ventricle is normal in size. Right ventricular systolic function is normal.

Atria: Left atrial size is normal. Right atrial size is normal. No Doppler evidence suggests an atrial septal defect.

Mitral valve: The mitral valve is normal. No evidence suggests mitral valve prolapse. No mitral valve stenosis is found. Trace mitral regurgitation is noted.

Tricuspid valve: The tricuspid valve is normal. Trace tricuspid regurgitation is noted. RVSP estimated at 26 mm Hg.

Aortic valve: The aortic valve is trileaflet. The aortic valve opens well. No valvular aortic stenosis is noted. No aortic regurgitation is present.

Pulmonic valve: Pulmonic valve leaflets are thin and pliable; valve motion is normal.

Great vessels: The aortic root is normal in size.

Pericardium/Pleura: No pericardial effusion.

Mode: 2D measurements and calculations:

IVSd	1.2 cm
LVIDd	4.7 cm
LVIDs	2.7 cm
LVPWd	1.3 cm
A0 root diam	3.5 cm
LA dimension	3.7 cm
LVOT diam	2.3 cm
LVOT area	4.2 cm

Doppler measurements and calculations:

MV E point	70 cm/sec
MV E/A	1.3
MV max PG	2.9 mm Hg
MV mean PG	1.3 mm Hg
A0 max PG	5.9 mm Hg
A0 mean PG	3.4 mm Hg
AVA (I,D)	3.9 cm^2
AVA (V,D)	3.9 cm^2
LV VI max	114 cm/sec
RVSP	29 mm Hg

History: 43-year-old man with HIV, cough, SOB, and CT changes suggestive of PCP.

Procedure description: The attending physician supervised the procedure and results. Airway inspection and lavage were performed without difficulty.

Impression: Normal airway examination.

Recommendations: Follow-up culture results.

Procedure data:

Preop status:
Aspirin within previous 7 days	No
History of excessive bleeding	No

Case medications:
Fentanyl (Sublimaze)	75 mcg IV
Lidocaine 1%	25 cc topical
Midazolam (Versed)	3 mg IV
Promethazine (Phenergan)	12.5 mg IV

General information: Insertion via left nare.
Scope model	BFIT160
Vocal cords	Normal
Trachea	Normal
Main carina	Normal
Right side airway	Normal
Left side airway	Normal

Specimens sent for analysis:
Bacteriology	Yes
Legionella studies	Yes
Mycobacteriology (AFB)	Yes
Parasitology	Yes
Mycology (fungal)	Yes
Virology	Yes

Diagnostic Bronchoscopy

Indications: Primary indication: Diffuse infiltrates.

Procedures:

	Procedure #1	Procedure #2
Procedure	Airway inspection	Alveolar lavage (BAL)
Location		Left lingual
Amt instilled, cc		120
Amt recovered, cc		38

Diagnosis: No diagnosis was obtained.

Thoracic CT: History: The patient has abdominal pain and HIV; the study is done for evaluation.

Chest CT: Lung fields were evaluated; the patient had patchy ground-glass infiltrates bilaterally that were best seen in the upper lung zones, although they involved mid and lower lung zones as well. The possibility of viral pneumonitis was suggested. The patient has small axillary nodes bilaterally and tiny mediastinal nodes.

Impression: Ground-glass infiltrates. In this patient with HIV, the differential would tend to center around CMV versus PCP pneumonia.

Abdomen CT: Thickening of the lower esophagus is seen as suspicious for esophagitis. On this noncontrast study, the liver and spleen are unremarkable. The left kidney is smaller than the right. Vascular calcification is noted in the abdominal aorta. Small nodes are present.

Pelvis CT: Scans through the pelvic region are unremarkable. No pelvic mass is seen. No other finding of note is seen.

Impression: No evidence of pelvic abscess is detected. No intra-abdominal abscess is noted. Small mesenteric nodes in this patient with history of HIV.

PA and lateral chest:

Indication: Cough.

Impression: Possible subtle interstitial infiltrate right lower lobe. Follow-up examination suggested. Moderate air distention left colon.

53

DAY 1

Afebrile. RR 36, P 96. No acute distress. Comfortable, speaking in full sentences. No thrush. Still has RLQ tenderness on palpation without rebound. +BS. Patient is hypoxic. Suspect that patient's CD4 count is low, and that he has advanced HIV disease with bilateral pneumonia and possible esophagitis. Pneumonia could be PCP. Trial fluconazole for dysphagia. Also has HTN and renal insufficiency, possibly due to HTN or HIVAN.

DAY 2

Complains of chest pain this morning. Says it began last night and has been constant since that time. He describes it as pressure and rates it 7/10. He has some SOB, but this is no worse than when he presented. CT suggests pneumonia consistent with PCP. Continue treatment with Bactrim and steroid. D/C vancomycin. Plan for bronch tomorrow (NPO after midnight). Presents with ARF, which is not resolving. If Cr remains elevated, will consider renal workup. Mild anemia.

DAY 3

Chest pain has resolved and shortness of breath is improving. ACS with cardiac enzymes and TTE ruled out. Will switch to captopril for antihypertensive management, given the patient's CKD. Patient presents in ARF, and Cr has stabilized at 1.7. Patient has nongap acidosis consistent with RTA. Will have bronch today.

DAY 4

Tolerates bronch well. Is eating well. Afebrile. Continue treatment for PCP and hypertension. Leukocytosis probably secondary to steroids for PCP.

DAY 5

Bronch is positive for PCP. Fungal culture negative. No other new issues. Creatinine is stable at 1.7. No further oxygen requirement. CD4 count is pending. Renal ultrasound shows renal scarring, so there is underlying renal disease. The patient is ready for discharge.

CASE STUDY QUESTIONS

9-2a. Admit diagnosis: _____

9-2b. Discharge disposition: _____

9-2c. Principal diagnosis: _____

9-2d. Secondary diagnoses (indicate POA status for secondary diagnoses):

_____

_____

_____

_____

_____

54

9-2e.   Principal procedure: _____

9-2f.   Secondary procedures: _____

_____

9-2g.   Assign MS-DRG: _____

9-2h.   Relative weight of MS-DRG: _____

9-2i.   Can this MS-DRG be optimized with the addition of a CC? Yes or No

Can this MS-DRG be optimized with the addition of an MCC? Yes or No

9-2j.   Is there a main guideline pertinent to selection of the principal diagnosis in this case study?

_____

_____

9-2k.   Is there another diagnosis that meets the definition for principal diagnosis? Yes or No

9-2l.   If yes, what is the other diagnosis? _____

9-2m. Is there any opportunity for physician query?

_____

_____

9-2n.   What is the drug Bactrim used to treat? _____

9-3. CASE STUDY

History and Physical

CC: *C. diff*

HPI: The patient is a 44-year-old woman status post laparoscopic left salpingo-oophorectomy, lysis of adhesions, and cytoscopy about 10 days ago who presents with right-sided abdominal pain and *Clostridium difficile* colitis. The patient had been admitted to the hospital, where she underwent an operative laparoscopy with left salpingo-oophorectomy, lysis of adhesions, and cystoscopy. The surgery was performed for a newly diagnosed irregular cystic structure within the ovary. Final pathology from the left adnexal mass consisted of hydrosalpinges and tubal ovarian adhesions. The patient's blood loss during surgery was minimal. Pertinent operative findings included adhesions, normal-appearing bladder, and left ovarian fallopian tube adherent to the left pelvic side wall. The patient was extubated and transferred to the recovery room in stable condition following her procedure. However, she reported pain rated 8 to 9 out of 10 that was most notable at the right lower quadrant trocar site. She was re-admitted because of poor pain control at night. The patient was discharged the next day with the pain well controlled with Tylox.

The patient says she began to experience right-sided abdominal pain shortly after she was discharged. She first presented to her local emergency department with right lower quadrant pain. A CT scan performed at that time showed postsurgical changes. The patient began to experience diarrhea, poor oral intake, and generalized weakness. She was admitted to another hospital and was subsequently given a diagnosis of colitis. She tested positive for the *C. difficile* toxin. Repeat CT scan

55

showed thickening of the colon wall that was new compared with the previous CT scan. While admitted, the patient was treated with intravenous Flagyl 500 mg every 8 hours. She was transferred to our facility for further treatment and evaluation because she had undergone surgery here.

Past medical history: Hypothyroidism and seizure disorder.

Past surgical history: TAH-RSO 2 years ago. LSO as described previously about 10 days ago.

Gyn-obstetric history: Menarche age, 16. The patient underwent hysterectomy. Her last Pap smear was performed a few months ago, and findings were within normal limits. The patient underwent cone biopsy and cryotherapy many years ago for cervical dysplasia. Her last mammogram was performed a few months ago, and findings were within normal limits. The patient is not currently sexually active. She has no history of oral contraceptive tablet use. The patient had three full-term spontaneous vaginal deliveries and two miscarriages.

Social history: The patient is divorced. She works full time and also attends college. She exercises by riding a bicycle and/or walking every day. She drinks 1 cup of coffee and does not do monthly breast self-examinations.

Family history: The patient has two great aunts on the maternal side with breast cancer, one maternal aunt with ovarian cancer. No history of colon or endometrial cancer was reported.

Allergies: Vancomycin and gentamicin.

Medications on admission: Synthroid, Trileptal, Lamictal, Klonopin, MOBIC, and Flagyl.

Review of systems: See HPI. All other systems negative.

PHYSICAL EXAMINATION:

Vitals: Temperature 36.7 degrees, heart rate 85, blood pressure 138/78, respiratory rate 18, and O_2 saturation 98% on room air.

General: NAD. Well nourished and well developed.

HEENT: Atraumatic, normocephalic. PERRL. EOMI. Neck is supple. Trachea is midline. Oropharynx is clear.

Chest: CTA.

CV: RRR. No M/R/G.

Abd: Soft and nontender with normoactive bowel sounds. A resolving hematoma is visualized in the right lower quadrant.

Ext: No edema. No clubbing or cyanosis.

GU/Rectal: Deferred.

Skin/Musculoskeletal: Benign.

Neuro: Alert and oriented ×3. Cranial nerves intact.

ASSESSMENT/PLAN:

Patient is admitted for treatment of *Clostridium difficile* colitis. Potassium supplements will be started for hypokalemia. IV fluids will be administered. Medications for hypothyroidism and seizure disorder will be continued.

DIAGNOSES/PROBLEMS:

1. *Clostridium difficile* colitis.

2. Seizure disorder.

3. Hypothyroidism.

4. Status post laparoscopic left salpingo-oophorectomy.

PROCEDURES:

1. Antibiotics.

2. Intravenous fluids.

HISTORY, MAJOR FINDINGS, AND HOSPITAL COURSE:

The patient is a 44-year-old woman status post laparoscopic left salpingo-oophorectomy, lysis of adhesions, and cytoscopy about 10 days ago who presents with right-sided abdominal pain and *Clostridium difficile* colitis. The patient had been admitted to the hospital, where she underwent an operative laparoscopy with left salpingo-oophorectomy, lysis of adhesions, and cystoscopy. The surgery was performed for a newly diagnosed irregular cystic structure within the ovary. Final pathology from the left adnexal mass consisted of hydrosalpinges and tubal ovarian adhesions. Blood loss during surgery was minimal. Pertinent operative findings included adhesions, normal-appearing bladder, and left ovarian fallopian tube adherent to the left pelvic side wall. The patient was extubated and was transferred to the recovery room in stable condition following her procedure. However, she reported pain rated 8 to 9 out of 10, most notably at the right lower quadrant trocar site. The patient was then admitted because of poor pain control at night. She was discharged the next day with pain well controlled with Tylox.

The patient says she began to experience right-sided abdominal pain shortly after she was discharged. She first presented to the local emergency department with right lower quadrant pain. CT scan performed at that time showed postsurgical changes. She also began to experience diarrhea, poor oral intake, and generalized weakness. The patient was admitted to another hospital and was subsequently diagnosed with colitis. She tested positive for the *C. difficile* toxin. Repeat CT scan showed thickening of the colon wall that was new compared with the previous CT scan. While admitted, the patient was treated with intravenous Flagyl 500 mg every 8 hours.

Admission labs: Notable at that time for a positive urine toxicology for barbiturates and leukopenia, with a white blood cell count of 3.1. The patient also had hypokalemia. The patient was transferred to our hospital for evaluation of her right-sided abdominal pain because she had recently undergone surgery here. On admission, the patient rated her right lower quadrant pain as 4 out of 10. The patient noted that her pain was worse after oral intake.

Past medical history: Hypothyroidism and seizure disorder.

Past surgical history: TAH-RSO 2 years ago. LSO as described above about 10 days ago.

Gyn-Obstetric history: Menarche, age 16. The patient underwent hysterectomy. Her last Pap smear was performed a few months ago, and findings were within normal limits. The patient underwent cone biopsy and cryotherapy many years ago for cervical dysplasia. Her last mammogram was performed a few months ago, and findings were within normal limits. The patient is not currently sexually active. She has no history of oral contraceptive tablet use. The patient had 3 full-term spontaneous vaginal deliveries and 2 miscarriages.

Social history: The patient is divorced. She works full time and also attends college. She exercises by riding a bicycle and/or walking every day. She drinks 1 cup of coffee and does not do monthly breast self-examinations.

Family history: The patient has two great aunts on the maternal side with breast cancer and one maternal aunt with ovarian cancer. No history of colon or endometrial cancer was reported.

Allergies: Vancomycin and gentamicin.

Medications on admission: Synthroid, Trileptal, Lamictal, Klonopin, MOBIC, and Flagyl.

PHYSICAL EXAMINATION ON ADMISSION:

Temperature 36.7 degrees, heart rate 85, blood pressure 138/78, respiratory rate 18, and O_2 saturation 98% on room air. The patient's physical examination is notable for an abdomen that is soft and nontender with normoactive bowel sounds. A resolving hematoma is visualized in the right lower quadrant. The patient was then admitted for evaluation of right lower quadrant pain. Following is the summary of her hospital stay by system:

Gyn/Oncology: The patient's final pathology showed a hydrosalpinx and adhesions. The patient was reassured about these benign findings.

Infectious disease: The patient was admitted with a *C. difficile* colitis that was diagnosed at an outside hospital 5 days prior to admission. At the outside hospital, the patient was treated with intravenous Flagyl. Upon transfer to our facility, the patient was started on oral Flagyl. The patient was afebrile during her hospital stay. She had no episodes of diarrhea during her hospital stay and believed that her *C. diff* colitis was improving symptomatically.

GI: The patient was admitted with abdominal pain with *C. diff* colitis, as described earlier. The patient reported on admission that her abdominal pain was actually resolving. Her pain during admission was well controlled with Motrin. The patient had been treated with MOBIC while at the outside hospital. This treatment was discontinued.

Neuro: The patient has a history of seizure disorder, and her home antiepileptic medications of Trileptal and Lamictal were continued.

Endocrine: The patient has a history of hypothyroidism and was continued on Synthroid. Fluid, electrolyte, and nutrition: The patient was tolerating a soft diet when admitted. She was continued on that diet as tolerated. Additionally, the patient was given intravenous fluids. The patient's electrolytes were checked on hospital day 2 and were found to be within normal limits. Of note, the patient's potassium was 4.2, which is well within normal limits. This is notable because the patient was diagnosed with hypokalemia on admission.

The patient was discharged home on hospital day 2, and on that day, the patient's abdominal pain was very much improved and was well controlled with Motrin. Symptoms of diarrhea had resolved. She was tolerating a general diet and was afebrile.

Condition on discharge: Good.

DISCHARGE MEDICATIONS:

Flagyl 500 mg by mouth 3 times a day.

Motrin 600 mg by mouth every 6 hours.

The patient is also instructed to continue her home medications, which include Synthroid, Lamictal, and Trileptal.

The patient is instructed not to take any antidiarrheal medications.

DISCHARGE INSTRUCTIONS:

Diet: The patient may follow a regular diet.

Activity: She is instructed not to lift more than 25 pounds.

FOLLOW-UP CARE:

The patient is to follow up with her surgeon at a scheduled postoperative appointment.

Progress Notes

DAY 1

The patient is feeling a little better. She is afebrile. Her abdominal pain is resolving, and she has had only one episode of diarrhea since admission. Advance diet. Repeat electrolytes.

DAY 2

The patient's abdominal pain and diarrhea have resolved. She is tolerating a regular diet. Electrolytes are within normal limits, including a potassium of 4.2. She is ready for discharge home.

CASE STUDY QUESTIONS

9-3a. Admit diagnosis: _____

9-3b. Discharge disposition: _____

9-3c. Principal diagnosis: _____

9-3d. Secondary diagnoses (indicate POA status for secondary diagnoses):

_____

_____

_____

_____

_____

_____

9-3e. Principal procedure: _____

9-3f. Secondary procedures: _____

_____

9-3g. Assign MS-DRG: _____

9-3h. Relative weight of MS-DRG: _____

9-3i. Can this MS-DRG be optimized with the addition of a CC? Yes or No

Can this MS-DRG be optimized with the addition of an MCC? Yes or No

9-3j. Is there a main guideline pertinent to selection of the principal diagnosis in this case study?

_____

_____

9-3k. Is there another diagnosis that meets the definition for principal diagnosis? Yes or No

9-3l. If yes, what is the other diagnosis? _____

9-3m. Is there any opportunity for physician query?

_____

_____

9-3n. What is the drug Flagyl used to treat? _____

10 Neoplasms (ICD-10-CM Chapter 2, Codes C00-D49)

ABBREVIATIONS/ACRONYMS

Without the use of reference materials, define the following abbreviations or acronyms.

1. CLL _____
2. FNA _____
3. BMT _____
4. AML _____
5. NSCLC _____
6. RCC _____
7. NHL _____
8. CML _____
9. HCC _____
10. DCIS _____

GLOSSARY DEFINITIONS

Match the glossary term to the correct definition.

1. _____ Benign
2. _____ Primary
3. _____ Metastasis
4. _____ Radiation treatment
5. _____ Chemotherapy
6. _____ Grading
7. _____ Neoplasm
8. _____ Carcinoma in situ
9. _____ Staging
10. _____ Debulking
11. _____ Adenocarcinoma
12. _____ Lymphoma
13. _____ Prophylactic surgery
14. _____ Sarcoma
15. _____ Myeloma
16. _____ Carcinoma
17. _____ Brachytherapy

A. Neoplasm or tumor that is not malignant

B. Cancer of the lymphatic system

C. Location at which the neoplasm begins or malignancy originates

D. Administration of cancer-killing drugs

E. Malignancy of epithelial glandular tissue such as that found in the breast, prostate, and colon

F. Pathologic examination of tumor cells and determination of a grade based on extent of abnormality of the cells

G. Neoplasm of fibrous connective tissue

H. Surgery that is performed to remove tissue that has the potential to become cancerous

I. Means of categorizing a particular cancer that will help the physician determine a patient's treatment plan and the need for further therapy

J. The spread of a cancer from one part of the body to another, as occurs when neoplasms appear in parts of the body separate from the site of the primary tumor

K. Placement of radioactive material directly into or near the cancer

Continued

18. _____ Melanoma

19. _____ Fine needle aspiration

20. _____ Fibroma

L. Abnormal growth of melanin cells

M. Procedure that is performed when it is impossible to remove the tumor entirely

N. Malignant tumor that originates from epithelial tissue (e.g., skin, bronchi, stomach)

O. Use of high-energy radiation to treat cancer

P. Abnormal tissue that grows by cellular proliferation more rapidly than normal tissue and continues to grow after stimuli that initiated the new growth have been eliminated

Q. Malignant growth of connective tissue (e.g., muscle, cartilage, lymph tissue, bone)

R. Malignant cells that remain within the original site with no spread or invasion into neighboring tissues

S. Malignancy that originates within the bone marrow

T. Procedure in which a very small needle is used; works best for masses that are superficial or easily accessible

CODING

Using the code book, code the following.

1. Malignant neoplasm, unknown primary with metastasis to liver _____

2. Neurofibroma abdominal wall skin _____

3. Lymphangioendothelioma _____

4. GIST of the stomach _____

5. Primary peritoneal carcinoma _____

6. Lymphocytic leukemia in remission _____

7. Pancytopenia due to myelodysplastic syndrome _____

8. Inoperable tumor right lung _____

9. Admission for immunotherapy for left renal cell carcinoma; infusion high-dose interleukin-2 via central vein _____

10. Neurofibromatosis, type I _____

11. Carcinoma in situ prostate _____

12. Hemangioma of the subcutaneous axillary region _____

13. Vulvular malignancy _____

14. Large diffuse B-cell lymphoma _____

15. Basal cell carcinoma of nose _____

16. Admission for CHOP-R regimen of chemotherapy for mantle cell lymphoma (via central vein) _____

17. Bilateral orchiectomy with retroperitoneal lymph node dissection in patient with stage II testicular cancer with hypersecretion of testicular hormones _____

18. Retroperitoneal angiosarcoma _____

19. Familial adenomatous polyposis colon _____

20. Lung cancer with mets to bone, liver, and brain _____

CASE SCENARIOS

Using the code book, code the following cases.

1. This 30-year-old female patient has multiple intramural fibroids. She has become more symptomatic with menorrhagia, resulting in anemia due to blood loss and urinary frequency. The patient would like to maintain fertility, so a myomectomy is performed.
   Final Diagnosis: Intramural uterine fibroids.
   Procedure: Myomectomy.

   _____

   _____

2. The patient was admitted to the hospital for removal of recurrent brain tumor in the posterior fossa. The patient was taken to the OR, where the previous craniotomy incision was entered and the tumor excised. Extensive vasogenic edema was observed to surround the neoplasm. The path confirmed that the tumor was a recurrence of the patient's glioblastoma multiforme. The patient must undergo another round of chemotherapy treatments and possibly radiation treatment. The patient was given Decadron to reduce cerebral edema.
   Final Diagnosis: Recurrent glioblastoma multiforme tumor.
   Procedure: Craniotomy with excision of posterior fossa tumor.

   _____

   _____

3. A 24-year-old man presented with a mediastinal mass and superior vena cava syndrome. He was diagnosed with large cell lymphoma, stage IIB, and was treated with CHOP followed by mediastinal irradiation. He was well until October 1997, when he was found to have recurrent disease with a large abdominal mass. The patient was treated with salvage chemotherapy with ESHAP. The disease then went into remission, and the patient was scheduled for stem cell transplantation. The patient's other medical problems include asthma during childhood with no attacks since age 10, for which he is no longer on medication, and a T&A at age 5. The patient underwent autologous stem cell transplantation during this admission with no complications.
   Final Diagnosis: Large cell lymphoma in remission.
   Procedure: Autologous stem cell transplant via central venous catheter.

   _____

   _____

4. The patient is currently undergoing chemotherapy for cancer of the sigmoid colon. Sigmoid tumor was removed 2 months ago with positive pelvic lymph nodes. The patient has had extreme nausea and vomiting caused by chemotherapy. When the patient arrived for scheduled chemotherapy treatment, it was decided that the patient should be admitted for intravenous fluids. Patient has a medical history of diverticulosis, hiatal hernia with GERD, and anxiety.
   Final Diagnosis: Dehydration due to chemotherapy.

   _____

   _____

5. The patient was admitted for chemotherapy for stage IIIA breast (left) cancer that has spread to the axillary lymph nodes. The patient takes medication for restless leg syndrome. The patient tolerated the chemotherapy regimen with no complications and will return as arranged for cycle 3.
   Final Diagnosis: Breast cancer, stage IIIA.
   Procedure: Chemotherapy via central vein.

   _____

   _____

6. This 50-year-old male patient was admitted for definitive treatment after a biopsy of his right tonsil showed squamous cell carcinoma. The patient has a history of GERD that is relieved with medication and had colon polyps removed 2 years ago. He is allergic to penicillin. The patient was taken to the OR, where he underwent bilateral tonsillectomy with radical dissection of the lymph nodes on the right side. Pathology showed metastasis to the lymph nodes. The patient will follow up with the oncologist.
Final Diagnosis: Squamous cell carcinoma of the right tonsil.
Procedure: Radical dissection of neck with bilateral tonsillectomy.

_____

_____

7. The patient was admitted for pain control. The patient has a history of prostate cancer and underwent radical prostatectomy a couple of years ago. His cancer has progressed by metastasizing to the bones. He has received palliative radiation in an attempt to sustain quality of life. Over the past couple of days, his pain has become unbearable. The patient was discharged to home once his pain was controlled.
Final Diagnosis: Metastatic prostate cancer.

_____

_____

8. The patient has a history of chronic hepatitis C. On routine ultrasonography, a suspicious mass of the liver was discovered. Biopsy confirmed hepatocellular carcinoma, and the patient was admitted for partial hepatectomy.
Final Diagnoses: Chronic hepatitis C.
                 Hepatocellular carcinoma.
Procedure: Partial hepatectomy for resection of HCC.

_____

_____

9. This is a 59-year-old male patient who is admitted from the ER for dyspnea and chest pain. Chest x-ray shows a large pleural effusion on the right. A thoracentesis is performed, and the patient's symptoms resolve. The cytology report shows that this was a malignant effusion. The patient has a history of colon cancer that was removed 5 years ago with no recurrence until now. The patient takes medications for CHF and CAD, and he has a history of CABG. The patient has an appointment with his oncologist next week.
Final Diagnosis: Colon cancer with metastasis to the pleura.
Procedure: Diagnostic thoracentesis.

_____

_____

10. This 67-year-old female is currently undergoing treatment for advanced uterine cancer. The patient presents for follow-up restaging CT, and a large pulmonary embolism is noted. The patient denies any shortness of breath, cough, or chest pain. She has a history of hydronephrosis and takes medications for hypertension and anemia caused by her cancer. CT scan shows ascites. Doppler of the lower extremities shows no DVT. The patient is treated with subcutaneous Lovenox, and Coumadin is started. She received two units of packed red cells (via peripheral vein) during her stay.
Final Diagnoses: Uterine cancer with spread to pelvic and peritoneal lymph nodes.
                 Pulmonary embolism.
                 Possible malignant ascites.

_____

_____

Using the code book, code and answer questions about the following case studies.

10-1. CASE STUDY

History and Physical

The patient is a 58-year-old female with a history of CNS lymphoma and systemic lymphoma who was admitted for high dose of methotrexate. She has a history of lymphoma treated with CHOP 6 to 7 years ago. She presented with confusion and central nervous system diffuse large B-cell lymphoma this past August. Biopsy was reviewed and confirmed the diagnosis. It is not clear whether this is a primary or a recurrent tumor. The patient was started on high-dose Decadron and was treated with high-dose methotrexate every 2 weeks. She has continued to improve on this regimen. She had a recent episode of left upper quadrant discomfort.

Family history: No lymphoma.

Social history: Nonsmoker, nondrinker.

REVIEW OF SYSTEMS:

Constitutional: No fevers, night sweats.

Eyes: No changes in vision, diplopia, blurring.

Ears, nose, throat: No tinnitus, epistaxis or rhinitis, pharyngitis.

Cardiovascular: No exertional pain, pedal edema, nocturnal dyspnea, cough, hemoptysis, chest pain.

Respiratory: Without shortness of breath, cough, chest pain.

GI: Without nausea, vomiting, reflux, abdominal pain, diarrhea, constipation, blood in stool.

Genitourinary: Without frequency, dysuria, hematuria, nocturia.

Skin: Without itching, rash.

Neuro: Without headache, seizure, syncope, paresthesias.

Psychiatric: Without depression, mood swings, memory problems.

Endocrine: Without temperature intolerance, weight change, bowel changes, polyuria, loss of consciousness, flushing.

Hematologic/Lymphatic: Without symptoms of bleeding, easy bruising, thrombosis.

Allergy: No allergies.

Musculoskeletal: Without arthritis or arthralgias or myalgias; she has had difficulty with stairs after starting steroids.

Meds: Decadron 2 mg.

Healthy appearing in no distress. Vital signs stable.

Eyes: Visual acuity grossly intact, conjunctivae moist.

Nose and mouth: Without rhinitis, oral mucosal lesions.

Integument: Without rash, raised lesions, jaundice, or cyanosis.

Musculoskeletal: Without skeletal deformity. Only 4 strength in proximal muscles.

Respiratory: Without special respiratory efforts, cough. Clear to auscultation.

Cardiac: Without murmur, rub, or gallop. No jugular venous distention or pedal edema. Heart rate regular.

Gastrointestinal: No hepatosplenomegaly. Abdomen soft, nontender without masses. Normal bowel sounds. Rectal exam deferred.

Genitourinary: No CVA tenderness, bladder not distended or tender.

Neuro: Patient alert and oriented. Affect appropriate. Memory intact.

Lymph nodes/Hematologic: No palpable submental, cervical, axillary, supraclavicular, inguinal lymphadenopathy. No signs of bleeding or bruising.

PROBLEMS:

1. High-dose methotrexate. The patient was hydrated overnight with alkalinization of urine. We will go ahead and start methotrexate with leucovorin rescue today.
2. CNS lymphoma. We will repeat MRI to assess continued resolution of her CNS lesions.
3. H/O systemic lymphoma. We will repeat chest and abdominal CT to be sure there is no evidence of systemic disease.
4. Steroids. She has been slowly tapered. We are discontinuing Decadron.
5. *Pneumocystis* prophylaxis (for high-dose steroids). We are holding during MTX infusion but will restart at discharge.

Discharge Summary

DIAGNOSES/PROBLEMS:

Primary CNS lymphoma.

PROCEDURES:

1. Administration of high-dose methotrexate.
2. CT scan of the chest, abdomen, and pelvis with contrast.

HISTORY, MAJOR FINDINGS, AND HOSPITAL COURSE:

The patient is a 58-year-old woman with a distant history of lymphoma, for which she was treated approximately 7 years ago; however, no details are available. Unfortunately, primary CNS lymphoma was diagnosed relatively recently, and the patient has been on therapy with high-dose methotrexate. She now is admitted for administration of 8 cycles of high-dose methotrexate.

The patient was admitted for administration of high-dose methotrexate. Upon admission, she was aggressively hydrated with intravenous fluids containing bicarbonate in order to alkalinize the urine. Once her urine had been appropriately alkalinized, the patient received methotrexate 8 g per meter squared, which she tolerated well. Serum methotrexate levels were measured 24 and 48 hours after administration of methotrexate. Serum methotrexate level 24 hours after administration was 4.17 micromoles per liter, and 48 hours after methotrexate, 0.13 micromoles per liter. Given that her methotrexate level was at a suitable level for discharge, we discharged her to home in good condition. Additionally, in order to restage her systemic lymphoma, a CT scan of the chest, abdomen, and pelvis was performed. A preliminary result, available at this time, shows no evidence of occult neoplasm or mass; however, a final reading is still pending. Additionally, we attempted to obtain an MRI of the head in order to assess for the status of her CNS lymphoma; however, we were unable to have one scheduled prior to the time of discharge.

DISCHARGE MEDICATIONS:

The patient will be given a prescription to take Leucovorin 25 mg 4 times a day for the next 3 days. She should continue all medications that she was taking prior to admission with the exception of dexamethasone, which was discontinued while she was in the hospital; she should remain off of this medication.

FOLLOW-UP CARE:

Follow-up appointment: The patient will be given an appointment for an outpatient MRI of the head. Additionally, she will follow up with her oncologist as an outpatient.

Progress Notes

DAY 1

The patient is tolerating methotrexate infusion without problem. Hydration is good. Her K is 3.3 and will be supplemented with oral KCL. Renal: Cr is stable. Patient has no complaints.

DAY 2

Methotrexate infusion is complete. We are continuing to hydrate and monitor levels. Also will obtain MRI to evaluate brain lesions and CT of chest and abdomen to evaluate possible recurrence of systemic tumor. We have recently discontinued daily Decadron. Case was discussed with the residents and nursing staff.

CASE STUDY QUESTIONS

10-1a. Admit diagnosis: _____

10-1b. Discharge disposition: _____

10-1c. Principal diagnosis: _____

10-1d. Secondary diagnoses (indicate POA status for secondary diagnoses):

_____

_____

_____

_____

_____

_____

10-1e. Principal procedure: _____

10-1f. Secondary procedures: _____

_____

10-1g. Assign MS-DRG: _____

10-1h. Relative weight of MS-DRG: _____

10-1i. Can this MS-DRG be optimized with the addition of a CC? Yes or No
        Can this MS-DRG be optimized with the addition of an MCC? Yes or No

10-1j. Is there a main guideline pertinent to selection of the principal diagnosis in this case study?

_____

_____

10-1k. Is there another diagnosis that meets the definition for principal diagnosis? Yes or No

10-1l. If yes, what is the other diagnosis? _____

10-1m. Is there any opportunity for physician query?

_____

_____

10-1n. What is the drug Decadron used to treat? _____

10-2. CASE STUDY

Clinic Note/Preoperative Evaluation

Reason for visit: This patient was seen for preoperative evaluation in anticipation of total thyroidectomy scheduled next week.

History of present illness: This 50-year-old woman has a history of coronary vasospasm and a thyroid follicular neoplasm. In 1995, the patient was evaluated for episodic chest pain. She underwent catheterization, which revealed no coronary artery disease, but coronary vasospasm could not be reproduced. Since then, she has been taking nitroglycerin and Cardizem regularly with complete resolution of her symptoms. She currently denies shortness of breath, PND, dyspnea on exertion, or palpitations. She also has a known left bundle branch block that was diagnosed in 1995. She has developed hoarseness of voice and occasional dysphagia without symptoms of aspiration. When lying supine, she does feel a "tightness" in her throat that makes it feel like she can't breathe, even though she continues to breathe without difficulty. Eventually, she is able to fall asleep and sleeps supine without difficulty. She does snore but has no symptoms of obstructive sleep apnea.

Past medical history: As above. Patient also has a history of breast cancer, for which a mastectomy was performed 5 years ago. There has been no recurrence.

Past surgical history includes right mastectomy.

Family history: No family history of thyroid cancers.

Social history: Nonsmoker. One glass of wine with dinner.

Review of symptoms: Per HPI. Otherwise negative.

Medications: Cardizem 240 mg PO qday; nitroglycerin SR 6.5 mg PO bid; Zetia 10 mg PO qday; Fosamax 70 mg PO qwk; Zyrtec 10 mg PO qday; mvi daily.

Allergies: NKDA; sensitive to cigarette smoke.

Physical Examination:

Vital signs stable. Weight stable at 125 pounds.

HEENT: Unremarkable. Trachea midline. Multinodular goiter. No carotid bruit.

Chest: Lungs clear to auscultation.

Abd: Soft, nontender.

Breasts: Absent right breast. No masses in left.

GU: Examination deferred.

Extremities: No cyanosis or edema. Good pulses.

Neurologic: Intact.

Assessments: This 50-year-old woman has a history of suspicious thyroid nodule, coronary vasospasm, left bundle branch block, and breast cancer. Her cardiac symptoms were probably due to Prinzmetal's angina, which has been under excellent control with a CCB and nitrate. She has excellent exercise tolerance and has had a recent EKG. She requires no further cardiac testing. Although she reports some choking sensations while lying supine, these do not seem to be due to mechanical obstruction of air flow, and we do not anticipate any airway problems.

DIAGNOSES/PROBLEMS:

1. Suspicious thyroid nodule, possible thyroid follicular cancer
2. Coronary vasospasm
3. Left bundle branch block
4. History of breast cancer

Plans: BMP, CBC, type and screen. Continue Cardizem and nitroglycerin.

Medication changes: NPO instructions given. Patient instructed to take Cardizem and nitroglycerin SR with sips of water on morning of surgery.

Discharge Summary

DIAGNOSES/PROBLEMS:

1. Hürthle cell adenoma
2. Hashimoto's thyroiditis
3. Coronary vasospasm
4. History of breast cancer

HISTORY, MAJOR FINDINGS, AND HOSPITAL COURSE:

The patient is a 50-year-old female whose past medical history is remarkable for breast cancer with mastectomy and subsequent chemotherapy. A few months ago, she developed upper arm pain and had an MRI of C-spine for workup. MRI noted a 1.5-cm nodule in the right lower lobe of the thyroid. This was confirmed by thyroid ultrasonography that revealed a heterogenous echotexture nodule at the medial aspect of the right lower pole, as well as two 7-mm nodules in the left lobe. Fine needle aspiration was performed and was notable for follicular cells and neoplasm with Hürthle cell features. The patient was subsequently referred for surgical evaluation. In addition to the above, her past medical history is notable for coronary spasms, occasional dyspepsia, occasional dysphagia, previously mentioned breast cancer, and subsequent chemotherapy.

Past surgical history is notable for left mastectomy with reconstruction and colonoscopy. The patient has no known drug allergies. She was taken to the Operating Room, and the above referenced procedure was performed. For additional details, please refer to the operative note. Pathology of the specimen was pending at the time of her discharge.

The patient tolerated the procedure well and was transferred and extubated to the regular floor. She remained hemodynamically stable. Incisions remained clean, dry, and intact. She denied perioral or extremity paresthesia. On postop day 1, ionized calcium was known to be 1.15. She was tolerating a regular diet and subsequently was discharged home in stable condition.

DISCHARGE MEDICATIONS:

Resume preoperative medications. Oxycodone 5 to 10 mg by mouth every 4 to 6 hours as needed for pain. Calcium 2 tablets by mouth 3 times a day and every 2 hours as needed for symptoms of hypocalcemia. Synthroid 125 mcg by mouth every 24 hours, to begin 11/18/06.

FOLLOW-UP CARE:

The patient will call for follow-up appointment next week.

Operative Report

Title of operation: Total thyroidectomy. Limited left central neck lymph node dissection. Intraoperative nerve monitoring.

Indications for surgery:

Clinical note: This patient has been given a diagnosis of multinodular goiter with a dominant nodule at the junction of the right thyroid lobe and isthmus, which, on needle biopsy, was suspicious with Hürthle cell features. Evidence revealed another nodule in the isthmus, small nodules in the left lobe of her thyroid, and two lymph nodes inferior to the left thyroid lobe. On the basis of these clinical findings, a total thyroidectomy was recommended, and the patient accepted this recommendation. Risks of the procedure, including bleeding, infection, nerve injury, hypoparathyroidism, voice change, and the requirement for a cervical skin incision, were explained to the patient. She wished to proceed.

Preoperative diagnosis: Hürthle cell nodule at junction of right thyroid lobe and isthmus with contralateral nodularity.

Postoperative diagnosis: Hürthle cell nodule at junction of right thyroid lobe and isthmus with contralateral nodularity.

Anesthesia: General endotracheal anesthesia.

Specimen (bacteriological, pathologic, or other): Total thyroidectomy. Left central neck lymph nodes.

Surgeon's Narrative

Operative findings: Total thyroidectomy was performed in standard fashion without complications. A nodule was noted at the junction of the right lobe of the thyroid and the isthmus. There were also some small lymph nodes inferior to the isthmus and inferior to the left lobe of the thyroid, as noted on ultrasonography, that were dissected as part of a limited central neck nodal dissection. Both recurrent laryngeal nerves were identified with the aid of the nerve stimulator and were stimulated normally at the completion of the procedure. A capsular dissection technique was used bilaterally to dissect the parathyroid glands off the thyroid.

Details of the procedure: With the patient in the supine position and the neck extended, the skin was prepped and draped in standard fashion. A cervical skin incision was fashioned, and superior and inferior skin flaps were raised. The superficial layer of the deep cervical fascia was incised at the midline, and dissection was begun on the right side by dissecting the strap muscles off the right lobe of the thyroid. A palpable nodule was noted on ultrasonography at the junction of the right lobe and the isthmus. The right lobe was retracted medially, and the middle thyroid vein was ligated and divided between 3-0 silk ties. Some small lymph nodes inferior to the thyroid isthmus were dissected and handed off for pathologic evaluation. The right recurrent laryngeal nerve was identified with the aid of a nerve stimulator deep in the neck and was carefully preserved. The right lower parathyroid gland was dissected laterally off the thyroid and was preserved on its blood supply. Superior pole vessels were then ligated and divided between 0 silk ties, with dissection proceeding lateral to the cricothyroid muscle directly on the upper pole of the thyroid to preserve the external branch of the superior laryngeal nerve. The lobe was retracted farther medially, and right upper parathyroid gland tissue was dissected laterally off the thyroid. The nerve was then reidentified, traced to its distal insertion, and carefully preserved with the secondary branches of the inferior thyroid artery ligated and divided between 3-0 silk ties, as were several small inferior thyroid veins. With the nerve in clear view, the ligament of Berry was divided with the use of bipolar electrocautery; dissection continued beneath the right lobe of the thyroid and the thyroid isthmus. We then began dissection on the left side by dissecting the strap muscles off the left lobe of the thyroid. The lobe was retracted medially and the middle thyroid vein ligated and divided between 3-0 silk ties. The left recurrent laryngeal nerve was identified with the aid of the nerve stimulator in the tracheoesophageal groove and was carefully preserved. The left lower parathyroid gland was identified and dissected laterally off the thyroid. Superior pole vessels were ligated and divided between 0 silk ties with dissection proceeding lateral to the cricothyroid muscle directly on the upper pole of the thyroid to preserve the external branch of the superior laryngeal nerve. The lobe was then retracted farther medially, and the left upper parathyroid gland tissue was dissected laterally off the thyroid. The recurrent nerve was then re-identified and traced to its distal insertion; it was carefully preserved with the secondary branches of the inferior thyroid artery ligated and divided between 3-0 silk ties. With the nerve in clear view, the ligament of Berry was divided with the use of bipolar electrocautery; dissection continued beneath the left lobe of the thyroid and the isthmus until the total thyroidectomy specimen was now free and was handed off for pathologic evaluation. Lymph nodes anterior to the recurrent laryngeal nerve, inferior to the left thyroid lobe, and anterior to the trachea were then dissected. Specifically, the area was noted on ultrasonography. A small lymph node was observed in the specimen, and this was also handed off for pathologic evaluation. Meticulous hemostasis was then assured in the left and right neck, and both recurrent laryngeal nerves were restimulated and were found to stimulate normally. Following assurance of hemostasis, the strap muscles were closed with a running 3-0 Biosyn suture, the platysma muscle was closed with interrupted 3-0 Biosyn sutures, and the skin was closed with a running 4-0 subcuticular Biosyn suture; Steri-Strips were applied.

Estimated blood loss during the procedure was minimal. No complications were reported. Sponge, needle, and instrument counts were correct, and the patient was transported to the recovery room in stable condition.

Pathology Report

1. Inferior to thyroid, node (excision): one (1) lymph node. Associated fibroadipose tissue, negative for tumor.
2. Thyroid (total thyroidectomy): Hürthle cell adenoma (1 cm) arising in a background of Hashimoto's thyroiditis. Two (2) lymph nodes and associated fibroadipose tissue, negative for tumor. Margins negative for tumor.
3. Left central lymph nodes (excision): one (1) lymph node and associated fibroadipose tissue, negative for tumor.

BRIEF OP NOTE

Preop diagnosis: Hürthle cell nodule.

Postop diagnosis: Hürthle cell nodule, pending pathology.

Procedure: Total thyroidectomy with central lymph node dissection.

Anes: ETGA.

IVF: 1000 cc.

EBL: Minimal.

Specimen: Thyroid gland and central lymph nodes.

Condition: Stable.

Complications: None.

UOP: Not measured.

Progress Note

DAY 1

Vitals stable. Patient alert, NAD. No numbness or tingling. Tongue midline. Incision looks good. Ionized calcium at 10 PM 1.05, and at 3 AM 1.15.

Anesthesiology Progress Note

Awake. VS stable. Alert and oriented ×3. Good recovery from anesthesia with no apparent anesthesia complication.

Progress Note

DAY 2

Vital signs stable. Doing well. Good pain management. No neck hematoma. Steri-Strips intact. Tolerating clear liquid diet. Advance diet and recheck calcium level. Ready for discharge.

CASE STUDY QUESTIONS

10-2a. Admit diagnosis: _____

10-2b. Discharge disposition: _____

10-2c. Principal diagnosis: _____

10-2d. Secondary diagnoses (indicate POA status for secondary diagnoses):

_____

_____

_____

_____

_____

10-2e. Principal procedure: ————————————————————————————————————

10-2f. Secondary procedures: ————————————————————————————————————

——

10-2g. Assign MS-DRG: ——————————

10-2h. Relative weight of MS-DRG: ——————————

10-2i. Can this MS-DRG be optimized with the addition of a CC? Yes or No
        Can this MS-DRG be optimized with the addition of an MCC? Yes or No

10-2j. Is there a main guideline pertinent to selection of the principal diagnosis in this case study?

——

——

10-2k. Is there another diagnosis that meets the definition for principal diagnosis? Yes or No

10-2l. If yes, what is the other diagnosis? ————————————————————————————

10-2m. Is there any opportunity for physician query?

——

——

10-2n. What is the drug Synthroid used to treat? ————————————————————————

10-3. CASE STUDY

Clinic Note/Preoperative Evaluation

Reason for visit: Hemoptysis. Right middle lobe mass.

The patient is a pleasant 56-year-old gentleman with a history of hemoptysis and a right middle lobe mass that suggests concern for malignancy. He presents for evaluation regarding diagnosis and management.

History of present illness: The patient is a very pleasant 56-year-old gentleman with a smoking history for the past 36 years who presented with hemoptysis. CT scan revealed what appeared to be a bulla or pneumatocele in the right middle lobe with a solid component. Bronchoscopy was performed with a BAL and transbronchial FNA that was nondiagnostic; this also showed atypical glandular proliferation, which could not exclude adenocarcinoma. PET study showed moderately increased FDG activity fusing to the soft tissue component of his right middle lobe pneumatocele, with an FEV maximum of 2.1. Overall, this patient has had minimal hemoptysis related to this and denies any fevers or chills. He also denies any recent pneumonic infections. Denies any history of TB or atypical mycobacterial infections in the past. He currently smokes 6 to 7 cigarettes per day and denies fever, chills, night sweats, or weight loss.

Past medical history is significant for gastroesophageal reflux disease, pyelonephritis, hypothyroidism, and a history of DVT in his left lower extremity.

Past surgical history is negative.

Social history: The patient has a 6 to 7 cigarette smoking history for about 36 years, which translates to roughly a 15-pack-year smoking history. Alcohol intake is 6 to 7 cans of beer per day.

Review of systems: The patient denies any history of cardiac problems such as heart valvular problems, myocardial infarction, or hypertension. Denies any airway problems or snoring-related problems, chronic wheezing or chronic cough, or sputum production. Denies any history of easy bleeding. The patient does report lower extremity DVT. He denies any chronic renal insufficiency and denies any liver disease. Exercise tolerance is excellent, with 2 to 3 flights of dyspnea on exertion.

Medications: Aspirin 81 mg by mouth every day, Prilosec 20 mg by mouth 2 times a day, Synthroid 25 mcg by mouth every day, and Tenormin 25 mg by mouth every day

Allergies: Penicillin, which causes lower extremity swelling

Physical examination: On examination, this is a very pleasant gentleman in no acute distress. He is very thin; his weight is 125 pounds, his temperature is 97.8, his blood pressure is 158/84, and his pulse is 77.

HEENT: No cervical or supraclavicular lymphadenopathy. Trachea is midline. Thyroid is normal.

Chest: Clear lung fields bilaterally with no wheezes and no rhonchi.

CV: Regular rate and rhythm.

Abd: Normal bowel sounds. Nontender. No guarding.

Neuro: No abnormality.

Extremities: No pedal edema.

Examination on CT scan reveals a pneumatocele in the right middle lobe with a solid component inferiorly and medially; this is certainly suspicious for a primary lung tumor. PET shows moderately intense FOG activity in this area.

Pulmonary function tests reveal an FEV1 of 1.92, which is 54% of predicted, an FVC of 3.24, which is 87% predicted, and an FEV1-to-FVC ratio of 59%.

Assessments: The patient is a 56-year-old gentleman with a smoking history and a positive mass in the right middle lobe in the setting of a pneumatocele. I discussed with him the differential diagnoses, which include a primary non–small cell lung cancer or potentially an inflammatory process related to the pneumatocele or bulla. We discussed the need for a definitive diagnosis, should this potentially be a non–small cell lung cancer, which would require resection with a lobectomy for therapy. Because no mediastinal adenopathy was observed and no PET activity was noted in the mediastinum, I did not think that mediastinoscopy is indicated if this was a non–small cell lung cancer. His incidence of mediastinal involvement would be less than 4%. I discussed with him the details of a VATS procedure, and we tried to do a VATS lobectomy of the right middle lobe. I discussed with him the indications, benefits, alternatives, and risks. He understands and agrees to proceed.

Plans: At this juncture, we will take him to the Operating Room for a bronchoscopy and a right middle lobectomy. We will attempt to do this with a VATS procedure. I do not think that an epidural catheter would be necessary. We could place one postoperatively, should thoracotomy become necessary. Please note that I spent approximately 30 minutes with the patient answering questions, counseling, and coordinating care.

DIAGNOSES/PROBLEMS:

1. Right middle lobe malignant with invasion of pleura.
2. Hx of GERD.
3. Hx of pyelonephritis.
4. Hx of hypothyroidism.
5. Hx of DVT LLE.
6. Allergy to PCN.

PROCEDURES:

1. VATS right middle lobectomy.
2. Fiberoptic bronchoscopy with therapeutic aspiration of secretions.
3. Video-assisted thoracoscopy.
4. Mediastinal lymphadenectomy.

HISTORY, MAJOR FINDINGS, AND HOSPITAL COURSE:

The patient is a 56-year-old male smoker who initially presented with hemoptysis. CT revealed a right middle lobe mass, with FOG uptake on PET. The patient was brought to the OR for a VATS right middle lobectomy. For further information, please refer to the operative report. Postoperatively, the patient recovered in the intensive care unit. Pain was well controlled. On POD #1, a pleural tube was removed and the patient was discharged.

DISCHARGE MEDICATIONS:

Oxycodone 5 to 10 mg PO q 4–6 hours pm pain, Colace 100 mg PO BID, Atenolol 25 mg PO q day, Protonix 40 mg PO q day, Levothyroxine 25 mcg PO q day, ASA 81 mg PO q day.

DISCHARGE INSTRUCTIONS:

No driving until follow-up with physician. No heavy lifting until follow-up with surgeon. May shower but no baths or submersion. Please call physician's office for fevers greater than or equal to 101.5, increasing incisional pain, incisional discharge or bleeding. Regular diet. Patient to take Colace twice a day because oxycodone may cause constipation.

FOLLOW-UP CARE:

Patient to follow up with surgeon in 2 weeks. Please call to schedule appointment.

Title of operation: Fiberoptic bronchoscopy with therapeutic aspiration of secretions. Right VATS lobectomy, right middle lobe. Mediastinal lymphadenectomy.

Indications for surgery: The patient is 56-year-old gentleman with a spiculated right middle lobe mass that is PET positive. He initially presented with hemoptysis and bronchoscopy; biopsy revealed some atypical cells that were a matter of concern in terms of malignancy. I discussed with the patient the details of a VATS lobectomy and possible open right middle lobectomy for diagnostic and therapeutic reasons, should this turn out to be a non–small cell lung cancer. We discussed the indications, benefits, alternatives, and risks, and he understood and agreed to proceed.

Preoperative diagnosis: Spiculated PET positive mass, right middle lobe.

Postoperative diagnosis: Spiculated PET positive mass, right middle lobe.

Anesthesia: General.

Surgeon's Narrative

Fluids: 1500 cubic centimeters of crystalloid
Estimated blood loss: 20 cubic centimeters

Findings: The mass was palpated in the right middle lobe. Specimens of the right middle lobe and lymph nodes from stations 2, 4, 7, 11, 10, and 12 were sent for permanent pathology.

Technical details: After informed consent was obtained, the patient was taken to the Operating Room and was placed in supine position on the Operating Room table; general endotracheal anesthesia was administered. Fiberoptic bronchoscopy revealed normal endobronchial anatomy. No endobronchial masses or lesions were noted. A double-lumen endotracheal tube was placed under direct vision, and the patient was placed in the right side-up left lateral decubitus position. The right chest was prepped and draped in usual sterile fashion. A 1-cm incision was made at about the 8th interspace in the anterior axillary line, and the thoracoscope was passed. A posterior axillary port was placed over the 8th interspace with a 1-cm incision; the working port access incision was repositioned directly over the mediastinum and the lower lobe vein. A 3-cm incision was made, and we placed the serratus anterior muscles and bovied the intercostal muscles at the top of the lower rib. The inferior and superior pulmonary veins were identified, and the middle lobe vein to the middle lobe was seen coming off the superior pulmonary vein. This was ligated and divided with an Endo GIA 2.5-mm stapling device.

We then dissected the bronchus and the artery, which were dissected out. We then dissected out the fissure, identified the PA in the fissure, and completed the major fissure between the middle and lower lobes. I continued my dissection of the right middle lobe bronchus off the main PA and circumferentially dissected throughout, freeing up the bronchus from the middle lobe pulmonary branch. We sequentially dissected up the right middle lobe bronchus and then with the Endo GIA 4.8-mm stapling device, we divided and sealed it. I circumferentially dissected up the middle lobe artery; again, this was similarly ligated and divided with the Endo GIA 2.5-mm stapling device. Once this had been completed, we freed up the middle lobe tissues of the pulmonary artery and completed the fissure between the upper and middle lobes with the Endo GIA 4.8-mm stapling device. Once this had been completed, we performed a mediastinal lymphadenectomy to take out any identifiable lymph node tissue in the subcarinal spaces and in the upper mediastinum corresponding to L2 and R4 levels. A 20-French chest tube was placed over the lower anterior port site and 0 silk U stitch was used to secure.

We inflated the lung and checked the bronchus under 20 cm of water pressure and found no leak. The upper and lower lobes came up nicely, and the wounds were then closed in layers with absorbable sutures. The wounds were cleaned, and dressings were applied. The patient awoke from anesthesia and was extubated and transferred to the recovery area in satisfactory condition. I was present and scrubbed for the entire procedure.

Chest AP Portable

Result: Chest x-ray frontal view, 7 AM.

History: Chest tube removed.

Findings: Right chest tube has been removed. No pneumothorax is seen. Stable postsurgical changes in the right hilar region with slight prominence of the right hilum. Right thoracic subcutaneous emphysema. Heart is normal in size. Atherosclerosis thoracic aorta. Healed left rib fractures.

THORACIC SURGERY OP NOTE

Preop diagnosis: RML mass + PET.

Postop diagnosis: Pending path.

Proc: R VATS lobectomy, right middle lobe; mediastinal lymphadenectomy.

Anes: General.

Fluids: 1500 cc.

EBL: 20 cc.

Patient tolerated well.

POST-OP DAY 1

Patient has some resp acidosis. Treat mild alcohol withdrawal with Ativan.

Chest: CTA; SQ air noted.

CV: RRR.

GI: Benign.

POST-OP DAY 2

Doing well. No pneumothorax. Wounds clean. Hemodynamically stable. Convert to PO narcotics. D/C RT, Foley. Advance diet.

CASE STUDY QUESTIONS

10-3a. Admit diagnosis: _____

10-3b. Discharge disposition: _____

10-3c. Principal diagnosis: _____

10-3d. Secondary diagnoses (indicate POA status for secondary diagnoses):

_____

_____

_____

_____

_____

_____

10-3e. Principal procedure: _____

10-3f. Secondary procedures: _____

_____

10-3g. Assign MS-DRG: _____

10-3h. Relative weight of MS-DRG: _____

10-3i. Can this MS-DRG be optimized with the addition of a CC? Yes or No
        Can this MS-DRG be optimized with the addition of an MCC? Yes or No

10-3j. Is there a main guideline pertinent to selection of the principal diagnosis in this case study?

_____

_____

10-3k. Is there another diagnosis that meets the definition for principal diagnosis? Yes or No

10-3l. If yes, what is the other diagnosis? _____

10-3m. Is there any opportunity for physician query?

_____

_____

10-3n. What is the drug oxycodone used to treat? _____

Diseases of the Blood and Blood-Forming Organs and Certain Disorders Involving the Immune Mechanism (ICD-10-CM Chapter 3, Codes D50-D89)

ABBREVIATIONS

Without the use of reference materials, define the following abbreviations.

1. WBC _____

2. Hgb _____

3. ASA _____

4. PT _____

5. Hct _____

6. CBC _____

7. PTT _____

8. ITP _____

9. DIC _____

10. GVHD _____

GLOSSARY DEFINITIONS

Match the glossary term to the correct definition.

1. _____ Sickle cell anemia

2. _____ Anticoagulant medication

3. _____ Apheresis

4. _____ Purpura

5. _____ Hemophilia A

6. _____ Autologous transfusion

7. _____ Bone marrow biopsy

8. _____ Leukocytosis

9. _____ Anemia

10. _____ Coagulation defect

11. _____ Hemophilia B

12. _____ Thrombocytes

13. _____ Pancytopenia

14. _____ Antiplatelet medications

15. _____ Disseminated intravascular coagulation

16. _____ Thalassemia

A. Another name for platelets

B. Decrease in the production of erythrocytes, leukocytes, and thrombocytes

C. Most common type of hemophilia; a deficiency of clotting factor VIII

D. Causative factor unknown

E. Disorder that results in depletion of clotting factors in the blood

F. Procedure that separates the various components of the blood and removes a certain part of the blood, such as in leukapheresis, plateletpheresis, and plasmapheresis

G. Transfusion of patient's own blood

H. Increase in the number of white cells in the blood. May be a sign of infection, or may indicate that stress is being placed on the body

I. Another name for Christmas disease, which is the result of a deficiency of factor IX

Continued

17. _____ Aplastic anemia

18. _____ Neutropenia

19. _____ Idiopathic

20. _____ Platelets

J. One of the most common hemolytic anemias, in which red blood cells change to a crescent shape, causing obstruction of small blood vessels and eventual damage throughout the body

K. Ecchymoses or small hemorrhages in the skin, mucous membranes, or serosal surfaces due to blood disorders, vascular abnormalities, or trauma

L. Abnormal decrease of granular leukocytes in the blood

M. Breakdown in the clotting process of the blood

N. Condition in which the hemoglobin drops and interrupts the transport of oxygen throughout the body

O. Medications that are used to prevent clumping of platelets or formation of an arterial thrombus

P. Diagnostic procedure that is used to identify types of anemia, cell deficiencies, and leukemia

Q. Reduction in new blood cells due to impairment or failure of bone marrow function

R. Medications that are used to prevent venous thrombi

S. Hereditary disease that is similar to sickle cell anemia

T. Another name for thrombocytes; they circulate in the blood and assist with the clotting process

CODING

Using the code book, code the following.

1. Autoimmune cold sensitivity _____

2. Postoperative anemia _____

3. Blackfan-Diamond syndrome _____

4. Lederer-Brill syndrome _____

5. Christmas disease _____

6. Marchiafava-Micheli syndrome _____

7. Imerslund's syndrome _____

8. Blood dyscrasia _____

9. Siderotic splenomegaly _____

10. Idiopathic allergic eosinophilia _____

11. Thrombocytopenia due to linezolid _____

12. Anemia due to blood loss _____

13. Schwachman's syndrome _____

14. Pernicious anemia _____

15. Anemia due to colon cancer _____

CASE SCENARIOS

Using the code book, code the following cases.

1. The patient was admitted to the hospital with usual pain symptoms for sickle cell/Hb-SS disease. The patient did not fill the pain medication prescription, and recent cold weather has brought on vaso-occlusive crisis. Chest x-ray was performed and revealed evidence of acute chest syndrome. The patient has had right hip replacement for avascular necrosis and is scheduled to have the left hip replaced next month because of avascular necrosis due to the patient's sickle cell disease.
   Final Diagnoses: Sickle cell crisis with acute chest syndrome.
                    Status post hip replacement.

   _____

   _____

2. The patient was admitted for transfusion of 2 units of red blood cells via peripheral vein because of anemia due to the patient's recent diagnosis of rectal cancer. The patient will be having surgery next week to remove the tumor. Her past medical history includes a family history of colon cancer. Other medical conditions include mitral valve prolapse, hypothyroidism, and diabetes type II.
   Final Diagnoses: Anemia due to rectal cancer.
                    Mitral valve prolapse.
                    Hypothyroidism.
                    Diabetes mellitus.

   _____

   _____

3. The patient is being admitted for neutropenic fever. The patient is currently receiving chemotherapy treatments for acute myelogenous leukemia (AML). CBC and blood and urine cultures are completed, and IV antibiotics are started. The patient became afebrile on hospital day 2. No infectious source could be identified, and the patient was discharged home.
   Discharge Diagnoses: Neutropenic fever.
                        Acute myelogenous leukemia.

   _____

   _____

4. A 5-year-old boy was noted to have abnormal blood counts on preschool examination and was sent for admission to the hospital. A bone marrow aspiration was performed. The mother stated that her son has been tired lately and does seem to bruise easily. He recently had an upper respiratory tract infection. The patient received red blood cell and platelet transfusions.
   Final Diagnoses: Idiopathic aplastic anemia.
   Procedure: Transfusion.
                    Bone marrow aspiration, left iliac crest.

   _____

   _____

5. Patient has severe combined immunodeficiency (SCID) and is being admitted for regular infusion of intravenous immune globulin (IVIG). Following the infusion, patient is discharged home and resumes her routine medications, including medications for seizure disorder.
   Final Diagnosis: Severe combined immunodeficiency.
   Procedure: IVIG administration.

   _____

   _____

           Chapter **11** **Diseases of the Blood and Blood-Forming Organs**

6. The patient was admitted with a deep vein thrombosis. Doppler examination was positive for thrombosis right tibial vein. The patient was treated for DVT a couple of years ago. Because of recurrent thrombosis, the patient was assessed for coagulation disorders and was found to have protein S deficiency.

Final Diagnosis: Deep vein thrombosis with edema lower leg.

Protein S deficiency.

History of previous DVT.

_____

_____

CASE STUDIES

Using the code book, code and answer questions about the following case studies.

11-1. CASE STUDY

History and Physical

CC: Vaso-occlusive crisis.

HPI: The patient is a 25-year-old African American gentleman with a history of sickle cell anemia who presents with right-sided pleuritic chest pain consistent with his previous episodes of vaso-occlusive pain crisis. He does have a history of acute chest syndrome. The patient was recently treated at an outside hospital but signed out AMA because of inadequate pain control. On the day of admission, he was seen in the clinic. Usual triggers include stress, infection, and cold weather. No sick contacts. The patient is not compliant with medications.

Past medical history: Multiple admissions for sickle cell SS anemia. Acute chest syndrome ×1. History of community-acquired pneumonia. Mild pulmonary hypertension. The patient has avascular necrosis of both hips, right greater than left due to sickle cell.

Past surgical history: Splenectomy.

ROS: No cough, no sputum, no dysuria, no fever or chills. Positive for SOB caused by pain on inspiration.

Medications: Methadone 80 mg 2 times a day, hydroxyurea 160 mg by mouth daily, Folate 1 mg by mouth daily, and Dilaudid 4 mg PO q4h prn for pain.

Social history: Smoke 1 ppd. No alcohol or drugs. Married with 1 kid.

Family history: Both parents have SS trait.

PHYSICAL EXAMINATION:

Vitals: T 36.7, HR 90, BP 126/66, R 18, and O_2 sats 99% on room air.

General: The patient was in moderate distress and was holding his right chest.

HEENT: PERRL, EOMI, sclera anicteric, MMM. No sinus tenderness. Neck is supple without masses or lymphadenopathy. No carotid bruits.

Chest: CTA bilaterally. Tender to palpation on right side.

Abd: Normal BS, soft, nontender, no masses or organomegaly.

Extremities: Normal.

Neuro: Intact.

A/P: Sickle cell vaso-occlusive crisis; acute pain similar to previous crisis. Concern for acute chest syndrome versus pneumonia. X-ray shows possible infiltrate left lower lobe. Treat with IV fluids, pain control, supplemental oxygen, and incentive spirometry. Labs and cultures have been ordered. Start moxifloxacin 400 mg PO for possible pneumonia.

Discharge Summary

DIAGNOSES/PROBLEMS:

1. Sickle cell SS disease.
2. Vaso-occlusive pain crisis.

PROCEDURES:

1. Chest x-ray normal.

HISTORY, MAJOR FINDINGS, AND HOSPITAL COURSE:

The patient is a 25-year-old African American gentleman with a history of sickle cell anemia who presents with right-sided pleuritic chest pain consistent with previous episodes of vaso-occlusive pain crisis. He has a history of acute chest syndrome. The patient was recently treated at an outside hospital but signed out AMA because of inadequate pain control. On the day of admission, he was seen in the clinic.

Examination at admission, temperature 36.7, heart rate 90, blood pressure 126/66, respirations 18 per minute, and saturation 99% on room air. The patient was in mild to moderate distress and is holding his right chest. Head and neck examination was within normal limits. The heart had a regular rate and rhythm. No murmurs, gallops, or rubs. The lungs were clear to auscultation bilaterally. The abdomen was soft, nontender, and nondistended without hepatomegaly. Extremities were warm and no clubbing, cyanosis, or edema. Neurologically, the patient was intact.

HOSPITAL COURSE:

The patient was admitted from the clinic for pain management in the setting of vaso-occlusive crisis. He was maintained on oxygen and incentive spirometry. He was started on PCA Dilaudid, which was titrated for pain relief. Over the course of his 2-day stay, the patient's symptoms improved significantly to the point where he was pain free at the time of discharge. He had no significant oxygen requirement during his stay.

Allergies: The patient has no known drug allergies.

DISCHARGE MEDICATIONS:

Moxifloxacin 400 mg by mouth daily for 7 days for possible pneumonia

Dilaudid 4 mg by mouth every 4 hours as needed for pain

Methadone 80 mg 2 times a day for chronic pain

Hydroxyurea 500 mg by mouth daily

Folate 1 mg by mouth daily

Dilaudid 4 mg pos q4h prn for pain

Progress Notes

DAY 1

Vitals: 97% on RA, resp 16, BP 126/67, temp 97.5, and HR 78. The patient is still reporting pain in the center of the chest and SOB. Chest x-ray shows LLL infiltrate. The patient is lying in bed.

Chest: Decreased breath sounds bilaterally.

CVS: RRR S1 and S2 normal.

Ext: WNL.

Continue treatments.

A/P: Sickle cell SS vaso-occlusive crisis with acute chest syndrome and possible pneumonia.

DAY 2

The patient is improving clinically. He has refused his incentive spirometry treatment.

Give influenza vaccination before the discharge. Repeat labs.

DAY 3

Scripts for pain medications and moxifloxacin have been written. The patient will follow up with primary care provider.

CASE STUDY QUESTIONS

11-1a. Admit diagnosis: _____

11-1b. Discharge disposition: _____

11-1c. Principal diagnosis: _____

11-1d. Secondary diagnoses (indicate POA status for secondary diagnoses):

_____

_____

_____

_____

_____

11-1e. Principal procedure: _____

11-1f. Secondary procedures: _____

_____

11-1g. Assign MS-DRG: _____

11-1h. Relative weight of MS-DRG: _____

11-1i. Can this MS-DRG be optimized with the addition of a CC? Yes or No

Can this MS-DRG be optimized with the addition of an MCC? Yes or No

11-1j. Is there a main guideline pertinent to selection of the principal diagnosis in this case study?

_____

_____

11-1k. Is there another diagnosis that meets the definition for principal diagnosis? Yes or No

11-1l. If yes, what is the other diagnosis? _____

11-1m. Is there any opportunity for physician query?

_____

_____

11-1n. What is the drug hydroxyurea used to treat? _____

11-2. CASE STUDY

Clinic Note

History of present illness: The patient is a 6-year-old male with active AML who is here for evaluation and platelet transfusions in preparation for LP with intrathecal chemotherapy tomorrow. He has been afebrile at home for the past several days with good appetite. He does not complain of nausea, vomiting, headache, or abdominal pain. Review of systems is otherwise negative, including review of eyes, ears, nose and throat, heart and lungs, GI, GU, skin, neurologic, extremity, and mental status systems. Past family and social history were reviewed and are unchanged.

Medications: His medications on recent discharge from the hospital are Bactrim 60 mg by mouth 2 times a day Saturday and Sunday; Zosyn 2 g intravenous every 8 hours through the 28th day of the month; AmBisome 75 mg intravenous Monday, Wednesday, and Friday, or this past 2 weeks, it has been Tuesday and Friday; Zofran 4 mg every 6 hours as needed for nausea; Benadryl 25 mg; and allopurinol.

Allergies: None.

Major Findings

PHYSICAL EXAMINATION:
_____

Temperature 36.6 degrees, pulse 95, respirations 24, blood pressure 122/77, weight 23.1 kg, height 126 cm, and PSA 0.90 square millimeter.

Skin: No rash and no induration.

Oropharynx: Benign.

Eyes: Clear.

Neck: Supple. No masses.

Chest: Clear. No abnormal breath sounds. Normal respiratory effort.

Cardiac: No murmur, rub, or gallop.

Abdomen: Soft. No masses. Nontender.

Extremities: Normal joints. Normal muscle bulk. Nontender.

Neurologic: Normal strength and sensation.

Adenopathy: None.

Laboratory: WBC 420, hemoglobin 9.7, hematocrit 26, and platelets 12,000 pretransfusion, ANC 0, creatinine 0.4, glucose 98, sodium 145, potassium 2.9, bilirubin 0.8, SGPT 57, and calcium 9.4.

ASSESSMENTS:

1. Oncology: We will start intrathecal chemotherapy tomorrow; due to start unrelated donor transplant early next month. We will continue allopurinol for persistent peripheral blast.

2. Infectious disease: We will continue AmBisome prophylaxis and Zosyn. We will consider extending Zosyn if ANC of 0 persists. We will also continue Bactrim for PCP prophylaxis; hematology will monitor platelet count again tomorrow and over the weekend if necessary to maintain a platelet count greater than 10,000 to prevent bleeding.

3. Potassium 2.9 will be evaluated again tomorrow. His potassium has been between 2.4 and 2.9 and has been stable over the past couple of weeks. The patient has good oral nutrition, which should help him to maintain his potassium level despite the AmBisome therapy, which may be raising the potassium.

History and Physical

CC: Fever, neutropenia.

HPI: The patient is a 6-year-old with refractory AML who is S/P BMT about 3 months ago, which relapsed about 45 days later, and donor lymphocyte infusion 15 days ago; patient still has blasts in the peripheral blood caused by fever and neutropenia. The patient underwent nonablative haploidentical BMT from his father. At 30-day restaging, t(5;11) persisted and donor chimerism was 64%. Therefore, all GVHD prophylaxis was stopped to stimulate GVHD and GVL. Unfortunately, he never showed evidence of GVHD, and peripheral blasts and BM blasts re-emerged. He received salvage chemotherapy of Cytoxan and clofarabine, but bone marrow aspirate approximately 1 month later still revealed blasts. After a single dose of Cytoxan, the patient received a donor lymphocyte infusion with hope of another BMT in the future.

A few weeks ago, the patient was seen for fevers while on home Zosyn. His coverage was expanded to meropenem for 48 hours, and then he was discharged home. The patient was seen in clinic yesterday and received platelets and AmBisome. After he went home yesterday, he had repeated fevers to 100.5 degrees. No sick contacts are available at home, but he does live with siblings who attend school. Mom denies coughing, runny nose, diarrhea, emesis, and rash. The patient has been on long-term Zosyn.

ROS: See HPI.

PMH: See HPI.

Echo h/o LV mild dysfunction: Urine + BK virus.

Medications: Bactrim 60 mg BID on Sunday and Monday; AmBisome 75 mg on Monday, Wednesday, and Friday; Zofran 4 mg PO q6 prn nausea; Benadryl 25 mg PO as AmBisome premed; allopurinol 100 mg PO TID.

All: NKDA.

FH: MGGM with breast cancer, MGGF with DM on dialysis, PGGM with breast cancer, PGGF with Alzheimer's.

SH: Patient lives with mother and stepfather and two siblings; also spends time with father, who lives in the area. The patient has finished second grade but took third grade reading, which is his favorite subject.

PHYSICAL EXAMINATION:

Vitals: T_{max} of 38, HR 109, R 20, BP 138/98, Wt 23.8 kg.

HEENT: PERRL, EOMI, anicteric sclera, no conjunctivitis, no palp cervical LAD, TMs shiny and gray.

Cardiovascular: RRR S1/S2, no murmurs/rubs/gallops.

Extremities: 2+ radial and DP pulses, <2 sec capillary refill.

Pulmonary: Clear to auscultation bilat, central line C/D/I.

Gastrointestinal: Full, +BS, soft nontender, nondistended.

Musculoskeletal: No deformities.

Neurologic: CN II to XI grossly intact.

Skin: No rashes, no petechiae.

A/P: 6-year-old with refractory AML M2 with relapsed BMT over 90 days ago and s/p donor lymphocyte infusion 15 days ago presents with severe neutropenia, 90% blasts on peripheral smear, and fever.

Onc: Patient is s/p donor lymphocyte infusion 15 days ago in an attempt to stimulate acute GVHD, but patient still has 90% blasts on his smear as of yesterday. Patient is scheduled for another BMT in a few months. We will continue allopurinol to help prevent tumor lysis syndrome.

Heme: Follow counts. Transfuse prn. Premedicate with Tylenol and Benadryl for blood products.

FEN/GI: NPO at MN for LP and intrathecal chemotherapy planned in the morning. Antiemetics prn.

ID: For fever and neutropenia, we will discontinue Zosyn and start meropenem.

Operative Report

Title of operation: Lumbar puncture with intrathecal chemotherapy.

Indications for surgery: CNS prophylaxis for refractory relapsed AML.

Preoperative diagnosis: Relapsed AML.

Postoperative diagnosis: Relapsed AML.

Anesthesia: General.

Specimen (bacteriologic, pathologic, or other): Two cubic centimeters of CSF went for special hematology, 1 cubic centimeter to hematology, and 1 cubic centimeter to chemistry.

Prosthetic device/implant: None.

Chapter **11 Diseases of the Blood and Blood-Forming Organs**

The patient was taken to Room 4 in the general Operating Room. There, he received general anesthesia via the anesthesia team. He was then placed in the left lateral position and was prepped and draped in the usual sterile fashion. He received 0.5 cubic centimeter of 1% lidocaine injected at the lumbar puncture site, which was L4-5. Approximately 5 cubic centimeters of CSF was obtained with a 22-gauge 1- to 1.5-inch lumbar puncture needle without complications. Following confirmation of free-flowing fluid, he then received Ara-C 70 mg intrathecally. The patient tolerated the procedure well; the procedure was supervised by the attending physician. The patient was taken to the pediatric recovery room in good condition.

Discharge Summary

DIAGNOSES/PROBLEMS:

1. Refractory acute myelogenous leukemia.

2. Immunosuppression.

3. Neutropenic fever.

PROCEDURE:

Administration of intrathecal cytarabine.

HISTORY, MAJOR FINDINGS, AND HOSPITAL COURSE:

The patient is a 6-year-old male with refractory AML who is status post haploidentical bone marrow transplantation; he relapsed 45 days later and received a donor lymphocyte infusion about 15 days ago, but the patient still has blasts in his peripheral blood and presents with fever and neutropenia. The patient underwent nonmyeloablative haploidentical bone marrow transplantation from his father. At his restaging, t(5;11) persisted, and donor chimerism was 64%; therefore, all GVHD prophylaxis was stopped to stimulate graft-versus-leukemia effect. However, the patient never showed any evidence of graft-versus-leukemia or graft-versus-host disease, and peripheral blasts and bone marrow blasts re-emerged. He received salvage chemotherapy of Cytoxan and clofarabine, but bone marrow aspirate approximately 1 month later still revealed blasts. After a single dose of Cytoxan, the patient received donor lymphocyte infusion with hopes of another bone marrow transplantation in the future. A few weeks ago, he was seen for fevers while on home Zosyn; his coverage was expanded to meropenem for 48 hours, and he was discharged home. The patient was seen in clinic the day before admission and received platelets and AmBisome. After he was sent home, he had repeated fevers to 100.5 degrees Fahrenheit. No sick contacts are available at home, but he does live with siblings who attend school. Mom denies coughing, runny nose, diarrhea, emesis, and rash.

On physical examination, temperature was 38 degrees Celsius, heart rate 109, respiratory rate 20, and blood pressure 38/98. He is a thin male in no acute distress.

HEENT examination: Pupils were equal, round, and reactive to light; sclerae anicteric. Mucous membranes were moist. Oropharynx was clear.

Cardiovascular: Regular rate and rhythm; no murmurs, rubs, or gallops.

Pulmonary: Clear to auscultation bilaterally. Central line was clean, dry, and intact.

Gastrointestinal examination: Soft, nontender, and nondistended with normal bowel sounds. Neurologic examination was grossly nonfocal.

The patient was admitted after cultures were obtained in clinic and was placed on meropenem. Admission CBC showed a white count of 6.37, hemoglobin of 8.9, and platelets of 68,000 with an ANC of 74. The next morning, he went to the OR and received LP and intrathecal cytarabine. The procedure was without complications.

Results of CSF analysis showed white cells and 0 red cells. After 48 hours, blood cultures were negative; patient appeared well, and it was determined that he was well enough to be discharged to home. The plan was to discharge him home and continue his Zosyn secondary to continued neutropenia.

Allergies: No known drug allergies.

Condition on discharge: Good.

DISCHARGE MEDICATIONS:

Potassium chloride oral supplements: 20-mEq tablet 2 times a day.

Bactrim: Take 60-mg tablet 2 times a day on Sundays and Mondays.

AmBisome 75 mg intravenous, Monday, Wednesday, and Friday.

Zofran 4 mg orally every 6 hours as needed for nausea.

Allopurinol 100 mg by mouth 3 times daily.

DISCHARGE INSTRUCTIONS:

Patient is instructed to report to the Oncology Clinic for follow-up appointment.

Progress Notes

DAY 1

Patient had lumbar puncture and intrathecal chemotherapy for relapsed AML. Receiving IV fluids with KCL. No emesis.

T_{max} 37.2, P 72-99, R 20, BP 94-121/44/70, no emesis.

HEENT: Anicteric sclera. Normal oropharynx.

CV: RRR.

Resp: CTA.

Abd: Soft.

Skin: No rashes.

Neuro: Grossly intact.

Psych: Good mood.

Laboratory data and cultures reviewed. No infectious process identified.

DAY 2

Continue with KCL for hypokalemia, convert from IV to oral supplements. No pain. Renal status is stable. Ready for discharge to Home Health.

11-2a. Admit diagnosis: _____

11-2b. Discharge disposition: _____

11-2c. Principal diagnosis: _____

11-2d. Secondary diagnoses (indicate POA status for secondary diagnoses):

_____

_____

_____

_____

_____

_____

11-2e. Principal procedure: _____

11-2f. Secondary procedures: _____

_____

11-2g. Assign MS-DRG: _____

11-2h. Relative weight of MS-DRG: _____

11-2i. Can this MS-DRG be optimized with the addition of a CC? Yes or No

Can this MS-DRG be optimized with the addition of an MCC? Yes or No

11-2j. Is there a main guideline pertinent to selection of the principal diagnosis in this case study?

_____

_____

11-2k. Is there another diagnosis that meets the definition for principal diagnosis? Yes or No

11-2l. If yes, what is the other diagnosis? _____

11-2m. Is there any opportunity for physician query?

_____

_____

11-2n. What is the drug AmBisome used to treat? _____

12 Endocrine, Nutritional, and Metabolic Diseases (ICD-10-CM Chapter 4, Codes E00-E89)

ABBREVIATIONS/ACRONYMS

Without the use of reference materials, define the following abbreviations or acronyms.

1. CF _____

2. DM _____

3. SIADH _____

4. TPN _____

5. MEN _____

6. BMI _____

7. SCID _____

8. TLS _____

9. DI _____

10. IDDM _____

GLOSSARY DEFINITIONS

Match the glossary term to the correct definition.

1. _____ Steroid-induced diabetes

2. _____ Exophthalmos

3. _____ Cushing's syndrome

4. _____ Hyperthyroidism

5. _____ Morbid obesity

6. _____ Bariatrics

7. _____ Goiter

8. _____ Hypothyroidism

9. _____ Hypertrophy

10. _____ Hyperparathyroidism

11. _____ Diabetes insipidus

12. _____ Malnutrition

13. _____ Hashimoto's disease

14. _____ Myxedema

15. _____ Hypoparathyroidism

16. _____ Graves' disease

A. Branch of medicine concerned with the management of obesity and allied diseases

B. Inflammation of the thyroid gland that often results in hypothyroidism

C. Bulging of the eyes

D. Condition caused by low pituitary hormone levels

E. Deficiency in the release of vasopressin by the posterior pituitary gland

F. Skin and tissue disorder usually due to prolonged hypothyroidism

G. Underactive parathyroid gland that results in decreased levels of circulating calcium

H. Enlargement of the thyroid gland

I. Chronic syndrome of impaired carbohydrate, protein, and fat metabolism caused by insufficient production of insulin by the pancreas or faulty utilization of insulin by cells

Continued

17. _____ Thyrotoxic crisis/storm

18. _____ Cystic fibrosis

19. _____ Diabetes mellitus

20. _____ Hypoplasia

J. Form of diabetes that is caused by the use of steroids

K. Atrophy, or when a gland becomes smaller

L. Person who is 50% to 100% or 100 pounds above ideal body weight; BMI of 40 or greater

M. Complication of hyperthyroidism with a sudden intensification of symptoms plus fever, rapid pulse, and delirium

N. Condition that results in excessive circulating cortisol levels due to chronic hypersecretion of the adrenal cortex

O. Enlargement of a gland

P. Nutritional disorder caused by primary deprivation of protein energy due to poverty, self-imposed starvation, or deficiency diseases such as cancer

Q. Genetic condition that affects the cells that produce mucus, sweat, saliva, and digestive juices

R. Abnormality of the thyroid gland in which secretion of thyroid hormone is usually increased and is no longer under the regulatory control of hypothalamic-pituitary centers

S. The most common form of hyperthyroidism; occurs as the result of an autoimmune response that attacks the thyroid gland, resulting in overproduction of the thyroid hormone thyroxine

T. Overactive parathyroid gland that secretes excessive parathyroid hormone, causing increased levels of circulating calcium that result from loss of calcium in the bone

CODING

Using the code book, code the following.

1. Beriberi _____

2. Vitamin D deficiency _____

3. Testicular dysfunction _____

4. Pickwickian syndrome _____

5. CO_2 retention _____

6. Hashimoto's disease _____

7. Porphyria cutanea tarda _____

8. Gangrene toe due to diabetes _____

9. Secondary hyperparathyroidism _____

10. Adrenoleukodystrophy _____

11. Mild protein energy malnutrition (PEM) _____

12. Phenylketonuria (PKU) _____

13. Nutritional deficiency _____

14. Kallmann's syndrome _____

CASE SCENARIOS

Using the code book, code the following cases.

1. This 30-year-old male has a history of type I diabetes mellitus since age 8. His diabetes is complicated by polyneuropathy. He has been noncompliant with glucose monitoring and insulin dosage. In the ER, the patient had hyperglycemia with blood glucose over 500. Patient was admitted for treatment of his out-of-control diabetes. Final Diagnosis: Diabetes mellitus, type I.

   _____

   _____

2. Patient is admitted for gastric banding procedure for treatment of morbid obesity. Patient has been obese most of her adult life and has failed all attempts at supervised diet; she has a BMI of 41.3. Patient has a family history of diabetes. She hopes to see improvement in her obstructive sleep apnea, asthma, and type II diabetes, with expected weight loss for bariatric surgery. Patient undergoes a laparoscopic gastric bypass with Roux-en-Y limb to jejunum and is put on the bariatric diet, which she tolerates without difficulty. She is discharged in satisfactory condition.
   Discharge Diagnoses: Morbid obesity.
                          Diabetes.
                          Asthma.
                          Obstructive sleep apnea.
                          Osteoarthritis of knees.
   Procedure: Laparoscopic gastric bypass with Roux limb.

   _____

   _____

3. This 80-year-old woman was admitted to the hospital because of hypoglycemic shock. She was confused about her insulin dosages and accidentally took twice the prescribed amount. Her past medical history includes coronary artery disease with stent placement last year, hyperlipidemia, and obesity.
   Final Diagnoses: Hypoglycemic shock.
                     Coronary artery disease.
                     Hyperlipidemia.
                     Obesity.
                     DM, type II.

   _____

   _____

4. Patient was admitted for a total thyroidectomy. Patient had been having progressive symptoms with a substernal goiter. She was having trouble swallowing, particularly breads and meats, with frequent coughing and trouble lying on her back. Past medical history includes TIA, osteoporosis, and sensorineural hearing loss. The procedure was performed as planned. Pathology showed a multinodular goiter. The patient's symptoms were relieved, and she was able to tolerate a solid food diet.

   _____

   _____

5. This 15-year-old male patient with cystic fibrosis diagnosed at the age of 2 has been admitted several times in the past for respiratory and intestinal complications. Patient needs a PEG tube to maximize his nutritional status. CF is stable at this time; a percutaneous gastrostomy tube is inserted, and feeds are initiated. The patient's mother is instructed on gastrostomy care and tube feedings.
   Final Diagnoses: Cystic fibrosis.
                        Moderate malnutrition.
   Procedure: Percutaneous endoscopic gastrostomy placement.

   _____

   _____

6. Patient was feeling fatigued, had nausea and vomiting, and felt her heart racing. She was worried that her Addison's disease was flaring up and reported to the ER. She was admitted from the ER for Addison's crisis. Lab results showed hyperkalemia, and serum sodium was low. Patient was treated with IV corticosteroids and IV fluids for low blood pressure. No evidence suggested that infection was responsible for this episode. Past medical history includes hypertension and chronic bronchitis. Her condition stabilized, and the patient was ready for discharge.
   Final Diagnoses: Addison's crisis.
                        Hypertension.
                        Chronic bronchitis.

   _____

   _____

7. This 3-year-old child has had several admissions for methylmalonic acidemia. Patient has had nausea and vomiting, has been unable to keep down any medications, and is unable to eat. Patient is currently being investigated for failure to thrive and global developmental delay. The parents are worried about the child's metabolic state and so reported to the ER. The patient's laboratory studies show severe acidosis and neutropenia. The patient is treated and by hospital day 2 is able to tolerate feeds and oral medications. The patient is discharged to the care of the parents.
   Discharge Diagnosis: Methylmalonic acidemia.

   _____

   _____

8. Patient is an elderly gentleman who was admitted from the ER with pain and swelling of his right knee. The pain is throbbing in nature, and the knee feels warm and is very tender to touch. The patient has a knee x-ray, and uric acid levels are elevated. Colchicine is started, and the patient's symptoms are much improved within 48 hours. The patient has diabetes, chronic renal insufficiency, and hypertension, and he is overweight. The patient is advised to limit alcohol consumption and to avoid dietary purines.
   Final Diagoses: Gouty arthropathy of right knee.
                        Diabetes mellitus, type II on insulin.
                        Chronic renal failure.
                        Hypertension.
                        Overweight.

   _____

   _____

9. Patient was admitted to the hospital with DKA. Labs showed glycosuria, ketonuria, and acidosis. Patient was admitted and was started on a sliding scale of insulin. Patient's past history includes diabetic retinopathy and kidney stones.
   Discharge Diagnosis: Diabetic (type I) ketoacidosis.

   _____

   _____

Using the code book, code and answer questions about the following case studies.

12-1. CASE STUDY

History and Physical

CC: Shortness of breath.

HPI: Patient is a 70-year-old female who presents with SOB ×1 day. She states that she was lying down when she felt SOB. SOB was not relieved by standing up. She decided to come to the ER because the SOB persisted. She denies chest pain. No N/V or diarrhea. No leg swelling. She has had a cough for the past couple of days with minimal sputum production. No sick contacts. No sore throat. Her last hemodialysis session occurred a couple of days ago.

Past medical history: ESRD on HD for 6 years. Diabetes mellitus with last Hgb A1C 6.8. Arthritis, chronic hepatitis C, dyslipidemia, hypertension, secondary hyperparathyroidism, and osteoporosis. Patient had a myocardial infarction a few years ago.

Social history: Patient has a history of cocaine and heroin use, none now. Patient smokes 3 to 5 cigarettes/day.

Allergies include oxycodone and Percocet, both of which cause itching.

Medications: See admission sheet.

PHYSICAL EXAMINATION:

VS: T 36.5, HR 84, BP 114/63, RR 24, Sao_2, 93% on 3L of oxygen.

General: Lying in bed sleeping. NAD.

HEENT: PERRL. Sclera anicteric. No elevated JVP.

Chest: Bibasilar crackles.

Heart: RRR. No murmur.

Abd: Soft, nontender, and no guarding.

Extremities: No edema.

Neuro: Alert and oriented ×3.

ASSESSMENT AND PLAN:

Patient is admitted with shortness of breath, which is likely due to volume overload secondary to missing dialysis session and dietary indiscrimination. Will consult Renal regarding dialysis. No fever, so not likely an infectious process.

DM: Patient on Lantus. Will continue.

HTN: Continue home medications.

Discharge Summary

DIAGNOSES/PROBLEMS:

1. End-stage renal disease, on dialysis, Monday, Wednesday, and Friday; missed dialysis on Wednesday and came in short of breath.

2. History of type II diabetes, but currently not clear whether she is on insulin therapy.

3. Hypertension.

4. Secondary hyperparathyroidism.

5. Hepatitis C.

6. Dyslipidemia.

7. History of non–ST-elevation myocardial infarction.

8. History of previous cocaine and heroin use.

9. History of osteoporosis.

10. Anemia due to ESRD.

11. Continual noncompliance with dialysis.

PROCEDURES:

1. Chest CT with intravenous contrast.

2. Chest x-ray.

3. Hemodialysis.

HISTORY, MAJOR FINDINGS, AND HOSPITAL COURSE:

History of present illness: The patient is a 70-year-old female with the above past medical history who presented with shortness of breath for 1 day. She states that she was lying down after her dialysis session on Friday and felt short of breath; the feeling was not relieved by standing up. So, she decided to come into the ED because of her shortness of breath. She denied any chest pain. She had no nausea, no vomiting, and no diarrhea. She has had no leg swelling. She reported a dry cough in the past couple of days with minimal sputum production. She had no sick contacts. She had no sore throat. She reported going to dialysis on Friday but missed her Wednesday dialysis session, and when I asked her specifically why she missed her Wednesday dialysis session, she said to me "Honey, I always miss my Wednesday dialysis session." In the emergency department, her temperature was 97.4 degrees. Blood pressure was 152/70. Heart rate was 96. Respiratory rate was 16. She was saturating 89% on room air and came up to 100% on 4 liters. She was given 400 mg of moxifloxacin by mouth, and she was given chest CT with intravenous contrast, which ruled out pulmonary embolism but did show diffuse ground-glass infiltrates, most consistent with pulmonary edema.

Past medical history is as described above.

Allergies include oxycodone and Percocet, both of which cause itching.

Her medications at home include Cozaar, Coreg 6.25 mg by mouth 2 times a day, Lantus 10 units every night (unclear if she is taking this), PhosLo, aspirin 81 mg daily, sevelamer 1600 mg with meals, pravastatin 20 mg daily, losartan 100 mg daily, Neurontin 300 mg every week after dialysis, Protonix 40 mg daily, Caltrate plus D, and calcitriol 0.25 mcg daily.

Social history: Smokes 3 or 4 cigarettes per day for the past 50 years. She denies any alcohol use. She denies any current illicit use but has a history of cocaine use. She lives with her daughter.

Family history is noncontributory.

PHYSICAL EXAMINATION:

Temperature was 36.5 degrees. Heart rate was 84. Blood pressure was 114/63. Respiratory rate was 24. Patient was saturating 92% on 3 liters. She was lying in bed sleeping, in no acute distress. HEENT examination was unremarkable. JVP was not markedly elevated. She had bibasilar crackles.

Heart sounds: Regular rate and rhythm. Normal S1 and S2. No murmurs, rubs, or gallops.

Abdomen: Soft, nontender, and nondistended with good bowel sounds. She had no lower extremity edema. She did wear a glove on her left hand, which was secondary to poor perfusion from her AV fistula. She had a left arm AV fistula with a good thrill and bruit. Neurologic exam was unremarkable.

HOSPITAL COURSE BY SYSTEM:

1. Shortness of breath: Patient was felt to be volume overloaded in the setting of missing her dialysis. She was dialyzed on hospital day number 2 with rapid resolution of symptoms. She was on room air and was ready to be discharged.

2. End-stage renal disease: She consistently misses her Wednesday session of dialysis, and at this time she has no plans of being compliant with Wednesday dialysis. She is hospitalized once every month to 2 months for volume overload in the setting of her dialysis noncompliance.

3. Diabetes: We attempted to contact her primary care doctor but were unable to verify her current insulin regimen. During hospitalization off insulin, she had no episodes of hyperglycemia. As such, she was discharged off insulin.

DISCHARGE MEDICATIONS:

Renagel 600 mg a day with meals.
Aspirin 81 mg daily.
Losartan 100 mg daily.
Carvedilol 6.25 mg by mouth 2 times a day.
Pravastatin 20 mg at bedtime.
Pantoprazole 40 mg daily.
Neurontin 300 mg weekly after dialysis.
Calcitriol 0.25 mcg.
Calcium carbonate.
Vitamin D 1 tablet daily.

FOLLOW-UP CARE:

Patient was given a follow-up appointment. She was given a Pneumovax and a flu vaccine during this admission.

Contrast CT

CHEST, ABDOMEN, AND PELVIS:

Clinical history: Diabetes, end-stage renal disease, and hemodialysis. Respiratory abnormality.

Technique: CT of the chest with IV contrast.

CT chest: Enlargement of the thyroid with bilateral nodules again noted. Extensive atherosclerotic disease is noted in the thoracic aorta and coronary arteries. Calcification along the region of the mitral valve also noted and unchanged. Mild mediastinal and hilar adenopathy. For example, prominent precarinal lymph node measuring 2 × 2.5 cm slightly increased from 1.8 × 2.2 cm. Cardiomegaly. No evidence of pulmonary embolus. Small right pleural effusion. Patchy bilateral ground-glass opacity lungs due to edema or infection. Mild superimposed linear atelectasis. Degenerative changes thoracic spine, and bony changes compatible with end-stage renal disease. Loss of height within several thoracic vertebral bodies.

Impression:

1. Patchy bilateral ground-glass infiltrate/edema. Small right pleural effusion.

2. Cardiomegaly. Extensive atherosclerotic disease.

3. Enlarged thyroid with multiple nodules.

Progress Notes

DAY 1

Patient with chronic kidney disease stage V on HD presents with acute SOB in the setting of hemodialysis noncompliance. Afebrile. VS stable. JVP elevated. Bibasilar crackles.

CT: Pulmonary edema consistent with fluid overload. No PE.

Imp: SOB due to fluid overload.

Plan: HD to reduce volume. If HD doesn't improve SOB, consider alternative dx.

Patient is less SOB. CVS: RRR. S1 and S2 normal.

Lungs: Still crackles.

Abd: Soft.

No lower extremity edema. Potassium is within normal limits. Check phosphorus. Follow Hgb.

Patient has no complaints. Vital signs are stable.

Gen: NAD, lying in bed.

Lungs: Mild bibasilar crackles.

Abd: BS, NT.

Plan: Dialysis today. SOB resolved. Discharge after dialysis.

CASE STUDY QUESTIONS

12-1a. Admit diagnosis: _____

12-1b. Discharge disposition: _____

12-1c. Principal diagnosis: _____

12-1d. Secondary diagnoses (indicate POA status for secondary diagnoses):

_____

_____

_____

_____

_____

_____

12-1e. Principal procedure: _____

12-1f. Secondary procedures: _____

_____

12-1g. Assign MS-DRG: _____

12-1h. Relative weight of MS-DRG: _____

12-1i. Can this MS-DRG be optimized with the addition of a CC? Yes or No

Can this MS-DRG be optimized with the addition of an MCC? Yes or No

12-1j. Is there a main guideline pertinent to selection of the principal diagnosis in this case study?

_____

_____

12-1k. Is there another diagnosis that meets the definition for principal diagnosis? Yes or No

12-1l. If yes, what is the other diagnosis?_____

12-1m. Is there any opportunity for physician query?

_____

_____

12-1n. What is the drug Renagel used to treat?

_____

12-2. CASE STUDY

History and Physical

CC: Referral for hyperparathyroidism.

HPI: The patient is a 26-year-old male whom you have referred with a diagnosis of hyperparathyroidism. His calcium was originally noted to be elevated during routine blood work and physical examination when he complained of some fatigue. He noted that he was feeling tired all of the time. There is no history of kidney stones. He does have some musculoskeletal aches and pains. There is no history of GI symptoms such as reflux, constipation, or pancreatitis, and no other neuropsychiatric symptoms other than the fatigue. He has no compressive symptoms such as hoarseness or dysphagia. There is no history of cervical irradiation. Lab work revealed his serum calcium to be elevated at 10.8 mg/dL. His ionized serum calcium was also elevated at 6.1 mg/dL, and concordant measurement of his parathyroid hormone level was also elevated at 111 pg/mL, consistent with a biochemical diagnosis of hyperparathyroidism. Notably, however, his 25-hydroxy vitamin D level was low at 12.9 ng/mL.

Past medical history: His past medical history is remarkable only for exercise-induced asthma, but this has not been a recent problem. His past surgical history is remarkable for an appendectomy.

Social history: He works as a restaurant manager. He is single and is a nonsmoker.

Family history: There is no family history of hyperparathyroidism, hypercalcemia, or multiple endocrine neoplasia syndromes.

Medications: He is on no medications.

Allergies: He has no allergies.

PHYSICAL EXAMINATION:

On examination, he is afebrile with a temperature of 98.4. His blood pressure is 154/67, pulse rate is 84, and weight is 223 pounds.

HEENT: There are no oral lesions. The thyroid gland is palpably normal. The trachea is midline. There is no cervical lymphadenopathy.

Chest: Clear to auscultation.

Abd: Soft, nontender. Active bowel sounds.

Extremities: No edema.

Skin: Warm and dry. No rashes.

Neurologic: Examination is grossly intact.

We had a detailed discussion about hyperparathyroidism in the clinic today and potential parathyroid surgery. I would like for him to have two localizing studies, including a parathyroid sestamibi scan and the thyroid and parathyroid ultrasound. He will return to the clinic to discuss these results and to plan for his surgery scheduling.

Discharge Summary

DIAGNOSES/PROBLEMS:

Hyperparathyroidism.

PROCEDURE:

Parathyroidectomy (left inferior and left superior).

HISTORY, MAJOR FINDINGS, AND HOSPITAL COURSE:

This 26 y/o male was referred with a diagnosis of hyperparathyroidism on routine blood work and physical examination in 01/06. Blood serum calcium was 10.8 mg/dL, ionized serum calcium was also elevated at 6.1 mg/dL, and PTH was 111 pg/mL. Patient did report feelings of fatigue and musculoskeletal aches and pains. Patient denied symptoms of kidney stones, reflux, constipation, pancreatitis, and neuropsychiatric symptoms. On neck ultrasound, the parathyroid glands were not visualized, and on SPECT parathyroid imaging, there was no evidence of parathyroid adenoma.

Patient was admitted for a parathyroidectomy. Please see operative note for further details.

Postoperatively, patient was extubated and transferred to PACU without difficulty. Patient advanced to regular diet and ambulated well; incision was clean, dry, and intact, with no redness, swelling, or discharge, and no difficulty with phonation. Patient denied symptoms of paresthesias, numbness, or tingling. Patient was deemed stable for discharge.

100

Oxycodone 5 mg PO q 4-6 hours prn pain
Colace 100 mg PO qd
Calcium carbonate 1300 mg PO tid q 2 hours prn symptoms of hypoparathyroidism

DISCHARGE INSTRUCTIONS:

Activity: Regular. Patient is able to shower but is advised not to submerge incision in water. Patient is able to return to normal activity but is advised not to lift more than 15 pounds. Patient is advised not to drive while on pain medication.

Diet: Regular.

Patient is to call and ask resident on call if he is having severe symptoms of hypoparathyroidism, fever >101, increasing swelling, pain, or discharge from incision; call 911 in case of an emergency.

FOLLOW-UP CARE:

Patient is to contact surgeon's office for follow-up appointment in 1 week.

Operative Report

Title of operation: Parathyroidectomy, four-gland identification. Intraoperative nerve monitoring.

Indications for surgery:

Clinical note: This patient has been given a diagnosis of hyperparathyroidism. A preoperative sestamibi scan was nonlocalizing; a preoperative ultrasound was also nonlocalizing. On the basis of this, a parathyroid four-gland exploration/identification was recommended, and the patient was accepting of this recommendation. Risks of the procedure, including bleeding, infection, nerve injury, persistent or recurrent hyperparathyroidism, hypoparathyroidism, voice change, and a requirement for cervical skin incision were explained to the patient, and he wished to proceed.

Preoperative diagnosis: Hyperparathyroidism.

Postoperative diagnosis: Hyperparathyroidism.

Anesthesia: General endotracheal anesthesia.

Surgeon's Narrative

Operative findings: The above-noted procedure was performed in standard fashion with no complication. The enlarged gland appeared to be the left lower parathyroid gland, which weighed 323 mg. Following resection of this gland, the intraoperative parathyroid hormone level decreased from a preoperative baseline of 91 down to 22. Frozen section examination confirmed cellular parathyroid tissue. The left upper gland was also identified at the posterior border of the left upper lobe of the thyroid. This gland was resected to potentially avoid any necessity for reexploration on the left side. The right lower gland was also identified and was of normal size in the thyrothymic ligament. The right upper gland was not clearly seen, but potential parathyroid tissue was seen in a subcapsular location on the right side.

Both recurrent laryngeal nerves were identified with the aid of the nerve stimulator and were stimulated normally at the completion of the procedure.

Details of procedure: With the patient in the supine position and the neck extended, the skin was prepped and draped in a standard fashion. The cervical skin incision was fashioned and superior and inferior skin flaps raised. The Joll retractor was inserted, and the superficial layer of the deep cervical fascia was incised in the midline. Dissection was begun on the left side by dissecting strap muscles off the left lobe of the thyroid. The left recurrent laryngeal nerve was identified in the tracheoesophageal groove with the aid of the nerve stimulator and was carefully preserved. The middle thyroid vein was ligated and was divided between 3-0 silk ties. Anterior to the nerve at the lower pole, the left lobe of the thyroid initially and an enlarged left lower parathyroid gland were identified. We identified the left upper parathyroid gland at the posterior pole of the left upper lobe. This appeared to be of more normal size. We then explored on the right side of the neck. Again, the strap muscles were dissected off the right lobe of the thyroid and the lobe retracted medially. The right recurrent laryngeal nerve was identified with the aid of the nerve stimulator and carefully preserved. The right lower parathyroid was also of normal size and was in the thyrothymic ligament on the right side. This was marked with a small clip. Exploration more superiorly did not definitively identify a right upper gland. However, there was potential parathyroid tissue in a subcapsular location at the posterior border of the right upper thyroid lobe. We thus returned to the left side and resected what then appeared to be the left lower parathyroid adenoma. It was somewhat surprising that this gland did not localize on sestamibi. This gland was resected and was confirmed to be cellular parathyroid tissue. It weighed 323 mg. Following resection of this gland, the intraoperative parathyroid hormone level was decreased from 91 down to 22, consistent with clinical and biochemical care. To avoid the potential necessity to reenter the left neck, the left upper gland on this side was also resected and handed off for pathologic evaluation.

Following this, meticulous hemostasis was ensured in the left and right neck. Both recurrent laryngeal nerves were reidentified and were stimulated normally with a nerve stimulator. The strap muscles were then closed with a running 3-0 Biosyn suture, the platysma muscle was closed with interrupted 3-0 Biosyn sutures, and the skin was closed with a running 4-0 subcuticular Biosyn suture; Steri-Strips were applied.

Estimated blood loss during the procedure was minimal.

There were no complications. Sponge, needle, and instrument counts were correct, and the patient was transported to the recovery room in stable condition.

Path Report

1. Left lower parathyroid (parathyroidectomy): Parathyroid tissue (323 mg).

2. Left upper parathyroid (parathyroidectomy): Parathyroid tissue (80 mg).

Progress Notes

BRIEF OPERATIVE NOTE

Preop dx: Hyperparathyroidism.

Postop dx: Same.

Procedure: Parathyroidectomy (L inferior and L superior).

Anes: GETA.

EBL: Minimal.

Findings: IPTH 91 to 43 immediately with gland removal, 43 to 22 at 10 minutes.

Complications: None.

Condition: Stable to PACU. Patient S/P parathyroidectomy.

Feels well. No N/V. No CP or SOB.

Vital signs are stable. Pain controlled.

No paresthesia, numbness, or tingling. Tongue is midline. No hoarseness.

Incisions C/D/I.

DAY 2

Doing well postop. Will advance diet in AM.

Patient ambulating. Normal voice with no hoarseness.

No numbness or tingling.

Incision C/D/I.

DAY 3

Regular diet. Discharge planning.

Patient S/P parathyroidectomy. No pain. Eating well. Calcium labs are stable.

Incision healing. Discharge home.

CASE STUDY QUESTIONS

12-2a. Admit diagnosis: _____

12-2b. Discharge disposition: _____

12-2c. Principal diagnosis: _____

_____

12-2d. Secondary diagnoses (indicate POA status for secondary diagnoses):

_____

_____

_____

_____

_____

_____

12-2e. Principal procedure: _____

12-2f. Secondary procedures: _____

_____

12-2g. Assign MS-DRG: _____

12-2h. Relative weight of MS-DRG: _____

12-2i. Can this MS-DRG be optimized with the addition of a CC? Yes or No

   Can this MS-DRG be optimized with the addition of an MCC? Yes or No

12-2j. Is there a main guideline pertinent to selection of the principal diagnosis in this case study?

_____

_____

12-2k. Is there another diagnosis that meets the definition for principal diagnosis? Yes or No

12-2l. If yes, what is the other diagnosis? _____

12-2m. Is there any opportunity for physician query?

_____

_____

12-2n. What is the drug calcium carbonate used to treat?

_____

12-3. CASE STUDY

History and Physical

Reason for visit: Follow-up of CF lung disease.

History of present illness: The patient is a delightful 17-year-old woman with cystic fibrosis with a baseline FEV_1 of about 40% who is seen now in clinic for follow-up of a prolonged exacerbation that has not been responding to IV antibiotics. Patient has been on home IV antibiotics and has received, at different times, amikacin/cefepime, colistin/Cipro, and now imipenem/tobramycin. Although her cough and sputum have finally improved, her PFTs have continued to plummet, and she has had progressive dyspnea and chest tightness. She returns now with continued progression of respiratory symptoms and the lowest PFTs she has ever had.

Medications: Her medications include Ultrase MT20 6 with meals and 4 with snacks; ADEK multivitamins once a day and a multivitamin with zinc once a day; azithromycin 500 mg 3 times per week; TOBI nebulized 300 mg 2 times a day every other month, which she is currently off; Advair 250/50 mcg 1 puff 2 times a day; Pulmozyme 2.5 mg nebulized every day; Flonase nasal spray 2 puffs to each nostril every day; aspirin 325 mg on Monday, Wednesday, and Friday; cetirizine 10 mg daily; and albuterol as needed. She is also on imipenem and every other day tobramycin IV.

Allergies: Allergies to meropenem cause hives; to piperacillin and tazobactam, fever. She has ototoxicity to aminoglycosides and difficulty tolerating inhaled colistin and hypertonic saline.

Major findings:

Physical examination: Weight is 95 pounds, temperature is 97.4 degrees, blood pressure 132/73, heart rate 150, and O_2 saturation is 94% on room air. She is a thin, Caucasian woman in no acute distress. Nasal mucosa is without lesions. Oral mucosa is pink and moist. Lungs are notable for few scattered crackles in both lungs, but no wheezing. Heart is tachycardic and regular with a normal S1 and S2, and no murmurs or gallops.

Abdomen: Patient has active bowel sounds, soft, nontender.

Extremities: Without edema.

Assessments: Patient underwent PFTs today, which showed another decline in FEV_1 to 24% of predicted. We walked her in the hall and she desaturated.

DIAGNOSES/PROBLEMS:

CF lung disease with progressive PFT decline. Despite 2 months of IVs, she continues to worsen. Patient has less sputum and cough, so I am not convinced that it is infection alone that is causing the decline. We have previously looked for atypical mycobacteria and evidence of ABPA without success. She may have a bronchiolitis obliterans syndrome that we have seen in a few young women with CF. Our plan is to admit her to the hospital, start her on 60 mg of oral prednisone a day, and do a rapid transplant evaluation. She should get 3 times a day chest PT and close monitoring of glucoses before and 1 hour after meals.

We will repeat her PFTs later this week to assess her response to prednisone. We will not start her on IVs immediately upon admission but will reassess as soon as we have her CBC and CT results. Upon admission, we will want to perform a noncontrast chest CT, echocardiogram (with bubble study), and other tests per the transplant team.

Discharge Summary

DIAGNOSES/PROBLEMS:

Cystic fibrosis.

PROCEDURES:

1. CT chest.

2. CT abdomen and pelvis.

3. V/Q scan.

4. Pulmonary function test.

5. Echocardiogram.

HISTORY, MAJOR FINDINGS, AND HOSPITAL COURSE:

The patient is a 17-year-old female with a history of cystic fibrosis (baseline FEV_1 40%) who was admitted to pulmonary service for a prolonged CF exacerbation; home IV antibiotic regimen over the past 2 months has failed, and pulmonary function tests have worsened. The patient complains of shortness of breath with minimal activity, has a cough productive of greenish/yellow sputum, and has significant fatigue. Her most recent antibiotic course includes imipenem and tobramycin. The patient was started on IV antibiotics and oral prednisone, especially because of concern about the development of bronchiolitis obliterans.

CT scan of the chest showed a tree-in-bud appearance in both lower lobes; voriconazole was instituted to cover for possible fungal processes. Later in her hospital stay, we isolated *Trichosporon* from her sputum. A decision was made to continue long-term voriconazole therapy. During her hospital stay, we also asked the lung transplant team to meet with the patient for evaluation of possible lung transplant. As part of the transplant workup, the patient had a cine-esophagogram done, as well as a V/Q scan and a CT of the abdomen and pelvis.

The patient's pulmonary status had improved significantly with oral corticosteroids, IV antibiotic therapy, and CF usual care. She was discharged home and was asked to continue with 60 mg of prednisone and to return to the pulmonologist next Tuesday. Her insulin regimen was modified accordingly, and it comprised a Humalog sliding scale and Lantus insulin.

DISCHARGE MEDICATIONS:

ADE 1 tablet orally daily
Cetirizine 10 mg orally daily
Dornase Neb Soln Inhalation (2.5 mg/2.5 mL) 2.5 mg inhalation daily
Fluticasone Nasal Spray (0.05 mg/inh), 2 spray nasal inhalation daily
Fluticasone-Salmeterol 500 mcg-50 mcg/puff 1 puff inhalation twice daily
Pancrelipase (Ultrase MT 20) 6 capsules orally with meals
Prednisone 60 mg orally daily
Regular Human Insulin Sliding Scale SubQ before meals and at bedtime
Vitamin, Multi 1 tablet orally daily
Voriconazole 200 mg orally every 12 hours
Azithromycin 500 mg PO 3×/week
ASA 325 g M,W, F
Nutren 2.0 2 cans 80 cc/hr
Tobi nebs 300 mg BID every other month, off month now
Ultrase MT20 4 tabs with snacks
Lantus 5 U sq hs

DISCHARGE INSTRUCTIONS:

Discharge to home. Resume CF diet and normal levels of activity.

Follow-up care: Appointment at the clinic.

Echocardiogram

Indication for study: worsening dyspnea, septal defect.

Interpretation summary:

Limited echo exam: 2D and Doppler.

The study was viewed and interpreted by the undersigned attending.

The study was technically difficult.

Limited views were obtained.

The study was technically limited.

Technically limited image quality precludes assessment (patent foramen ovale with agitated saline). No obvious defects noted by color Doppler.

Patient weight: 95 lbs.

Heart rate: 125 bpm.

Left ventricle: The left ventricle is normal in size. There is normal left ventricular wall thickness. Left ventricular systolic function is normal. EF estimated at 65%. Left ventricular wall motion is normal.

Right ventricle: The right ventricle is normal in size. Right ventricular systolic function is normal.

Atria: Left atrial size is normal. Right atrial size is normal. There is no Doppler evidence for an atrial septal defect.

106

Mitral valve: The mitral valve is normal. No mitral valve stenosis and no mitral regurgitation noted.

Tricuspid valve: The tricuspid valve is not well visualized but is grossly normal. No tricuspid regurgitation.

Aortic valve: The aortic valve is not well visualized. Trace aortic regurgitation.

Pulmonic valve: The pulmonic valve is not well visualized.

Great vessels: The aortic root is normal size.

Pericardium/Pleural: There is no pericardial effusion.

Consultation

Reason for visit: Patient was seen in consultation for irritation at the gastrostomy tube site.

History of present illness: This is a 17-year-old woman with cystic fibrosis who underwent placement of a One Step button. She is complaining of redness and itching underneath the gastrostomy device.

Major findings: Examination reveals a circular area of excoriation underneath the gastrostomy tube spacer device.

Plans: The patient was advised to put some Desitin or similar barrier cream on the erythematous area, and to call back if further rash or irritation develops.

Progress Notes

DAY 1

Patient complains of SOB with minimal activity. Increasing fatigue. She has failed antibiotic treatment. Worsening PFTs. Check sputum culture.

Continue chest PT 3× a day.

DAY 2

Sputum culture + budding yeast.

Chest CT: Bronchiectasis.

CV: Echo done.

Endo: Continue vitamins/Ultrase.

GI: Protonix.

DAY 3

Patient feels better.

Gen: NAD.

Resp: Crackles diffusely.

CV: RRR, no murmur.

Abd: Soft. No tenderness.

Continue voriconazole for empiric fungal coverage.

Continue transplant evaluation.

Day 4

Afeb. VSS.

Lungs: Diffuse crackles.

CV: RRR.

Abd: Soft.

Extr: No edema.

Sputum culture + trichosporin.

Day 5

No complaints. Patient is feeling better.

Gen: NAD.

Chest: Crackles bibasilar.

Heart: Tachy.

Abd: Soft. Bowel sounds present.

Continue steroids.

Watch her diabetes due to CF; may be worse on steroids; is receiving diabetic education and insulin use instructions.

CT abd shows fatty infiltrate of the pancreas.

Day 6

Patient is much improved. Lung transplant evaluation is ongoing. Discharge patient to Home Health Care.

CASE STUDY QUESTIONS

12-3a. Admit diagnosis: _____

12-3b. Discharge disposition: _____

12-3c. Principal diagnosis: _____

12-3d. Secondary diagnoses (indicate POA status for secondary diagnoses):

_____

_____

_____

_____

_____

12-3e. Principal procedure: _____

12-3f. Secondary procedures: _____

_____

12-3g. Assign MS-DRG: _____

12-3h. Relative weight of MS-DRG: _____

12-3i. Can this MS-DRG be optimized with the addition of a CC? Yes or No

Can this MS-DRG be optimized with the addition of an MCC? Yes or No

12-3j. Is there a main guideline pertinent to selection of the principal diagnosis in this case study?

_____

_____

12-3k. Is there another diagnosis that meets the definition for principal diagnosis? Yes or No

12-3l. If yes, what is the other diagnosis? _____

12-3m. Is there any opportunity for physician query?

_____

_____

12-3n. What is the drug Pancrelipase used to treat?

_____

12-4. CASE STUDY

History and Physical

CC: Diabetic ketoacidosis.

HPI: 12½ y/o female admitted after recent episodes of vomiting, diarrhea, decreased energy, and hyperglycemia. Patient's mother had a 12-hour history of gastroenteritis on Sunday, which patient's mother feels she passed on to her daughter and then provoked diabetic ketoacidosis. Patient had episodes of vomiting and diarrhea on Monday. On Tuesday, the patient was not eating and was sleeping all day, and sugars continued in the 200s. Wednesday early hours of the morning, patient had labored breathing and shivering. Sugars persisted and were elevated to close to 500. Mom used a sliding scale; however, despite this, glucose was still 500. Patient had large quantities of ketones and glucose in the urine. Last hospital admission was a few months ago. Mom attributes this to her daughter taking control over her treatment: Mom also states that since that time, she has been motivated and on top of her medications; the last hospitalization gave her a scare. Prior to this, her last admission had occurred 2.5 years ago.

In the ED, patient was started on IVF and insulin drip.

PMHx: Seizures diagnosed at 6 years of age.

Diabetes type I diagnosed at age 4.

PSHx: None.

Medications: Lantus 25 units AM

Zonegran

Sliding scale: 1 unit: 100-151, 2 units: 152-200, 3 units: 201-250, 4 units: 251-200, 5 units: 301-350, 6 units: 351-400

Allergies: NKDA.

Family history:

Family heart: Uncle with pphn.

Asthma: Brother.

Rheumatic heart: None.

Diabetes: None.

Jaundice/liver disease: None.

Epilepsy: Maternal great uncle.

Tuberculosis: None.

ROS:

Neuro: Patient less responsive.

CV: nL.

Resp: nL.

GI: Currently no diarrhea and no vomiting.

Derm: No rashes.

Endo: Currently glucose 86.

Vitals: HR 98, RR 18, BP 114/62, 99% on RA.

HEENT: Neck supple, pupils equal and reactive, nares patent.

CV: S1–S2, m, cr <2 sec.

Resp: Clear bilateral air entry, no wheeze, no creps.

GI: Soft, nontender, +BS.

Neuro: Reflexes ++, decreased responsiveness.

Ext: Moving all four limbs.

A/P: 12½-year-old female admitted with DKA and background history of seizures.

Endo: Insulin drip, IVF, q-d sticks each hour. Tomorrow, resume home meds (Lantus, Humalog, and sliding scale).

Dispo: PMD.

Ophthal: Yearly eye checks.

Derm/Wound: Teaching regarding ulcers.

DIAGNOSES/PROBLEMS:

Type 1 diabetes mellitus, diabetic ketoacidosis.

PROCEDURES:

None.

HISTORY, MAJOR FINDINGS, AND HOSPITAL COURSE:

The patient is a 12½-year-old female with a history of type I diabetes mellitus diagnosed at 4 years of age who presented to the ER in the early morning hours in diabetic ketoacidosis. She developed nausea, vomiting, and diarrhea a few days prior to admission, which resolved 24 hours later, but she was subsequently noted by her mother to be excessively fatigued over the next 2 days. Over this course, there was no history of polyuria or polydipsia, but on the morning of the day prior to admission, she awoke with blood glucose in the mid-300s; she was given Humalog insulin correction doses over the course of the day (23 units in total over the first 12 hours), and by bedtime, her blood sugar was reportedly in the 140s. However, at approximately 0130 on the day of admission, she was noted by her sister to have developed labored respirations, and by 0330 was noted to be unresponsive with a blood glucose of 499. She was subsequently brought to the ED, where initial blood sugar was 504 with large urine ketones, a bicarbonate of 9, and a pH of 7.24. She received 2 normal saline IV boluses and was started on an insulin drip at 0.1 unit/kg/hr; over the first 5 hours of therapy, her blood glucose dropped from the mid-500s to 68, and the insulin drip and all IV fluids were discontinued. On admission, pH was 7.27 with bicarb of 9, BG 153, and large urine ketones. Insulin drip was restarted at 0.1 u/kg/hr, and dextrose-containing IV fluids were started at 1.5 × maintenance. On physical examination, she was noted to be difficult to arouse and not appropriately answering questions; therefore a CT of the head was ordered to rule out cerebral edema; this was reported as normal. By the next morning, her sensorium was normal and her anion gap had closed with trace-small urine ketones. She was transitioned back to her basal-bolus insulin regimen with Lantus and NovoLog, and insulin drip and IV fluids were discontinued after her first dose of NovoLog and upon resumption of a regular diet. The patient was able to tolerate her diet and maintained euglycemia through lunch on her first hospital day. She was discharged to home with her mother on her usual insulin regimen.

DISCHARGE MEDICATIONS:

Lantus 25 u SQ qAM NovoLog bolus dose 1 u for every 10 g of carbohydrate consumed; correction factor 1 unit for every 50 BG points above 150

DISCHARGE INSTRUCTIONS:

Resume home insulin regimen.

for addressograph plate

Date	Time	
		Peds Endo
12/14	10:00	S: MS much improved this am, asking for breakfast, wants
		to go home. Overnight BG ~ 60s-80s, insulin gtt ↓'d
		to 0.8 u/kg/hr, nausea ↑ to yesterday. Foley d/c'd
		O: 36.5 91 14 109/67
		Gen - comfort, sleepy HEENT: PERRL, EOMI mmm, oro-
		chest - CTAB CV - RRR, no m/r/g Abd - soft nt nd ext - wwp
		BG trend
		0000 76 → return gtt 1.0 u/kg/hr
		0300 57 → ↓ 0.8 u/kg/hr (gtt held: ○)
		0400 93
		0600 86 138 | 109 | 15 ⟨ 81
		3.9 | 19 | 0.5
		0800 86 vBG: 7.41/34/52/21
		A/P 12 mo/o ♀ c̄ DM1, resolved DKA. Appears ready for
		transition to breakfast insulin, right PO today
		① Will restart home insulin regimen:
		- Give 25 u Lantus SQ this am
		- Start diet now; give u Novolog: 10 g CHO
		prior to breakfast
		- CF Novolog: 1u for every 50 BG >150
		- Please d/c IVF/insulin gtt ~ 1 hr p̄ Novolog dose
		② Will consult d/c to home this afternoon
		if no issues
		③ Pls ✓ BG qAC, qHS

for addressograph plate

Date	Time	
12/14	10²⁵	Peds Endo Attending
		_____ looking much better today, answering questions appropriately, hungry this AM. CO_2 19 @ 4³⁰ AM, BG 60-80's.
		PE: VSS. mmm
		Lungs CTA CV RRR ∅ (m)
		Abd NT
		Ext ∅ edema
		A/P: 12 y.o. ♀ c̄ type 1 DM, DKA now resolved. Still c̄ mod ketones in urine
		① Can d/c insulin gtt, Δ to home regimen for insulin.
		② Encourage fluids
		③ If urine ketones cleared, anticipate D/C home this evening.

for addressograph plate

Date	Time	
12/14	0620	S— improvement in mental status, awakes and easier wants to eat, no headache, no complaints
		O— Tm
		I/o— 2200 / 750 since 8pm
		PE: D/o @ 75 D20 ½ NS + 20 kcl @ 25
		gen— sleepy, oriented to place, not time, following directions
		HEENT— slightly, dry mm, eyes
		cv— RRR w/o m
		lungs— CTAB, no distress
		abd— soft, nontender
		neuro— alert, drowsy, following commands
		labs:
		7.38 / 37 / 52 137 / 110 / 12 \ 64 u/A— lrg ketones 35 / 16 / 0.5
		dstx 36-90-82, 62-93-82-86
		CT— unremarkable, acute sinusitis
		A/P 12½ yo hx of DM type I, presents in DKA, gap now cleared
		① FEN/GI— NPO am, likely transition to taking PO today, likely gastroenteritis that precipitating this episode

for addressograph plate

Date	Time	
12/14/...	1600	S: MS back to baseline, answers questions appropriately, A+O x3. Resolved N&V/pain, wish app as pr bone regimen; wish gtt/IVF & lytes BG resolved
		1005 66 → Normal lytes (K+ 3.5, gluc 40), labs ↓↓↓
		1115 → less gtt/IVF LLC%
		1255 55 → Normal 4u; 40 gtt/min
		1415 48
		A/P 18 y/o F c DM1, resolved DKA; gluc/ketoacidosis resolved, tolerated back to bone wish app
		① OK for d/c to home c:
		labs ↓↓↓ sx gtt/min
		Normal K+: 10 gluc/c+o; K+: 50 BG >150
		⊗ Attend to keep well hydrated, √ urine ketones c ↑ BG

Chapter **12** **Endocrine, Nutritional, and Metabolic Diseases**

History: Headache.

Technique: Axial CT scan images were performed from the foramen magnum to the vertex without administration of intravenous contrast.

Comparison: None available.

Findings: There is no evidence of acute intracranial hemorrhage. No evidence of abnormal intra-axial or extra-axial fluid collections. The ventricles are symmetric in size and unremarkable, given the patient's stated age. No evidence of mass, mass effect, or midline shift. The gray-white matter differentiation is intact and unremarkable.

The bony calvarium is unremarkable. The visualized paranasal sinuses and mastoid air cells are clear, except for fluid within the left sphenoid sinus and a tiny amount of fluid within the right sphenoid sinus. The globes and orbits are symmetric and grossly unremarkable.

Impression: Unremarkable noncontrast CT of the brain. Small amounts of fluid within the sphenoid sinus, possibly due to acute sinusitis.

CASE STUDY QUESTIONS

12-4a. Admit diagnosis: _____

12-4b. Discharge disposition: _____

12-4c. Principal diagnosis: _____

12-4d. Secondary diagnoses (indicate POA status for secondary diagnoses):

_____

_____

_____

_____

_____

_____

_____

12-4e. Principal procedure: _____

12-4f. Secondary procedures: _____

_____

12-4g. Assign MS-DRG: _____

12-4h. Relative weight of MS-DRG: _____

12-4i. Can this MS-DRG be optimized with the addition of a CC? Yes or No

Can this MS-DRG be optimized with the addition of an MCC? Yes or No

12-4j. Is there a main guideline pertinent to selection of the principal diagnosis in this case study?

_____

_____

12-4k. Is there another diagnosis that meets the definition for principal diagnosis? Yes or No

12-4l. If yes, what is the other diagnosis? _____

12-4m. Is there any opportunity for physician query?

_____

_____

12-4n. What is the drug Lantus used to treat? _____

Mental Disorders and Behavioral Disorders (ICD-10-CM Chapter 5, Codes F01-F99)

13

ABBREVIATIONS/ACRONYMS

Without the use of reference materials, define the following abbreviations or acronyms.

1. OBS _____

2. MR _____

3. IQ _____

4. ADD _____

5. PTSD _____

6. DTs _____

7. ADHD _____

8. LD _____

9. DSM-IV-TR _____

10. CC _____

GLOSSARY DEFINITIONS

Match the glossary term to the correct definition.

1. _____ Organic brain syndrome

2. _____ Bipolar disorder

3. _____ Posttraumatic stress disorder

4. _____ Dementia

5. _____ Phobia

6. _____ Schizophrenia

7. _____ Mood disorder

8. _____ Detoxification

9. _____ Mental retardation

10. _____ Psychosis

11. _____ Affective disorders

12. _____ Depression

13. _____ Panic disorder

14. _____ Oppositional defiant disorder

15. _____ Generalized anxiety disorder

A. General term used to describe the decrease in mental function due to other physical diseases

B. Brain disorder that causes unusual shifts in a person's mood, energy, and ability to function; different from the normal ups and downs that everyone goes through; symptoms are severe

C. Category of mental health problems that includes depressive disorders/mood disorders

D. Affective disorder that is characterized by sadness, lack of interest in everyday activities and events, and a feeling of worthlessness

E. Terrifying experience that occurs suddenly without any warning; physical symptoms include pounding heart, chest pains, dizziness, nausea, shortness of breath, trembling, choking, fear of dying, sweating, feelings of unreality, numbness, hot flashes or chills, and a feeling of going out of control or "crazy"

F. Chronic, exaggerated worry, tension, and irritability that may be without cause, or that is more intense than the situation warrants

Continued

G. Disorder in which a person's overall intellectual functioning is well below average, with an intelligence quotient (IQ) around 70 or less

H. Anxiety disorder that is triggered by memories of a traumatic event

I. Change in mood for a prolonged time

J. Pattern of uncooperative, defiant, and hostile behavior toward authority figures that does not involve major antisocial violations, is not accounted for by the child's developmental stage, and results in significant functional impairment

K. Irrational anxiety or fear that can interfere with one's everyday life or daily routine

L. Impairment of mental state in which perception of reality has become distorted

M. Progressive deterioration of mental faculties characterized by impairment of memory and one or more cognitive impairments such as in language, reasoning and judgment, calculation, or problem-solving ability

N. Active management of withdrawal symptoms in a patient who is physically dependent on alcohol or drugs

O. Disorder of the brain characterized by trouble differentiating between real and unreal experiences, logical thinking, normal emotional responses to others, and appropriate behavior in social situations

CODING

Using the code book, code the following.

1. Korsakoff's alcoholic psychosis   _____

2. Drug-seeking behavior   _____

3. Patient feigning illness   _____

4. Munchausen's syndrome   _____

5. Voyeurism   _____

6. Schizoid personality   _____

7. Chronic pain with psychogenic factors   _____

8. Shoe fetish   _____

9. Erectile dysfunction with psychogenic factors   _____

10. Laxative abuse   _____

11. Grief reaction due to son's suicide   _____

12. Female sexual arousal disorder   _____

13. Night terrors   _____

CASE SCENARIOS

Using the code book, code the following cases.

1. This 45-year-old female was brought to the Emergency Room following a seizure. While she was being evaluated, she had another seizure and was admitted to the hospital. Family members state that she has been drinking heavily. She was started on detox protocol. Psychiatric evaluation revealed that she has drunk 6 beers a day for the past 10 years and smokes 1 pack of cigarettes per day. She was discharged to an outpatient rehabilitation program on hospital day 2.
Final Diagnosis: Alcohol withdrawal.
Procedures: Alcohol detoxification.

_____

_____

2. This 28-year-old male was brought to the ER by a friend who stated that the patient had been acting bizarrely. The patient has been irritable, pacing the apartment, and talking nonstop. He was admitted to the psychiatric unit for management of his manic symptoms.
Final Diagnosis: Bipolar affective disease, severe manic phase, recurrent episode with psychosis.

_____

_____

3. Patient was admitted with delirium tremens due to alcohol withdrawal. Patient has had a bout of acute gastroenteritis and has not had a drink for a couple of days. Patient was admitted and was started on IV fluids and a banana bag. Patient is hypokalemic with a potassium of 3.0 and is also dehydrated. Patient's potassium was repleted with oral medication.
Final Diagnoses: Acute gastroenteritis.
           Alcohol withdrawal.
           Hypokalemia.

_____

_____

4. Patient was brought to the ER because of disorganized speech and thought patterns. He has a history of schizophrenia, and further questioning revealed that he has not taken his medications for 1 month. Patient was admitted to the psychiatric unit for stabilization and monitoring.
Final Diagnosis: Exacerbation of chronic schizophrenia.

_____

_____

5. Patient was admitted to the psychiatric floor for evaluation of mood disorder. After extensive testing and evaluation, it was determined that patient was suffering from major depression that is severe in nature, and that some psychotic features are present.
Final Diagnosis: Major depressive disorder, severe with psychosis.

_____

_____

Chapter **13** **Mental Disorders and Behavioral Disorders**

6. Patient presented to the ER requesting detox. Patient had a previous admission for heroin dependence 2 years ago. Patient's drug use cost about $50.00 per day and he occasionally smoked cocaine. Patient is unemployed. Routine labs were within normal limits, and the detoxification protocol was implemented. The patient did experience some mild withdrawal symptoms. The patient was discharged after 3 days and was instructed to attend 90 NA meetings in 90 days and to find a sponsor.
Discharge Diagnoses: Heroin dependence with withdrawal.
          Cocaine abuse.

_____

_____

7. Patient was admitted to the hospital for cocaine-induced chest pain. After undergoing evaluation, the patient was stable for transfer to the psychiatric floor for treatment of his cocaine abuse. Patient has an antisocial personality disorder and uses cocaine almost daily. Patient occasionally smokes marijuana. A detoxification and rehabilitation program (12-step group counseling) was implemented. After day 5, patient signed out AMA.
Final Diagnoses: Cocaine abuse.
          Antisocial personality disorder.
Procedure: Detoxification and rehabilitation.

_____

_____

8. Patient was admitted to the psychiatric unit for treatment of anorexia nervosa. Patient's weight has fallen by 30%, and she has evidence of moderate malnutrition. Patient was hypokalemic, and she has a history of osteoporosis. Patient was hospitalized for intensive therapy, and her medical conditions were evaluated and treated.
Final Diagnoses: Anorexia nervosa with moderate malnutrition.
          Hypokalemia.
          Osteoporosis.
Procedure: Total parenteral nutrition (via peripheral vein).

_____

_____

9. Patient was admitted to the psychiatric unit for worsening symptoms of posttraumatic stress disorder. Patient was the victim of a violent crime. Patient has been having increasing nightmares, insomnia, flashbacks, and feelings of anxiety. Patient felt like he was going crazy and had suicidal ideation upon presentation. Patient participated in individual and group therapies, and some medication adjustments were made. He had been noncompliant with his medications, and the importance of medication compliance was stressed.
Discharge Diagnosis: Chronic posttraumatic stress disorder.

_____

_____

10. Patient was brought to the hospital with a seizure-like attack. Neurology evaluated the patient, and EEG was normal. Following thorough evaluation and monitoring, no medical reason could be found for the patient's symptoms. Patient has been under a great deal of stress lately, and a psychiatric consult was obtained. Psychiatry felt that the patient's symptoms may be due to conversion disorder.
Final Diagnosis: Conversion disorder with seizure.

_____

_____

Using the code book, code and answer questions about the following case studies.

13-1. CASE STUDY

History and Physical

CC: Seizure

HPI: The patient is a 45-year-old male with a history of multiple admissions for alcohol withdrawal seizures. He presented to the ED via EMS after a witnessed seizure at his house. He was recently released from jail after a 1-month stay, during which he abstained from alcohol. He then drank heavily for 3 days but could not recall when he took his last drink.

Past medical history: He has had severe alcohol withdrawal in the past, requiring intubation and Ativan drip.

Social history: Positive for tobacco, daily alcohol, and occasional cocaine (nasal). Lives with sister.

Review of systems: Positive for headache, seizures, visual changes. No chest pain, shortness of breath, abdominal pain.

Medications: None.

Allergies: NKDA.

Physical examination:

Vitals: T 100.3, P 100, BP 144/86, RR 16.

General: NAD.

HEENT: Poor dentition. Dry mucous membranes. PERRL. Trachea is midline.

Chest: CTA.

CV: RRR.

Abd: Soft. No distention. No hepatomegaly.

Ext: No telangiectasia.

Neuro: No hallucination. Slight tremor.

A/P: Patient admitted for alcohol withdrawal seizure. Seizure precautions and alcohol withdrawal protocol. Substance abuse consult.

Discharge Summary

DIAGNOSES/PROBLEMS:

1. Alcohol withdrawal seizure with fall and laceration to forehead.
2. Hypertension.
3. Alcoholism.
4. Cocaine use.

PROCEDURES:

Suture forehead laceration.

1. CXR: hyperinflated lungs.
2. Head CT: no hemorrhage, minimal scalp edema. No acute abnormality.
3. L-spine x-ray: degenerative changes.

History, Major Findings, and Hospital Course:

The patient is a 45-year-old male with a history of multiple admissions for alcohol withdrawal seizures. He presented to the ED via EMS after a witnessed seizure at his house. The patient was recently released from jail after a 1-month stay, during which he abstained from alcohol. He then drank heavily for 3 days but could not recall when he had taken his last drink. He has had severe alcohol withdrawal in the past, requiring intubation and Ativan drip.

ROS: +Headache, seizures, visual change. No chest pain, shortness of breath, abdominal pain.

In the ED, the patient had two additional seizures. Received Ativan, Versed, and Dilantin.

SH: Positive for tobacco, alcohol, cocaine (nasal). Lives with sister.

Physical examination: Temp 100.3, pulse 100, BP 144/86, RR 16, sat 100% on 2L NC sleeping. +Laceration on forehead. Poor dentition. No meningismus. Chest clear to auscultation. Heart regular and rhythm.

Abdomen: Soft, nontender, nondistended.

Ext: No telangiectasias. No hallucinations.

Neuro: Alert and oriented ×3, slight tremor, unable to walk straight.

EKG: Sinus tachycardia.

Hospital course: The patient's alcohol withdrawal seizures did not recur on the inpatient ward. He was treated with Ativan 2 mg IV q2h PM, as well as with chlordiazepoxide 50 mg PO. He never had delirium tremens. The patient improved back to baseline within the next 24 hours. He was also given thiamine and folate. BP was normal, and the patient required no antihypertensives. Therefore, his home nifedipine XL was not restarted.

Discharge medications: Thiamine enteral, 100 mg PO daily folic acid enteral, and Ativan 1 mg by mouth every 8 hours as needed for tremors.

Follow-up Care:

Strongly encourage alcohol cessation. Please consider attending rehab or AA.

Chest:

Indication: Seizures. Alcohol abuse. Shortness of breath.

Impression: Vascular congestion gone since prior examination. Increased inflation. No other changes or abnormalities.

Brain Without IV Contrast, CT

Results:

History: Laceration on head.

Technique: Axial CT scan images were performed from the foramen magnum to the vertex without administration of intravenous contrast.

Findings: These images exhibit no evidence of mass lesion ventricles, and sulci are appropriate for age. Shift of midline structures is noted. The brain is not evident. Minimal scalp edema is noted in the right frontoparietal region. Visualized portions of the bones are unremarkable. Vascular calcification is apparent in the bilateral distal vertebral arteries.

124

Impression: No evidence of acute intracranial abnormality.

CT C-spine Without Contrast Complex

Results:
Indication: Trauma.

Technique: Multiple contiguous axial CT scans were performed through the cervical spine without contrast, with coronal and sagittal 2D reformations.

Findings: Straightening of the normal cervical lordosis is seen. Alignment is otherwise normal. No evidence of fracture or subluxation is apparent. Visualized soft tissues are unremarkable, and the prevertebral fat stripe is preserved. Degenerative joint disease is noted in the cervical spine, along with anterior and less prominent posterior osteophytes.

At the C3-4 level, bilateral posterior osteophytes and uncovertebral hypertrophy result in bilateral moderate to severe foraminal narrowing. Mild narrowing of the central canal is evident. Flattening of the ventral thecal sac is seen, with no evidence of cord compression.

At C4-5 level, bilateral posterior osteophytes and left uncovertebral hypertrophy are noted. Moderate left foraminal narrowing and mild to moderate right foraminal narrowing are apparent. Mild narrowing of the central canal is evident, without cord compression and flattening of the ventral thecal sac.

At the C5-6 level, right uncovertebral hypertrophy and foraminal osteophytes result in moderate to severe right foraminal narrowing. Left uncovertebral hypertrophy results in moderate left foraminal narrowing. Mild narrowing of the central canal is noted. No evidence of cord compression is found.

At the C6-7 level, left uncovertebral hypertrophy and posterolateral osteophytes result in moderate left foraminal narrowing. Right neural foramen is patent. Mild central canal narrowing is noted.

Impression: No acute injury to the cervical spine. Degenerative spondylosis, particularly from C3-4 to C6-7 levels, with mild central canal narrowing and moderate bilateral foraminal narrowing, as described previously.

Progress Notes

DAY 1

No further seizures. No evidence of delirium tremens. Patient has improved quickly and is asking to be discharged. BP has been normal without medications.

DAY 2

Patient has been seen by the substance abuse counselor and was given a listing of AA meetings in the area. Patient remains seizure free and is ready for discharge home.

CASE STUDY QUESTIONS

13-1a. Admit diagnosis: _____

13-1b. Discharge disposition: _____

13-1c. Principal diagnosis: _____

13-1d. Secondary diagnoses (indicate POA status for secondary diagnoses):

_____

_____

_____

_____

_____

_____

13-1e. Principal procedure: _____

13-1f. Secondary procedures: _____

_____

13-1g. Assign MS-DRG: _____

13-1h. Relative weight of MS-DRG: _____

13-1i. Can this MS-DRG be optimized with the addition of a CC? Yes or No
       Can this MS-DRG be optimized with the addition of an MCC? Yes or No

13-1j. Is there a main guideline pertinent to selection of the principal diagnosis in this case study?

_____

_____

13-1k. Is there another diagnosis that meets the definition for principal diagnosis? Yes or No

13-1l. If yes, what is the other diagnosis? _____

13-1m. Is there any opportunity for physician query?

_____

_____

13-1n. What is the drug thiamine used to treat? _____

CC: OxyContin dependence.

HPI: Patient is 26-year-old male who showed up at the ER requesting admission for detox. Patient was admitted for detoxification protocol.

Past medical history: Patient was detoxed at this facility 2 years ago. He was clean until 2 months ago; he relapsed after breaking up with his girlfriend.

Past surgical history: None.

Social history: OxyContin dependence, relapsed with daily use. No alcohol. Smokes ½ pack of cigarettes a day.

Medications: None.

Allergies: NKDA.

Review of systems:

Constitutional: No fevers, chills, or sweats. A 10-pound weight loss over the past 2 months.

Neuro: No headache, seizures, or syncope.

HEENT: No vision changes, no diplopia or hearing loss. No sore throat. No polyuria or polydipsia.

CV: No chest pain or palpitations.

Resp: No SOB, wheezing, cough, sputum production, or hemoptysis.

GI: No abdominal pain. No N/V/D.

GU: No dysuria or frequency.

Skin: No rashes.

Musculoskeletal: No myalgias or joint pain.

Physical examination:

Vitals: Stable.

General: No acute distress. Appears anxious.

HEENT: Erosions of the nasal septum. Otherwise negative.

Chest: CTA.

CV: RRR.

Abd: Soft.

Extremities: WNL.

Neuro: Intact.

A/P: Admit for detoxification protocol.

This 26-year-old male patient with no significant past medical history presented to the ER requesting detoxification. Patient has been treated for OxyContin dependence in the past and has recently relapsed. Patient did have some mild withdrawal symptoms. Labs were within normal limits, and no other problems were identified. Patient has agreed to attend 90 NA meetings in 90 days and will be attending an outpatient drug rehab program.

Diagnosis: OxyContin dependence.

Procedure: Detoxification.

DAY 1
_____

Detoxification protocol was initiated. Patient has some mild withdrawal symptoms. Patient is eating well.

DAY 2
_____

Patient's withdrawal symptoms are clearing. No medical problems. Continue detox.

DAY 3
_____

Patient is ready for discharge to an outpatient drug program.

CASE STUDY QUESTIONS

13-2a. Admit diagnosis: _____

13-2b. Discharge disposition: _____

13-2c. Principal diagnosis: _____

13-2d. Secondary diagnoses (indicate POA status for secondary diagnoses):

_____

_____

_____

_____

_____

_____

13-2e. Principal procedure: _____

13-2f. Secondary procedures: _____

_____

13-2g. Assign MS-DRG: _____

13-2h. Relative weight of MS-DRG: _____

13-2i. Can this MS-DRG be optimized with the addition of a CC? Yes or No
Can this MS-DRG be optimized with the addition of an MCC? Yes or No

13-2j. Is there a main guideline pertinent to selection of the principal diagnosis in this case study?

_____

_____

13-2k. Is there another diagnosis that meets the definition for principal diagnosis? Yes or No

13-2l. If yes, what is the other diagnosis? _____

13-2m. Is there any opportunity for physician query?

_____

_____

Diseases of the Nervous System, Diseases of the Eye and Adnexa, and Diseases of the Ear and Mastoid Process (ICD-10-CM Chapter 6, Codes G00-G99, Chapter 7, Codes H00-H59, Chapter 8, Codes H60-H95)

14

ABBREVIATIONS/ACRONYMS

Without the use of reference materials, define the following abbreviations or acronyms.

1. VPS _____

2. CNS _____

3. IOP _____

4. SZ _____

5. EEG _____

6. NPH _____

7. CSF _____

8. PDT _____

9. SIRS _____

10. CVA _____

GLOSSARY DEFINITIONS

Match the glossary term to the correct definition.

1. _____ Congenital
2. _____ Hemiplegia
3. _____ Vertigo
4. _____ Hydrocephalus
5. _____ Lumbar puncture
6. _____ Tremor
7. _____ Quadriplegia
8. _____ Plasmapheresis
9. _____ Senile
10. _____ Electrode

A. Pertaining to old age
B. Occurring at birth
C. Paralysis of half the body
D. Unintentional or involuntary movement that affects the muscle
E. Accumulation of fluid on the brain
F. Dizziness
G. Wire that emits, controls, or receives electricity
H. Process of separating certain cells from the plasma
I. Test used to evaluate the spinal fluid
J. Paralysis of all four limbs

CODING

Using the code book, code the following.

1. Meniere's disease _____
2. Intracranial abscess _____

131

3. Congenital nystagmus   _____

4. Chalazion, right upper eyelid   _____

5. Presbyopia   _____

6. Cervical root lesion   _____

7. Trigeminal neuralgia   _____

8. Bell's palsy   _____

9. Cluster headache   _____

10. Anoxic brain damage   _____

11. Restless legs syndrome (RLS)   _____

12. Cerebral palsy   _____

13. Acute post-thoracotomy pain   _____

14. Obstructive sleep apnea   _____

15. Cognitive impairment, mild   _____

CASE SCENARIOS

Using the code book, code the following cases.

1. Patient presents to the ER with high fever and headache. Meningitis is suspected. A lumbar puncture is performed and reveals bacterial meningitis.

2. Patient presents to the hospital after an episode of vertigo and word slurring. An MRI is performed and reveals cerebral hemorrhage. Patient is discharged home with mild hemiplegia on the right.

3. Patient is admitted with NPH with dementia; a ventriculoperitoneal shunt is inserted.

4. A patient is admitted following a seizure. Laboratory work reveals that the patient is dehydrated and hyponatremic. The final diagnosis lists seizure due to dehydration.

5. A patient with Parkinson's disease is admitted for insertion of an intracranial neurostimulator, leads, and a generator. Generator is inserted subcutaneously in the chest

6. Patient is admitted with epilepsy that is resistant to control. An EEG is performed.

_____

_____

7. Patient is admitted with Morton's neuroma of the left lower limb. She has severe mental retardation, so an overnight stay is warranted. Surgery is performed to remove the neuroma.

_____

_____

8. A patient with trigeminal neuralgia is admitted for a rhizotomy.

_____

_____

9. The deaf child was brought into the hospital to receive a bilateral multichannel cochlear implant.

_____

_____

10. Patient is admitted to the hospital for pain management. Patient suffers from severe chronic back pain. A single array spinal neurostimulator will be inserted.

_____

_____

CASE STUDIES

Using the code book, code and answer questions about the following case studies.

14-1. CASE STUDY

History and Physical

CC: Seizure following change in meds.

HPI: The patient is a 72-year-old man with a history of intractable epilepsy with complex partial seizures and bipolar disorder. He presented to the emergency department on the day of admission following two typical complex partial seizures. Per his nephew, he has 1 to 2 seizures approximately every other week or so and has been highly refractory to medications. The patient has been maintained on Trileptal 600 mg twice a day, Zonegran 200 mg twice a day, and Lamictal 50 mg twice a day. His Lamictal was decreased to 25 mg twice a day on the day prior to admission. In the past, he has been very sensitive to changes in his antiepileptic medications, which have precipitated seizures.

Past medical history:

1. Intractable epilepsy with complex partial seizures.
2. Bipolar disorder.
3. Status post CVA in the left cerebellar PICA distribution.
4. Multifactorial gait disturbance.

Family history: The patient's father died at the age of 89 with dementia. No other family history of dementia, seizures, or epilepsy is known.

Social history: The patient graduated from high school and served in the armed forces. He no longer smokes; he quit 15 years ago. He denies alcohol or illegal drug use. He is married and lives at home with his wife, who is his primary caregiver.

Medications on admission:

1. Oxcarbazepine 600 mg twice a day.
2. Zonisamide 200 mg twice a day.
3. Lamotrigine 25 mg twice a day.
4. Levothyroxine 150 µg daily.
5. Aspirin 325 mg daily.
6. Memantine 10 mg daily.
7. Quetiapine 200 mg in the AM and 300 mg in the PM.

Allergies: No known drug allergies.

REVIEW OF SYSTEMS:

Constitutional: No change in weight. No fevers or chills.

Neuro: Seizures. No headache or syncope.

HEENT: No changes in vision. Positive for hearing loss. No sore throat.

CV: No chest pain or palpitation. No diaphoresis or claudication.

Respiratory: No cough, hemoptysis, or SOB.

GI: Negative. No N/V/D. No abdominal pain. No dysphagia or reflux.

GU: Nocturia ×2.

Skin/Skeletal: No joint stiffness. Skin is WNL.

Physical examination:

Vitals: T 35.2, HR 58, BP 131/67, RR 16, and SaO_2 97% on RA.

General: Awake. NAD.

HEENT: Normocephalic, atraumatic. Oropharynx clear. MMM. Neck is supple, no palpable nodes.

Chest: CTA.

Resp: Crackles on the right.

Abd: Soft. Bowel sounds present. No organomegaly.

GU/Rectal: Deferred.

Neuro: Patient is oriented to person and place. Not oriented to date and year. Thinks he has been in the hospital for 5 days. Unable to test gait.

Assessment/Plan: Patient is admitted for monitoring of seizure activity. May need to adjust patient's medications.

Discharge Summary

DIAGNOSES/PROBLEMS:

1. Intractable epilepsy with complex partial seizures.
2. Bipolar disorder.

PROCEDURES:

Electroencephalograph.

134

The patient is a 72-year-old man with a history of intractable epilepsy with complex partial seizures and bipolar disorder. He presented to the emergency department on the day of admission following two typical complex partial seizures. Per his nephew, he has approximately 1 to 2 seizures every other week or so and has been highly refractory to medications. He has been maintained on Trileptal 600 mg twice a day, Zonegran 200 mg twice a day, and Lamictal 50 mg twice a day. His Lamictal was decreased to 25 mg twice a day on the day prior to admission. In the past, he has been very sensitive to changes in his antiepileptic medications, which have precipitated seizures.

Past medical history:

1. Intractable epilepsy with complex partial seizures.
2. Bipolar disorder.
3. Status post CVA in the left cerebellar PICA distribution.
4. Multifactorial gait disturbance.

Family history: The patient's father died at the age of 89 with dementia. No other family history of dementia, seizures, or epilepsy is known.

Social history: The patient graduated from high school and served in the armed forces. He no longer smokes; he quit 15 years ago. He denies alcohol or illegal drug use. He is married and lives at home with his wife, who is his primary caregiver.

Medications on admission:

1. Oxcarbazepine 600 mg twice a day.
2. Zonisamide 200 mg twice a day.
3. Lamotrigine 25 mg twice a day.
4. Levothyroxine 150 µg daily.
5. Aspirin 325 mg daily.
6. Memantine 10 mg daily.
7. Quetiapine 200 mg in the AM and 300 mg in the PM.

Allergies: No known drug allergies.

Problem-oriented hospital course:

1. Neurology: The patient was admitted to the general neurology service status post two complex partial seizures that were typical in nature. He was not back to his baseline and was admitted for monitoring of his postictal state. An EEG was obtained to rule out subclinical status because the patient had several lapses of attention during examination on the morning following admission. This EEG was unchanged from his previous EEG and showed slowing of the posterior basic rhythm, consistent with a diffuse cerebral disturbance. No seizures or localizing signs were noted. By the next day, the patient had recovered entirely to his baseline. He was, however, maintained in the hospital secondary to hyponatremia as detailed below. His Lamictal was increased back to his previous level of 50 mg twice a day immediately upon admission. Given the occurrence of the staring episodes witnessed on the day after admission, his zonisamide was also increased from 200 mg twice a day to 300 mg twice a day. He was maintained on the discharge medications on the following page and had no other clinical seizures during his hospitalization.
2. Hyponatremia: Two days after admission, the patient was noted to be hyponatremic, with a nadir of 124. He had no seizure activity or other symptoms associated with this hyponatremia. This was followed closely, and he was fluid restricted. Laboratory testing was consistent with SIADH. His hydrochlorothiazide was discontinued, and he was started on salt tablets. His sodium was followed. At the time of discharge, his sodium was 129. Sodium should be rechecked in 1 week. Salt tablets may be withdrawn if sodium remains greater than 130 with withdrawal of HCTZ and fluid restriction.
3. Psychiatry: Patient was continued on his standing medications. He was discharged to home in the care of his wife. He will continue with the psychiatry day program.

135

Discharge medications: Oxcarbazepine 600 mg by mouth twice a day, zonisamide 300 mg by mouth twice a day, lamotrigine 50 mg by mouth twice a day, levothyroxine 150 µg by mouth daily, aspirin 325 mg by mouth daily, memantine 10 mg by mouth daily, and quetiapine 200 mg by mouth in the AM and 300 mg by mouth in the PM.

Discharge instructions: Recheck sodium in 1 week. Goal >130. Fluid restriction.

Follow-up care: The patient will follow up in clinic.

Report of Electroencephalogram

Referral reason: Changes in mental status.

Medications: Keppra, Trileptal.

Technique: 21 electrodes and EKG. International placement, bipolar and referential technique. Agitated, confused, mental stimulation.

Brief history: 72-year-old male weaning from lamotrigine had seizures and changes in mental status.

ICD-9 Diagnosis Codes:

780.99 = Change in Mental Status.

RVU: 9903.30 (EEG Awake and Sleep 20 to 40 mins).

The record showed the following:

Overall voltage: Overall medium voltage.

Posterior background activity: Medium voltage, 7 to 8 Hz activity, rhythmic in appearance. Within normal limits of symmetry. Occurring continuously in the awake resting state, although waxing and waning in amplitude. The posterior background was reduced by eye opening.

Background slow activity: Medium voltage. 3 to 7 Hz activity. Semirhythmic in appearance. Occurring diffusely. Within normal limits of symmetry.

Background fast activity: Low voltage. 15 to 25 Hz activity. Rhythmic in appearance. Occurring in the frontocentral regions. Within normal limits of symmetry. Occurring continuously.

Sleep activity: Medium voltage. Approximately 3 to 7 Hz activity with drowsiness and sleep. Semirhythmic in appearance. Within normal limits of symmetry. Lasting about 10 minutes. Vertex sharp transients were apparent.

Summary: A minimally abnormal EEG because of posterior basic rhythm slowing.

Comment: The EEG suggests the presence of a diffuse cerebral disturbance. No seizure discharges or localizing signs are evident.

Progress Notes

DAY 1

This 72-year-old man, who is known to have complex partial seizures and bipolar disorder, was seen on rounds. He was admitted with recurrence of seizures on the right side with slurred speech and altered mental status. This occurred in the setting of lowering of his dose of Lamictal by outside physicians. He requires day program care. Any changes in his medications or infection have not been tolerated well. This current seizure occurred in the setting of changing his Lamictal dose. His other medications include Zonegran and Trileptal. He was partially responsive and had relatively intact antigravity strength, although he was not fully cooperative. Reflexes appeared symmetric.

During the examination, the patient appeared to doze off, and it was not clear whether he was having seizures. An immediate EEG was ordered. For now, his Lamictal dose has been increased back to 50 mg two times a day. Lamictal and Zonegran are being continued.

Day 2

This 72-year-old man with complex partial seizures was seen. The patient has complex partial seizures and bipolar disorder. He is currently on zonisamide, Lamictal, and Trileptal. His sodium is 125 today. Fluids are being restricted. The plan is to check sodium again. He should be discharged to a nursing home placement on Tuesday or Wednesday.

Day 3

This 72-year-old man with complex partial seizures and a history of bipolar disorders was seen on rounds. The patient appears alert and interactive, although he is only partially oriented. He is able to take a few steps but appears unsteady. He knows he is in the hospital. He appears brighter and more cheerful than at his evaluation yesterday. He did not show any active seizures, although with increases in zonisamide and Lamictal doses, he appears to have improved. The sodium level is normalizing. The plan is to discharge him if his family is agreeable.

CASE STUDY QUESTIONS

14-1a. Admit diagnosis: _____

14-1b. Discharge disposition: _____

14-1c. Principal diagnosis: _____

14-1d. Secondary diagnoses (indicate POA status for secondary diagnoses):

_____

_____

_____

_____

_____

_____

14-1e. Principal procedure: _____

14-1f. Secondary procedures: _____

_____

14-1g. Assign MS-DRG: _____

14-1h. Relative weight of MS-DRG: _____

14-1i.   Can this MS-DRG be optimized with the addition of a CC? Yes or No
         Can this MS-DRG be optimized with the addition of an MCC? Yes or No

14-1j.   Is there a main guideline pertinent to selection of the principal diagnosis in this case study?

_____

_____

14-1k.   Is there another diagnosis that meets the definition for principal diagnosis? Yes or No

14-1l.   If yes, what is the other diagnosis? _____

14-1m. Is there any opportunity for physician query?

_____

_____

14-1n.   What is the drug Lamictal used to treat? _____

14-2. CASE STUDY

History and Physical

CC: R facial droop.

HPI: The patient is a 35-year-old female with no significant past medical history who has had 15-minute to 1-hour episodes of diplopia, visual field deficits, and vertigo in the past week. Had a URI the week prior. After taking a hot bath at 9:30 PM, noticed right facial droop and continued to have blurriness. Also complains of some RUE weakness and numbness with numbness of the right face.

No headache. No fever or chills. No dysphagia. No dysarthria or language problems. No gait abnormalities. No prior history of neurologic symptoms. No migraines. She denies tick exposure and rash, reports some joint pain in one of her fingers, denies use of OCPs, and denies any miscarriages.

Past medical history: Pregnant once, with twins, via IVF. No other medical history.

Past surgical history: No surgeries.

Medications: None. No OTC medicines.

Social history: No alcohol, tobacco, or drugs. Patient is married with twin sons.

Family history: Mother has breast cancer. Father has prostate cancer. No siblings.

Allergies: NKDA.

REVIEW OF SYSTEMS:

Constitutional: No change in weight. No night sweats.

Neuro: No migraines. Positive for vertigo and numbness.

HEENT: See HPI.

CV: No chest pain.

Respiratory: No SOB.

GI: No dysphagia.

GU: No dysuria or urgency.

138

Skin/Skeletal: No rashes, bruising, or lymphadenopathy.

Psych: No depression.

PHYSICAL EXAMINATION:

VS: T 96.1, HR 86, BP 141/52, RR 18.

General: NAD. Well developed and well nourished.

HEENT: Atraumatic. MMM. Oropharynx clear. Sclera anicteric. Neck is supple.

Chest: Clear bilaterally.

Heart: RRR.

Abd: Normal bowel sounds.

Ext: No cyanosis.

Neuro: Alert and oriented ×3. Intact language and memory. Cranial nerves: PERRLA. EOMI. Hearing intact. Right peripheral seventh nerve palsy. On motor examination, she had 5 out of 5 strength. On sensory examination, she had no deficits to sensations. On coordination examination, she had normal finger-to-nose and heel-to-shin. Her gait was normal. Her reflexes were 3 plus in the upper extremities, 3 at the patellar, 2 at the ankles, and her plantar response was flexor bilaterally.

Assessment/Plan: Patient with no past medical history admitted with transient attacks of diplopia, visual field deficits, vertigo, and now right peripheral facial weakness and RUE weakness/numbness. Differential diagnoses include stroke, TIA, dissection, basilar migraine or infectious origin, such as viral encephalitis, or demyelinating disease. Admit for further investigation and monitoring.

Neurology consult: The patient is an otherwise healthy 35-year-old woman admitted 12/30 with right facial weakness and right arm numbness; she was seen this morning on rounds. She has had transient episodes of vertigo, diplopia, and then facial droop in the past week; it was the facial droop and sensation that her eyes were moving that brought her into the hospital. She was noted to have a peripheral right facial droop and nystagmus, worsening in the direction of gaze. She denies headache and had a mild DRI a few weeks ago but no other recent illness. She denies tick exposure and rash, reports some joint pain in one of her fingers, denies use of OCPs, and denies any miscarriages (has been pregnant once, with twins, via IVF).

On examination today, the patient has a right peripheral seventh nerve palsy, although per report, this is somewhat improved from yesterday. Hearing is intact. She has nystagmus toward the left in the left eye only with abduction of that eye, and less marked but still present nystagmus toward the right in the right eye only with abduction of that eye. No clear vertical nystagmus is seen this morning, but some was present on admission. No diplopia is noted. She does have significant overshoot of the left eye with saccades to the left, and less so in equivalent movement of the right eye. There is a hint of a possible right afferent pupillary defect. Strength is full, sensation is normal, reflexes are brisk but symmetric, and there is also a brisk jaw jerk; coordination and gait are normal.

Plan: The patient is a 35-year-old female with no prior neurologic symptoms who has had three isolated episodes in the past week, including, most recently, a facial droop with associated nystagmus, not quite consistent with a bilateral INO (given good adduction of the contralateral eye) but possibly suggestive of a prior lesion of this type. CTA (which I personally reviewed) does not show any basilar stenosis, as was initially a matter of concern; I agree that we need an MRI stroke protocol to evaluate this further, but I am also concerned about a possible demyelinating process, including MS or Lyme disease, or an autoimmune-mediated process. She will get an LP today to evaluate for some of these processes, as well as blood work, including HIV. If she has a stroke by MRI, we will perform an echocardiogram.

DIAGNOSES/PROBLEMS:

Facial nerve palsy.

PROCEDURES:

1. Head CT.
2. MRI.
3. MRA.
4. CT angiogram.
5. Lumbar puncture.

HISTORY, MAJOR FINDINGS, AND HOSPITAL COURSE:

Reason for admission is right facial palsy.

History of present illness: The patient is a 35-year-old woman who presented with a 15 minute to 1 hour episode of diplopia, left visual field cut, and vertigo that occurred within the past week. Of note, the patient had an upper respiratory infection prior to starting to have these symptoms. After taking a hot bath at 9:30 PM, she noticed a right facial droop and continued to have left visual field blurriness. She came to the Emergency Room and complained of some right upper extremity weakness and numbness, and some right face numbness. Of note, the patient had an episode of neck pain 2 weeks ago during a cough that resolved immediately after coughing. She did not have any headache, fevers, chills, dysphagia, dysarthria, language problems, or gait abnormalities. She did not have any history of prior neurologic symptoms. No history of migraines. Her past medical history is unremarkable.

Allergies: She has no known drug allergies. She is currently on no medications.

Social history: The patient is married. She has twin boys whom she conceived through IVF. She denies use of tobacco, alcohol, or illicits.

Family history: Her mother had breast cancer. Her father had prostate cancer.

Her examination on admission: Temperature was 96.1°. Heart rate was 86. Blood pressure was 141/52. Respiratory rate was 18. In general, she is a pleasant woman in no acute distress. HEENT examination showed an atraumatic and normocephalic head with moist mucous membranes and clear oropharynx. Her neck was supple. Her chest was clear to auscultation bilaterally. On cardiac examination, she had a regular rate and rhythm with no murmurs, rubs, or gallops. On abdominal examination, she had good bowel sounds and was nondistended and nontender; no hepatosplenomegaly was noted. On extremity examination, she had no clubbing, cyanosis, or edema. On neurologic examination of her mental status, she was alert and oriented ×3 with normal speech, normal fluency, and normal comprehension. On cranial nerve examination, pupils were equal, round, and reactive to light. Extraocular movements were intact, except that she had nystagmus in all gaze directions with increased pathways on lateral left gaze. The patient was noted to have a mild right peripheral VII nerve palsy. Hearing was intact, and sensation in her face was also intact. Her tongue, uvula, and palate were midline. The patient was noted to have a jaw jerk. On motor examination, she had 5 out of 5 strength. On sensory examination, she had no deficits to sensations. On coordination examination, she had normal finger-to-nose and heel-to-shin. Gait was normal. Reflexes were 3 plus in the upper extremities, 3 at the patellas, and 2 at the ankles; plantar response was flexor bilaterally.

Problems: Facial palsy. The patient was admitted to the neurology unit for evaluation for an acute stroke. The patient had a head CT, which was unremarkable. A CT angiogram was performed, which was also unremarkable for any stenosis. The patient had an MRI, which showed no acute intracranial pathology but did show punctate foci in the corona radiata bilaterally that appeared nonspecific. The cause may have been vasculitis, Lyme disease, or migraines. After MRI revealed no acute abnormality, the patient underwent several laboratory examinations, including a lipid profile with cholesterol of 192, LDL of 85, triglycerides of 91, HDL of 89, erythrocyte sedimentation rate of 9, and CRP of less than 0.1. The patient underwent lumbar puncture, which revealed glucose of 61, protein of 26, and cell count of 3:1 white cells and 9:1 red blood cells; most cells were mononuclear. At the time of dictation, the following tests are pending: Lyme antibody test in her blood, vitamin B_{12}, TSH in the blood, ANA screen, RPR screen, anticardiolipin and IgG panel in the blood, CSF and IgG indices, oligoclonal bands, EBV PCR, CMV PCR, VZV PCR, HSV PCR, and HIV. The patient also underwent HIV testing, results of which are also pending at this time. Because the patient appeared to have the symptoms of a peripheral facial droop that was isolated, but with nystagmus, it was felt that she may have some form of a peripheral facial palsy similar to Bell's palsy. The patient was started on Valtrex and prednisone therapy for this.

Discharge condition: Good.

Discharge medications: Prednisone 70 mg by mouth every day for 1 week, Valtrex 1 g by mouth every 8 hours for 1 week, and aspirin 325 mg by mouth every day.

DISCHARGE INSTRUCTIONS:

Patient should follow up with PMD in 1 to 2 weeks.

FOLLOW-UP CARE:

Patient should follow up in Neurology clinic in 1 to 2 months.

MRI, Brain with and Without Contrast with Diff

History: 35 y/o with episodes of diplopia, vertigo, left VF cut, right facial and upper extremity weakness, and nystagmus.

Technique: Sagittal T1-weighted, axial T2-weighted, axial FLAIR, axial diffusion weighted scans, and postgadolinium contrast-enhanced scans after administration of 0.1 mmol per kilogram of a gadolinium-based contrast agent were performed through the brain. No immediate complications were noted. ADC maps were constructed from axial diffusion-weighted scans after 3D post processing from raw data. MR angiographic images with 3D reconstructions of axial data were also performed. No prior studies were available for comparison.

Findings: A few punctate foci of FLAIR and T2 hyperintensity were noted in the corona radiata bilaterally and in the left periatrial corona white matter; these appear nonspecific. No acute ischemia is noted on diffusion-weighted sequences.

Ventricles, cisterns, and sulci are normal in size and configuration. No signal abnormality on diffusion-weighted images and on corresponding ADC map suggests an acute infarct. No evidence is noted of mass, mass effect, midline shift, or abnormal enhancement. Normal flow voids are visualized in major intracranial vascular territories.

Visualized orbits and paranasal sinuses are unremarkable, except for retention cysts in the bilateral maxillary sinuses (larger on the left side) and minimal mucosal thickening in the right posterior ethmoid and sphenoid sinuses.

3D MRA of the circle of Willis reveals normal flow-related enhancement of the intracranial circulation. The intracranial internal carotid artery and the proximal anterior, middle, and posterior cerebral arteries are normal. No aneurysm, flow gap, or stenosis is identified. The vertebrobasilar system is intact with no flow gap, vascular malformation, or aneurysm. The vertebral arteries are codominant.

Impression: No acute intracranial pathology seen. Punctate foci of T2/FLAIR hyperintensity in the corona radiata bilaterally appear nonspecific. Vasculitis, Lyme's disease, and migraineur changes may have this appearance.

Normal 3D-TOF intracranial MRA. No hemodynamically significant stenosis or aneurysm in the anterior and posterior circulation.

Brain Without IV Contrast CT

Technique: Unenhanced axial CT scans were obtained from the foramen magnum to the vertex.

Findings: No evidence of acute intracranial hemorrhage, mass, mass effect, or midline shift. The gray-white junction is preserved. Ventricles and sulci are normal. Basilar cisterns are unremarkable. The calvarium is intact. The frontal sinuses are hypoplastic. Visualized paranasal sinuses and mastoid air cells are normally aerated. Orbits and globes are unremarkable.

Impression: Unremarkable noncontrast CT examination of the head.

Progress Notes

DAY 1

Patient was admitted with episodes of diplopia, R facial droop, and nystagmus. Head CT shows no abnormality. UA is negative. Pregnancy test is negative. Will do LP. Appreciate neurology consult and recommendations.

Procedure note: Informed consent was obtained. Patient was sterilely prepped and draped. Area was anesthetized with 1% lidocaine. With a 22-gauge needle, 12 cc of CSF was obtained.

DAY 2

All studies have been negative so far. It appears that the patient has a Bell's palsy–like condition that should resolve. Patient is ready for discharge.

CASE STUDY QUESTIONS

14-2a. Admit diagnosis: _____

14-2b. Discharge disposition: _____

14-2c. Principal diagnosis: _____

14-2d. Secondary diagnoses (indicate POA status for secondary diagnoses):

_____

_____

_____

_____

_____

_____

14-2e. Principal procedure: _____

14-2f.　Secondary procedures: _____

_____

14-2g.　Assign MS-DRG: _____

14-2h.　Relative weight of MS-DRG: _____

14-2i.　Can this MS-DRG be optimized with the addition of a CC? Yes or No
　　　　Can this MS-DRG be optimized with the addition of an MCC? Yes or No

14-2j.　Is there a main guideline pertinent to selection of the principal diagnosis in this case study?

_____

_____

14-2k.　Is there another diagnosis that meets the definition for principal diagnosis? Yes or No

14-2l.　If yes, what is the other diagnosis? _____

14-2m.　Is there any opportunity for physician query?

_____

_____

14-2n.　What is the drug Valtrex used to treat? _____

14-3. CASE STUDY

Admission History and Physical Examination

CC: The patient is a 67-year-old gentleman with CIDP who is being directly admitted to the Neurology Service for initiation of plasmapheresis.

HPI: The patient initially developed CIDP about 5 to 6 years ago. His initial symptoms were left leg weakness and sensory changes, with occasional sensory changes in his left arm. A couple of years ago, he received 5 rounds of plasmapheresis, which resulted in significant improvement in his strength. He had no complications during that hospitalization, other than a brief episode of hypertension, which he attributes to "hospital panic."

The patient has generally been doing very well. He was able to walk his daughter down the aisle and dance at her wedding. He exercises on a stationary bike every day. At a recent clinic visit, it was decided that it may be feasible to repeat the phoresis treatments, because they had been successful previously. His most recent EMG/NCV suggested active disease; therefore, his physician felt that there is room for improving his immunotherapy. The patient does not wish to pursue high-dose Cytoxan treatment at this time. At that appointment, a decision was made to schedule the current admission, and his Imuran dose was increased to 225 mg once daily; prednisone was decreased to 25 mg every other day. Dosages previously had included prednisone 30 mg every other day and Imuran 200 mg once daily.

Review of systems: As per HPI above. He denies recent fevers, chills, headache, head injury, vertigo, dizziness, vision changes, hearing loss, chest pain, shortness of breath, nausea, vomiting, diarrhea, constipation, dysuria, rashes, mood changes, recent illnesses, or sick contacts. Review of 11 different systems is otherwise negative.

Past medical history: Postherpetic neuralgia after an episode of zoster 3 years ago, still with significant residual pain that waxes and wanes. He is status post resection of Dukes C2 colon cancer, reportedly with no recurrence seen on recent colonoscopy and PET scan. Also, hypertension, hyperlipidemia, status post bilateral knee surgery, history of benign prostatic hypertrophy, and mild arthritis in his knees.

Medications: Prednisone 25 mg every other day, Imuran 225 mg once daily, pravastatin 20 mg once daily, Flomax 0.4 mg once daily, Neurontin 300 mg twice daily, glipizide 2.5 mg once daily, Flonase 1 to 4 puffs once daily, Boniva 150 mg once monthly, Claritin PRN, Ultram 50 mg PRN shingles pain, Lomotil PRN, Imodium PRN, econazole nitrate cream 3 times/week to toenails, valium 5 mg PRN, Motrin PRN, and Centrum Multivitamin once daily.

Allergies: Penicillin caused swelling of the bottoms of his feet and his hands. No trouble breathing. He also has seasonal allergies ("hay fever").

Social history: Lives with his wife. Retired 2 years ago. Still works part time, 1 day a week. Has a daughter who visits frequently. Quit smoking 30 years ago. Had smoked one pack per day for 20 years. Currently does not drink any alcohol. Previously was a heavy drinker. No illicits or other drugs.

Family history: His mother died from complications of Alzheimer's disease and had diabetes. His father died from complications of lung cancer (he was a smoker). He had a brother who had a stroke and cardiovascular disease. His son died at the age of 28 from hypertrophic cardiomyopathy. His daughter is 32 years old and healthy.

PHYSICAL EXAMINATION:

Vitals: Temp 35.7, pulse 103, BP 165/90, resp 16, and SaO_2 95% on room air.

General: Well-developed, well-nourished gentleman in no acute distress.

HEENT: Normocephalic and atraumatic. Sclera anicteric. Mucous membranes moist. Oropharynx clear.

Neck: Supple, no masses. No nodes. No carotid bruits appreciated.

Chest: Clear to auscultation bilaterally.

Heart: Regular rate and rhythm. No murmurs appreciated.

Abdomen: Soft, nontender, nondistended. Normal bowel sounds. No organomegaly.

Extremities: Warm. No edema.

Neuro: Alert and oriented ×3. Language and comprehension intact, including naming and repetition. No dysarthria. Normal attention span. Appropriate fund of knowledge. Pupils are equal, round, and reactive to light, constricting from 3 mm to 2 mm bilaterally. Extraocular movements are full. Pursuits are smooth, with no nystagmus. Saccades are normal. Visual fields are full to confrontation. Facial sensation is intact and normal in VI, V2, and V3. Face is symmetric, with symmetric smile. Tongue is midline, with no atrophy or fasciculations. Hearing is grossly intact to finger rub bilaterally. Palate rises symmetrically. Shoulder shrug is strong bilaterally.

Motor examination reveals normal tone. Atrophy of the intrinsic hand muscles is noted bilaterally, most noticeable in the first dorsal interossei. Flexion deformities of the fourth and fifth digits are apparent bilaterally. He has bilateral hammertoes, worse on the left. Strength testing reveals weakness in bilateral finger abduction (4/5) and extension of the 4th and 5th digits (2/5). In the lower extremities, he is weak in ankle dorsiflexion bilaterally (4/5), worse on the right than the left. Per the patient, this is a change (i.e., he is usually weaker on the left). Plantar flexion and inversion are strong (5/5). Ankle eversion is slightly weak bilaterally (5/5). Great toe dorsiflexion is 3/5 bilaterally. The rest of his strength examination is within normal limits. No pronator drift is observed. Upper extremity orbit testing is normal. Reflexes are absent at all sites and toes are mute. Vibration is absent at the great toes bilaterally, almost absent at the ankles, and normal at the knees. Vibration is also decreased at the fingers

144

bilaterally. Temperature is decreased on both lower extremities to the mid calf, as is light touch. No dysmetria is noted on finger-nose-finger testing. Rapid alternating movements are normal. Gait was not tested.

Discharge Summary

DIAGNOSES/PROBLEMS:

1. Chronic immune demyelinating polyneuropathy (CIDP).
2. Postherpetic neuralgia after an episode of zoster in 2004, still with significant residual pain that waxes and wanes.
3. Status post resection of Dukes C2 colon cancer; no recurrence seen on recent colonoscopy and PET scan.
4. Hypertension.
5. Hyperlipidemia.
6. Status post bilateral knee surgery.
7. Benign prostatic hypertrophy.
8. Mild arthritis in his knees.

PROCEDURES:

1. Pheresis catheter placement
2. Plasmapheresis

HISTORY, MAJOR FINDINGS, AND HOSPITAL COURSE:

The patient is a very pleasant 67-year-old gentleman who has had severe CIDP for the past 5 to 6 years, which has generally shown gradual improvement despite a few exacerbations. His recent EMG/NCS suggested active disease, and he previously had a very good response to plasmapheresis. He therefore is being admitted for initiation of a course of five plasmapheresis treatments. Please see the Admission H&P for full details of his history and current presentation.

Neuro examination on admission showed him to be alert and oriented ×3, with intact language and comprehension. Cranial nerve examination is entirely normal. Findings are significant for atrophy of the intrinsic hand muscles bilaterally, most noticeably in the first dorsal interossei. Flexion deformities of the fourth and fifth digits are noted bilaterally. He has bilateral hammertoes, worse on the left. Strength testing reveals weakness in bilateral finger abduction (4/5) and extension of the fourth and fifth digits (2/5). In the lower extremities, he is weak in ankle dorsiflexion bilaterally (4/5), worse on the right than the left. Per the patient, this is a change (i.e., he is usually weaker on the left). Plantar flexion and inversion are strong (5/5). Ankle eversion is slightly weak bilaterally (5/5). Great toe dorsiflexion is 3/5 bilaterally. The rest of his strength examination is within normal limits. No pronator drift is noted. Upper extremity orbit testing is normal. Reflexes are absent at all sites and toes are mute. Vibration is absent at the great toes bilaterally, almost absent at the ankles, and normal at the knees. Vibration is also decreased at the fingers bilaterally. Temperature is decreased in both lower extremities to the mid calf, as is light touch. No dysmetria is seen on finger-nose-finger testing. Rapid alternating movements are normal. Gait was not tested.

Hospital course: The patient was admitted to Neurology Service. During the first course of plasmapheresis, he had some mild nausea and vomiting. He was given Anzemet; this resolved and did not recur. He received his first two courses of plasmapheresis as an inpatient, then was discharged to receive the remaining three treatments as an outpatient. He experienced no adverse effects and no complications during this hospitalization.

Discharge medications: Patient was instructed to resume all home medications: Atacand (unknown home dose; given 16 mg once daily while hospitalized), prednisone 25 mg every other day, Imuran 225 mg once daily, pravastatin 20 mg once daily, Flomax 0.4 mg once daily, Neurontin 300 mg twice daily, glipizide 2.5 mg once daily, Flonase

145

1 to 4 puffs once daily, Boniva 150 mg once monthly, Claritin PRN, Ultram 50 mg PRN shingles pain, Lomotil PRN, Imodium PRN, econazole nitrate cream 3 times/week to toenails, valium 5 mg PRN, Motrin PRN, and Centrum multivitamin once daily.

DISCHARGE INSTRUCTIONS:

Discharge to home, resume normal activity. Patient given pheresis catheter flushing instructions.

FOLLOW-UP CARE:

Follow up with Neurology as an outpatient. Follow up in pheresis center for remaining three treatments, then will have catheter removed.

Procedure Note

Following administration of IV sedation, a pheresis catheter was placed with the tip in the cavoatrial junction. It is okay for use. Flush per protocol.

DAY 1

The patient's lower extremity weakness has worsened lately, and he was admitted for plasmapheresis. The catheter was placed today and pheresis will start tomorrow.

DAY 2

Patient with CIDP for plasmapheresis. Line placed yesterday. First pheresis session this morning. BP was high overnight. Patient forgot to mention that he takes Atacand (will start this morning). Other vitals are stable.

Pulmonary: No issues.

Renal: No issues.

GI: No issues.

Plan: Will receive a second pheresis session as an inpatient, then will discharge home to receive remaining three sessions as an outpatient.

DAY 3

Patient has an episode of nausea and vomiting ×2 during the plasmapheresis session. The procedure was paused and symptoms relieved. Postprocedure nausea is now resolved. BP 124/80 with pulse of 76.

DAY 4

Patient has undergone second procedure for his CIDP. He feels good and is going to be discharged today. His vitals are stable. His BP is well controlled. No issues. He will return for remaining sessions as an outpatient.

CASE STUDY QUESTION

14-3a.   Admit diagnosis: _____

14-3b.   Discharge disposition: _____

14-3c.   Principal diagnosis: _____

14-3d. Secondary diagnoses (indicate POA status for secondary diagnoses):

_____

_____

_____

_____

_____

_____

14-3e. Principal procedure: _____

14-3f. Secondary procedures: _____

_____

14-3g. Assign MS-DRG: _____

14-3h. Relative weight of MS-DRG: _____

14-3i. Can this MS-DRG be optimized with the addition of a CC? Yes or No
        Can this MS-DRG be optimized with the addition of an MCC? Yes or No

14-3j. Is there a main guideline pertinent to selection of the principal diagnosis in this case study?

_____

_____

14-3k. Is there another diagnosis that meets the definition for principal diagnosis? Yes or No

14-3l. If yes, what is the other diagnosis? _____

14-3m. Is there any opportunity for physician query?

_____

_____

14-3n. What is the drug Neurontin used to treat? _____

15 Diseases of the Circulatory System (ICD-10-CM Chapter 9, Codes I00-I99)

ABBREVIATIONS/ACRONYMS

Without the use of reference materials, define the following abbreviations or acronyms.

1. CHF _____

2. AF _____

3. MI _____

4. PTCA _____

5. CABG _____

6. CAD _____

7. MVR _____

8. TPA _____

9. RHD _____

10. PPH _____

GLOSSARY DEFINITIONS

Match the glossary term to the correct definition.

1. _____ Regurgitation of heart valve

2. _____ Atherosclerosis

3. _____ Capillaries

4. _____ Blood pressure

5. _____ Stenosis

6. _____ Insidious

7. _____ Aphasia

8. _____ Cognitive defect

9. _____ Interventionalist

10. _____ Thoracentesis

11. _____ Conduction disorder

12. _____ Insufficiency of a heart valve

A. Incomplete closure of a heart valve causing a leaky valve

B. Abnormal narrowing

C. Force that blood puts on the arterial walls when the heart beats

D. Backward flowing of blood between the heart chambers

E. Process of draining fluid from the chest cavity; also known as pleurocentesis

F. Disorder in thinking, learning, awareness, and/or judgment

G. Impairment in speech expression and/or word understanding

H. Physician trained in disease treatment via the use of catheter-based technique

I. Abnormalities of cardiac impulses

J. Type of arteriosclerosis where fatty substances such as plaque block or clog the arteries

K. Smallest blood vessel in which material passes to and from the bloodstream

L. Harmful

149

CODING

Using the code book, code the following.

1. Hypertension secondary to renal artery occlusion   _____
2. Ischemic cardiomyopathy   _____
3. Acute pulmonary edema with CHF   _____
4. Dressler's syndrome   _____
5. NSTEMI   _____
6. USA   _____
7. Gonococcal endocarditis   _____
8. Hypertensive cardiovascular disease with CHF   _____
9. Paroxysmal VT   _____
10. Mobitz type II heart block   _____
11. Atrial fibrillation and flutter   _____
12. Mitral and aortic insufficiency   _____
13. HTN and chronic renal insufficiency   _____
14. CVA   _____
15. Old CVA with residual hemiparesis of the left side   _____

CASE SCENARIOS

Using the code book, code the following cases.

1. Patient is admitted with chest pain and rules in for an anterolateral MI. There is a family history of CAD.

    _____

    _____

2. Patient is admitted with syncope. After tests are performed, it is determined that the patient has bradycardia due to first degree AV block. The patient has a pacemaker inserted. Generator is inserted into the chest with leads inserted into right atrium and right ventricle.

    _____

    _____

3. Patient is admitted in ARF. The patient has a history of HTN, CRI, and DM. The patient is treated with multiple sessions of dialysis because the CRI has progressed to end-stage renal disease.

    _____

    _____

4. Patient comes into the ER after fainting at work. The physician determines that the fainting was caused by elevated blood pressure due to extreme stress.

    _____

    _____

5. Patient is admitted with CHF and known hypertensive heart disease.

_____

_____

6. A patient is found down in the street. Upon admittance to the hospital, the patient is determined to be intoxicated and suffers from alcohol dependence. An MI is suspected. CPK and serial troponins are performed, as well as an EKG, and an inferoposterior wall MI is confirmed. Patient is taken to the cath lab for a left heart cath, ventriculography, and angiography, using one catheter and high osmolar contrast.

_____

_____

7. Patient is transferred from hospital A where the subendocardial MI was identified and the cardiac cath performed to hospital B for a CABG. CABG is performed for underlying CAD by a left greater saphenous vein to LAD on the day of admit. The patient subsequently develops CHF. After 5 days in the hospital, the patient is discharged home.

_____

_____

8. Patient presents to the hospital with pulmonary edema and CHF, is admitted, and given IV Lasix.

_____

_____

9. Patient presents to the ER with left-sided weakness and trouble speaking. After completion of the MRI, it is determined that the patient has had an ischemic stroke. The speech problem is resolved before discharge, but the patient has residual left-sided weakness.

_____

_____

10. Patient with extreme stomach pain presents to the ER. Patient is discharged with a diagnosis of ruptured abdominal aortic aneurysm that is repaired by clipping during this admit.

_____

_____

11. The patient is a 10-year-old female who was admitted to rule out appendicitis. The patient presented with fever, abdominal pain, nausea, and diarrhea. CT scan showed no evidence of appendicitis. The patient was observed overnight and felt fine the next day and was able to tolerate lunch. The patient was discharged with instructions to return if any more symptoms occur.

Final Diagnosis: Mesenteric lymphadenitis.

_____

_____

Chapter **15** **Diseases of the Circulatory System**

Using the code book, code and answer questions about the following case studies.

15-1. CASE STUDY

History and Physical

CC: Intractable chest pain.

HPI: The patient is a very pleasant 80-year-old man who was admitted because of intractable chest pain in the setting of a new ischemic EKG finding and a positive troponin of 28. While in the Emergency Room, he was given sublingual nitroglycerin and experienced partial relief of chest burning. EKGs at the time of admission were significant for ST depressions in the precordial leads and ST elevations in the inferior leads (leads III and aVF). Initial cardiac enzymes measurements were significant for initial troponin of 1.71. The patient was admitted to the cardiac intensive care unit.

Past medical/surgical history: Previous MI 20 years ago, PVD with right carotid endarterectomy, COPD with chronic bronchitis, gout, BPH, hypertension, hearing impairment, CAD with stent in circumflex coronary artery.

Social history: Widower. Retired. No alcohol or tobacco use. Family in the area.

Family history: No significant family history.

Allergies: NKDA.

Review of systems:

Constitutional: No fever or chills. Appetite is good. No change in weight.

Neuro: No headaches, seizures, or syncope.

HEENT: No vision changes. Hearing impairment and has hearing aids.

CV: Per HPI.

Respiratory: Mild SOB. No hemoptysis. Chronic bronchitis.

GI: No abdominal pain, dysphagia, or heartburn.

GU: Nocturia ×2.

Skin/Skeletal: Benign.

PHYSICAL EXAMINATION:

Vitals: Afebrile. HR 120, BP 109/62, RR 20.

General: In obvious distress from chest pain.

HEENT: PERRL, EOMI. Trachea is central. Neck is supple without masses.

Chest: Bibasilar crackles.

CV: RRR.

Abd: Bowel sounds present. No suprapubic tenderness.

Ext: WNL.

GU/Rectal: Deferred.

Skin/Musculoskeletal: Benign.

Neuro: A&O ×3.

ASSESSMENT/PLAN:

Patient is admitted to CCU to rule out MI.

Discharge Summary

DIAGNOSES/PROBLEMS:

1. Coronary artery disease.
2. Previous myocardial infarction 20 years ago.
3. Peripheral vascular disease, status post right carotid endarterectomy.
4. Chronic obstructive pulmonary disease/chronic bronchitis.
5. Gout.
6. Benign prostatic hypertrophy.
7. Hearing impairment, requiring hearing aids.
8. Nonsystolic heart failure.
9. Hypertension.
10. Stent in circumflex coronary artery.

PROCEDURES:

Transthoracic echo.

HISTORY, MAJOR FINDINGS, AND HOSPITAL COURSE:

Brief history: The patient is a very pleasant 80-year-old man with the above-stated medical history who was admitted because of intractable chest pain in the setting of a new ischemic EKG finding and a positive troponin of 28. While in the Emergency Room, he was given sublingual nitroglycerin and experienced partial relief of chest burning. EKGs at the time of admission were significant for ST depression in the precordial leads and ST elevation in the inferior leads (leads III and aVF). Initial cardiac enzyme measurements were significant for initial troponin of 1.71. At this point, the patient was admitted to the cardiac intensive care unit. Chest pain was completely resolved with aspirin, Plavix, heparin, and a nitroglycerin drip.

In addition, when antiplatelet agents were initiated, the patient developed frank hematuria through his Foley catheter. He was started on continuous bladder irrigation and ultimately was followed in the cardiac intensive care unit.

The CCU course was significant for a peak troponin of 48.43. In addition, a lipid profile revealed total cholesterol of 99, along with triglycerides of 108, HDL of 45, and LDL of 32. The patient was treated appropriately with aspirin, high-dose statin, ACE inhibitor, and intravenous heparin, as well as a glycoprotein IIb/IIIa inhibitor, for approximately 18 hours. The initial 24-hour CCU course was significant for sinus bradycardia alternating with junctional bradycardia; discontinuation of beta blockers was required, as was close observation for possible transvenous pacemaker placement. However, intrinsic heart rate improved such that no device was necessary.

In addition, hematuria continued such that urology consult was called and continuous bladder irrigation was continued. This hematuria was interpreted by the urologic consultant as secondary to traumatic Foley catheter placement. Close monitoring revealed a stable hematocrit that required no transfusions of packed red blood cells.

In addition, hospital course was complicated by minor congestive heart failure exacerbation, which required the use of intravenous diuresis; this was tolerated very well. The patient's laboratory data were significant for marked hyponatremia with sodium in the 120s. Workup for this hyponatremia included CAT scan of the chest and the head, which was unremarkable for any thoracic masses or lung masses and provided no evidence of intracranial disease that could explain the possible diagnosis of syndrome of inappropriate ADH secretion. Urine sodium was found to be 13 with urine osmoles of 362, serum osmoles of 280, and serum sodium of 130.

153

The patient had a transthoracic echo that revealed an estimated left ventricular ejection fraction of 45% to 50% with inferior wall akinesis. Posterior wall akinesis was also noted, as was severe lateral wall hypokinesis. The septum was noted to be mildly hypertrophied and measured 1.6 cm. No evidence of intracavitary obstruction was found. The patient's CCU course was significant for the development of atrial fibrillation that required recontinuation of Coumadin prior to discharge.

Condition at discharge: Stable.

Adverse drug allergies: None.

Allergies: No known drug allergies.

Complications of procedure: None.

DISCHARGE MEDICATIONS:

Aspirin 325 mg by mouth daily
Atorvastatin 80 mg by mouth at bedtime
Clopidogrel 75 mg by mouth daily
Doxazosin 2 mg by mouth at bedtime
Nitroglycerin sublingual 0.4 mg every 5 minutes whenever necessary ×3 for chest pain
Senna 1 tablet by mouth daily
Toprol XL 100 mg by mouth daily
Gemfibrozil 600 mg by mouth daily
Coumadin 5 mg by mouth daily

DISCHARGE INSTRUCTIONS:

Diet: The patient was seen by Nutrition, who gave explicit advice and instructions regarding a cardiac-friendly diet that is low fat, low cholesterol, and low sodium.

Activity: As tolerated.

FOLLOW-UP CARE:

The patient was given a follow-up appointment with Cardiology.

Electrocardiogram Report

Indication for study: N/A.

Ventricular rate:	45 bpm
Atrial rate:	45 bpm
PR interval:	142 ms
QRS duration:	113 ms
QT interval:	496 ms
QTc interval:	429 ms
P axis:	−49 degrees
R axis:	89 degrees
T axis:	111 degrees

JUNCTIONAL BRADYCARDIA.
LATERAL INFARCT, AGE UNDETERMINED.
INFERIOR-POSTERIOR INFARCT, POSSIBLY ACUTE.
ACUTE MI.
ABNORMAL EKG.

Transthoracic Echocardiogram

Indication for study: Acute MI, anterior wall.

Interpretation summary: A two-dimensional transthoracic echocardiogram was performed. The study was technically limited. Limited views were obtained. The study
154

was viewed and interpreted by the undersigned attending with the resident/fellow. Limited study for LVF. Left ventricular systolic function is mildly reduced. Estimated LVEF is 45% to 50%. Inferior wall akinesis is present, as are posterior wall akinesis and severe lateral wall hypokinesis. Transmitral Doppler pattern cannot be evaluated because of absence of atrial contraction. The septum is moderately hypertrophied, measuring 1.6 cm. No evidence of intracavitary obstruction is apparent.

Heart rate: 84 bpm.

Left ventricle: The left ventricle is normal in size. There is no thrombus. The septum is moderately hypertrophied, measuring 1.6 cm. No evidence of intracavitary obstruction is found. Estimated LVEF is 45% to 50%. Unable to evaluate transmitral Doppler pattern because of absence of atrial contraction. Left ventricular systolic function is mildly reduced. Posterior wall akinesis is present, as are severe lateral wall hypokinesis and inferior wall akinesis.

Right ventricle: The right ventricle is normal in size and function.

Atria: Left atrial size is normal. Right atrial size is normal.

Mitral valve: The mitral valve is normal. No mitral valve stenosis is evident.

Tricuspid valve: The tricuspid valve is normal. No tricuspid stenosis is noted. Trace tricuspid regurgitation is apparent. Unable to estimate RVS.

Aortic valve: Mild focal aortic valve calcification is seen. The aortic valve is trileaflet, and the aortic valve opens well. No valvular aortic stenosis.

Pulmonic valve: Pulmonic valve leaflets are thin and pliable; valve motion is normal. No pulmonic valvular stenosis is noted.

Pericardium/Pleura: Trace pericardial effusion. No pleural effusion.

M-mode 2D measurements and calculations:
IVSD: 1.6 cm
LVEDD: 5.2 cm
Lids: 4.2 cm
LVP WD: 0.93 cm

Chest AP Portable

Reason for examination: Dyspnea.

Comparison: None.

Discussion: Cardiac silhouette is enlarged. Perihilar opacities and increased interstitial markings within both lungs likely related to pulmonary edema. Portions of both lung bases are not included on today's study. Apical pleural thickening is noted. Defibrillator pad overlies the left hemithorax.

Thoracic CT

Reason for examination: Chest pain and mediastinal fullness.

Technique: The study was done without intravenous contrast.

Findings: Dilated aorta with aortic arch measuring 4.4 cm in diameter. Borderline pulmonary hypertension with main pulmonary artery measuring 36 mm and right pulmonary artery measuring 32 mm. Mild congestive changes with small bilateral effusions. No evidence of pulmonary neoplasm. No evidence of pleural abnormality. No evidence of pneumonia.

Impression: Widened mediastinum due to arteriosclerosis of the aorta.

Addendum: The patient also has calcification of coronary arteries with stent in circumflex coronary artery.

Impression: No evidence of a neoplasm. Arteriosclerosis.

DAY 1

Patient was admitted because of intractable chest pain and new ischemic EKG changes. Patient has been ruled in for an NSTEMI. Evidence of hematuria is present in Foley. This is likely due to traumatic Foley placement. Irrigate Foley. Check lipid panel and order echo.

DAY 2

Patient no longer has chest pain. Chest x-ray shows pulmonary edema that is likely due to mild exacerbation of his congestive heart failure. Will diurese. Also noted per labs is low sodium at 127. Continue medical management of NSTEMI.

DAY 3

Overnight, patient went into atrial fib. No chest pain. COPD is stable. Echo results are in the chart. Discontinue Foley. Begin Coumadin.

DAY 4

Patient admitted with NSTEMI. No complaints. Tolerating regular diet. Chest with a few bibasilar crackles. Hyponatremia is improved, likely secondary to CHF. No evidence of SIADH. Patient is ready for discharge home with his family.

CASE STUDY QUESTIONS

15-1a.   Admit diagnosis: _____

15-1b.   Discharge disposition: _____

15-1c.   Principal diagnosis _____

15-1d.   Secondary diagnoses (indicate POA status for secondary diagnoses):

_____

_____

_____

_____

_____

15-1e.   Principal procedure: _____

15-1f.   Secondary procedures: _____

_____

15-1g.   Assign MS-DRG: _____

15-1h. Relative weight of MS-DRG: _____

15-1i. Can this MS-DRG be optimized with the addition of a CC? Yes or No
        Can this MS-DRG be optimized with the addition of an MCC? Yes or No

15-1j. Is there a main guideline pertinent to selection of the principal diagnosis in this case study?

_____

_____

15-1k. Is there another diagnosis that meets the definition for principal diagnosis? Yes or No

15-1l. If yes, what is the other diagnosis? _____

15-1m. Is there any opportunity for physician query?

_____

_____

15-1n. What is the drug nitroglycerin used to treat? _____

15-2. CASE STUDY

History and Physical

CC: Atrial fib.

HPI: The patient is a 55-year-old male with symptomatic atrial fibrillation for at least the past 5 years. Patient can tell when he is in AF. He gets SOB and feels his heart pounding. This has limited his exercise tolerance. In total, he has undergone seven cardioversions. He has been in permanent atrial fibrillation for the past 6 months. However, when seen in clinic about a month ago, he was started on sotalol at 160 mg 2 times a day and underwent cardioversion that resulted in maintenance of sinus rhythm until the date of the procedure. The patient is therefore now referred for pulmonary vein isolation.

Past medical history: Atrial fibrillation, hypercholesterolemia, and ruptured disc with transient spinal injury.

Past surgical history: Discectomy.

Social history: No tobacco and rare alcohol use.

Family history: No family history of cardiac arrhythmias.

Allergies: NKDA.

Medications:
Lipitor 10 mg a day
Sotalol 160 mg 2 times a day
Coumadin dosed by INR results

REVIEW OF SYSTEMS:

Constitutional: No signs or symptoms of systemic infection. No fever or chills.

Neuro: Occasional headache. No weakness or numbness.

HEENT: No changes in vision.

CV: See HPI. No symptoms suggestive of CHF. No chest pain.

Respiratory: See HPI. No cough or hemoptysis.

GI: No abdominal pain, dysphagia, or N/V.

GU: No dysuria. Nocturia ×1.

Skin/Skeletal: No rashes or joint pain.

PHYSICAL EXAMINATION:

Vitals: Afebrile. HR 72, BP 108/74, RR 12.

General: NAD.

HEENT: Normocephalic, atraumatic, sclera anicteric, and MMM. Neck is supple with no masses.

Chest: CTA.

CV: RRR.

Abd: Obese. Soft, nontender, positive bowel sounds.

Ext: No cyanosis, clubbing, or edema.

GU/Rectal: Deferred.

Skin/Musculoskeletal: Benign.

Neuro: Alert and oriented ×3. Cranial nerves intact. Normal gait.

CT chest: Clear.

ASSESSMENT/PLAN:

Patient was admitted with symptomatic atrial fibrillation that has required multiple ablations. Patient will undergo pulmonary vein isolation.

PROCEDURES PERFORMED:

1. Anesthesia.
2. Vascular access.
3. Electrophysiology study.
4. Transseptal catheterization.
5. Transseptal catheterization.
6. Endomyocardial mapping: Ablation.

Arrival condition: Stable.

Case priority: Elective.

BSA: 2.3600.

Estimated blood loss (cc): 20.

Height (in/cm): 72.0/182.9.

Weight (lb/kg): 255.0/116.0

Fluoro time (min): 90.2.

Intravenous fluid volume (cc): 2000.

PAST MEDICAL HISTORY:

The patient is a 55-year-old man with a history of persistent atrial fibrillation for the past 5 years. He has undergone seven cardioversions in total and has been maintained on sotalol 160 mg twice daily. When in atrial fibrillation, he is symptomatic with palpitations and fatigue. He is now referred for pulmonary vein isolation.

158

PROCEDURE DESCRIPTION:

After informed consent was obtained and the usual sterile prep and drape was performed, the right femoral site was locally anesthetized, and three venous sheaths (8 Fr × 2, 11.5 Fr × 1, middle) and one arterial vascular sheath (4 Fr) were inserted via modified Seldinger technique.

With routine hemodynamic and electrocardiographic monitoring, electrophysiology catheters were advanced under fluoroscopic guidance to the HIS bundle and coronary sinus. Intracardiac electrocardiograms and conduction were measured at rest and after ablation.

A guidewire and a transseptal sheath were advanced to the superior vena cava under fluoroscopic guidance. The guidewire was withdrawn, the sheath was vigorously flushed, and the needle assembly was advanced to the end of the sheath. Under fluoroscopic guidance, the sheath was withdrawn until its tip engaged the fossa ovalis of the interatrial septum. The fossa ovalis was crossed with the needle. Localization within the left atrium was confirmed. The needle and sheath assembly then was advanced as a unit a short distance into the left atrium, and the needle was withdrawn. This procedure was repeated for the second transseptal puncture.

Pulmonary venous angiograms were then obtained for each of the four pulmonary veins. An endocardial map of the left atrium was created and was superimposed upon the preexisting CT image of the chamber.

With routine hemodynamic and electrocardiographic monitoring, an ablative thermocouple was advanced under fluoroscopic guidance to the left atrium. Circumferential radiofrequency lesions were applied around the pulmonary veins until complete isolation was achieved. A lasso catheter was used to confirm and guide complete isolation of all four pulmonary veins by identifying sites of earliest activation within the ostia.

After a waiting period of 1 hour, repeat lasso mapping was performed. The catheters were then withdrawn to the right atrium and were removed from the body. Systemic anticoagulation with heparin was maintained during the transseptal portion of the case. The attending physician performed the procedure and interpreted the results.

IMPRESSION:

1. Baseline: Sinus rhythm with normal HV conduction.
2. Two transseptal punctures were performed without complication.
3. Pulmonary venous angiograms were obtained for each of the four pulmonary veins.
4. A 3D left atrial map was created.
5. Circumferential linear ablation lesions were made around the left- and right-sided pulmonary veins with the use of a 4-mm tipped irrigated ablation catheter.
6. Lasso mapping after creation of circumferential lesions revealed remaining potentials in all pulmonary veins.
7. Continued ablation along circumferential lesions resulted in isolation of all pulmonary veins.
8. After a 30-minute waiting period, lasso mapping revealed recovery of pulmonary vein potentials in the left inferior pulmonary vein. Continued ablation led to reisolation of all four veins.
9. The catheters were then pulled to the right atrium and were removed from the body.
10. Final: Sinus rhythm with preserved HV conduction.

Summary: Successful atrial fibrillation ablation with electrical isolation of all four pulmonary veins.

RECOMMENDATIONS:

1. Heparin with bolus per 30/12 (U/kg) dose protocol started 4 hours after the sheath pull.
2. Starting 4 hours after sheath pull, please remove 10 cc of air per 2 hours from the pressure balloon. The adhesive may be removed after 16 total hours.
3. Restart Coumadin tonight at usual outpatient dose. On the morning of discharge and 4 hours after discontinuation of heparin, please start Lovenox at 0.6 mg/kg SC twice daily until INR >2.0 has been reached.
4. Continue sotalol at 160 mg twice daily.
5. Restart all other medications.
6. Avoid vigorous activity ×48 hours.
7. Please set up a follow-up INR check 2 to 3 days post discharge with the patient's primary care physician or cardiologist.
8. Follow up in 3 months with Cardiology.
9. We anticipate early recurrences of atrial fibrillation during the healing phase following ablation. This healing phase may last 3 months. The efficacy of the procedure will be assessed beginning 3 months post ablation.
10. Given the potential for asymptomatic episodes of atrial fibrillation post ablation, we recommend 24-hr Holter monitoring of all patients, regardless of symptoms, every 3 months (i.e., at 6, 9, and 12 months) during the first year and every 6 months thereafter. Please arrange this monitoring with your primary cardiologist.

Complications: No immediate complications were evident.

Procedure Data

CASE MEDICATIONS:

General anesthesia
Heparin 22,000 U IV
Protamine 30 mg IV
Contrast: Visipaque 40.0 cc, vascular

VITAL SIGNS:

	Pre-case	Post-case
Pulse, beats/min	58	63
SBP (auto cuff), mm Hg	106	122
DBP (auto cuff), mm Hg	68	69
Respiration rate	16	16
Arterial O_2 Sat, %	100	100

EPS/ABLATION METHODS:

Mapping method: 3D

LA recording/stimuli: Yes, transseptal puncture

ANESTHESIA:

Anesthesia detail: Observation

Indication for anesthesia: Patient preference

Anesthesia type: General inhalation

Airway control: Endotracheal intubation

VASCULAR ACCESS:

Vessel: Vein, femoral

Access type: Percutaneous puncture

Sheath count: 3

Vessel side: Right

Sheath size: 8.0

Vascular closure: Manual compression

GUIDANCE METHODS, NEEDLES, AND WIRES:

Guidance method: Palpation successful

Needle type: 5 Fr micropuncture, attempted 3 times: successful

Wire type: 0.035 J: successful

Vascular access:

Vessel: Art, femoral

Access type: Percutaneous puncture

Sheath count: 1

Vessel side: Right

Sheath size: 4.0

Vascular closure: Manual compression

GUIDANCE METHODS, NEEDLES, AND WIRES:

Guidance method: Palpation successful

Needle type: 5 Fr micropuncture attempted 1 time: successful

Wire type: 0.035 J: successful

ELECTROPHYSIOLOGIC STUDY:

Indications:

Primary indication: Atrial fibrillation

Native conduction:

State	Obs #1	Obs #2
	Baseline	Post ablation
Systolic BP, mm Hg	110	122
Diastolic BP, mm Hg	75	65
Native CL ms	1235	1000
Rhythm	Sinus	Sinus
PR interval, ms	160	180
AH interval, ms	100	
HV interval (His bundle study), ms	33	
QRS duration, ms	73	75
QRS morphology	Normal	Normal
QT interval, ms	530	470

TRANSSEPTAL CATHETERIZATION:

Method: Observation

Needle type: Brockenbrough

Sheath type: SR 0

Sheath size: French 8

Number of puncture attempts: 1

Left atrial oxygen saturation: 100.0

Contrast injected in LA? Yes

Catheter placement successful? Yes

LA Hemodynamics:

Observation:

Hemodynamic state: Baseline

Left atrial mean pressure, mm Hg: 10

Transseptal Catheterization:

Method: Observation

Needle type: Brockenbrough

Sheath type: SR 0

Sheath size: French 8

Number of puncture attempts: 1

Contrast injected in LA? Yes

Catheter placement successful? Yes

LA Hemodynamics:

Observation:

Hemodynamic state: Baseline

Left atrial mean pressure, mm Hg: 10

Pulmonary Angiograms

Pulmonary venous angiograms were performed to establish the fluoroscopic location of the venous ostia. Two left-sided and two right-sided pulmonary veins were localized.

Endomyocardial Mapping (Biosense):

An endocardial map of the left atrium was created with electroanatomic mapping system and was superimposed upon a preacquired CT image of the chamber.

Ablation:

Indications:
Primary indication: Atrial fibrillation.
Ablation: Observation.
Ablation type: Atrial fibrillation (linear).
Ablation history: Initial attempt.
Ablation approach: Transseptal.
Special guidance methods: 3-dimensional mapping.
RF mode: Standard.
Target temperature, C: 60.
Number of energy applications: 90.
Number of sites: 30.
Total ablation duration mm, ss: 79:53.
Ablation successful? Yes.
Resulting rhythm: Sinus.
Resulting AV conduction: Normal.
QRS morphology: Normal.

DIAGNOSES/PROBLEMS:

1. Atrial fibrillation.
2. Hypercholesterolemia.
3. History of ruptured disc with transient spinal injury. S/P discectomy.

PROCEDURES:

1. Pulmonary vein isolation, transesophageal echocardiography.
2. Computer tomography of the chest.

HISTORY, MAJOR FINDINGS, AND HOSPITAL COURSE:

The patient is a 55-year-old man with history of atrial fibrillation for the past 5 years requiring multiple cardioversions. In total, he has undergone seven cardioversions. He has been in permanent atrial fibrillation for the past 6 months. However, when seen in clinic about a month ago, he was started on sotalol at 160 mg 2 times a day and underwent cardioversion, resulting in maintenance of sinus rhythm until the date of the procedure. The patient is symptomatic with palpitations and fatigue during bouts of atrial fibrillation and is therefore now referred for pulmonary vein isolation.

On review of systems, he denies any signs or symptoms of systemic infection. He denies symptoms of congestive heart failure. He otherwise feels well.

Past medical history: Atrial fibrillation, hypercholesterolemia, and ruptured disc with transient spinal injury and discectomy.

Allergies: None.

Medications:
Lipitor 10 mg a day
Sotalol 160 mg 2 times a day
Coumadin dosed by INR results

Social history: Significant for lack of any smoking or alcohol use.

Family history: Significant for lack of any arrhythmia.

The patient first underwent computed tomography of the chest. The CT chest portion was thought to show normal left atrial and pulmonary vein anatomy with mildly dilated left ventricle and normal left ventricle systolic function with an EF of 62%. The thoracic portion was read by the radiologist and was thought to be unremarkable except for minimal degenerative changes in the mid and lower thoracic spine. The cardiac portion was imported into the electron atomic system for the purposes of mapping and ablation.

Physical examination: On presentation to the cardiovascular diagnostics laboratory, the patient's blood pressure was 106/62 with a heart rate of 58, respiratory rate of 16, and oxygen saturation of 100%. Jugular venous pressure was flat. Lungs were clear to auscultation bilaterally. Cardiac examination revealed regular rate and rhythm with normal S1, S2 and no murmurs or rubs. No peripheral edema.

Review of his laboratory data was significant for sodium of 141 mL/L with a creatinine of 1.1 mg/dL. Hematocrit was 44%. Platelets were 208,000/cubic millimeter. White count was 5240/cubic millimeter. INR was 0.9.

The patient then underwent transesophageal echocardiography. The final report of this procedure is pending at the time of dictation; however, the preliminary report indicated no left atrial thrombus.

The patient was brought to the electrophysiology laboratory after informed consent was obtained. The baseline rhythm was sinus with normal HV conduction. Two transseptal punctures were performed without complications. Pulmonary venous angiograms were obtained for each of the four pulmonary veins. A three-dimensional left atrial map was created with the electron atomic mapping system and the preacquired CT image. Circumferential linear ablation lesions were made around the left and right sides of the pulmonary veins with a 4-mm tip to irrigate the ablation catheter. Laser mapping after creation of circumferential lesions revealed the remaining potentials in all pulmonary veins. Continued ablation along circumferential lesions resulted in isolation of all pulmonary veins. After a 30-minute waiting period, laser mapping revealed pulmonary vein potentials in the left inferior pulmonary vein and continued ablation via isolation of all four veins. The catheters were then pulled to the right atrium and were removed from the body. The final rhythm was sinus with preserved HV conduction.

In summary, the patient underwent successful atrial fibrillation ablation with electrical isolation of all four pulmonary veins. He was admitted to an inpatient monitoring unit and was observed overnight. He was started on anticoagulation on the night of the procedure in the form of IV heparin and was transitioned to Lovenox as a transition to a fully therapeutic INR and Coumadin the day after the procedure. Notably, he was given a dose of Coumadin on the night of the procedure. In the morning, there was no sinus bleeding. The patient retained sinus rhythm. He was continued on sotalol 160 mg 2 times a day. He was discharged home in stable condition on the same medications as at admission, which included the following.

DISCHARGE MEDICATIONS:

Lipitor 10 mg a day
Sotalol 160 mg 2 times a day
Coumadin dosed by INR in addition to Lovenox at 0.6 mg/kg subcutaneous 2 times a day until a therapeutic INR has been reached

CT Thorax with Contrast

History: Cardiac CT of the heart and vessels for preablation procedure for atrial fibrillation.

Technique: Contrast-enhanced CT scan, limited evaluation of the chest. Heart and vessels reported separately.

Comparison: None.

Findings: The lungs are clear bilaterally. No significant mediastinal, hilar, or axillary lymphadenopathy. No evidence of pleural or pericardial effusions. The heart appears normal in size. Minimal degenerative changes mid and lower thoracic spine. No evidence of suspicious osseous lesions.

Impression: Unremarkable chest CT except for minimal degenerative changes mid and lower thoracic spine.

Progress Notes

POSTOP NOTE

Patient is S/P pulmonary vein isolation for atrial fib. He tolerated the procedure well. Begin heparin at 10 PM as long as the groin continues to look okay. Tylox prn for pain. IVF overnight. Resume Coumadin tonight. Check INR.

DAY 1

Patient feels well. Groin site looks good without hematoma. Feels slightly congested but no other symptoms. Maintaining sinus rhythm. Discharge home later today.

CASE STUDY QUESTIONS

15-2a.   Admit diagnosis: _____

15-2b.   Discharge disposition: _____

15-2c.   Principal diagnosis: _____

15-2d.   Secondary diagnoses (indicate POA status for secondary diagnoses):

_____

_____

_____

_____

_____

_____

15-2e.   Principal procedure: _____

15-2f.   Secondary procedures: _____

_____

15-2g.   Assign MS-DRG: _____

15-2h.   Relative weight of MS-DRG: _____

15-2i.   Can this MS-DRG be optimized with the addition of a CC? Yes or No
         Can this MS-DRG be optimized with the addition of an MCC? Yes or No

15-2j.   Is there a main guideline pertinent to selection of the principal diagnosis in this case study?

_____

_____

15-2k.   Is there another diagnosis that meets the definition for principal diagnosis? Yes or No

15-2l.   If yes, what is the other diagnosis? _____

15-2m.   Is there any opportunity for physician query?

_____

_____

15-2n.   What is the drug sotalol used to treat? _____

Chapter **15** **Diseases of the Circulatory System**

CC: Abnormal adenosine myocardial perfusion SPECT study.

HPI: This 80-year-old man with known coronary artery disease who is status post bypass surgery and subsequent balloon angioplasty and angioplasty with stent procedures was referred for cardiac catheterization because of recurrent chest pain. His last coronary interventional procedure about 8 years ago involved the deployment of two 3.0-mm Duet stents in the proximal right coronary artery. Recently, he developed recurrent angina. An adenosine perfusion SPECT study showed a left ventricular ejection fraction of 38% and evidence of reversible ischemia in the inferolateral and anterolateral walls. On the basis of these findings, he was referred for cardiac catheterization. He was admitted to the hospital for cardiac cath and possible intervention.

Past medical history: CAD, previous MI, dyslipidemia, GERD, gout, and hypertension. He had a stroke 3 years ago.

Past surgical history: CABG, PTCA, left total knee replacement, and left carotid endarterectomy.

Social history: History of tobacco many years ago. Social alcohol.

Family history: Positive family history for CAD.

Allergies: NKDA.

REVIEW OF SYSTEMS:

Constitutional: No fever or chills. No change in weight. Appetite is good.

Neuro: No headache, seizures, or syncope. No dizziness.

HEENT: No diplopia or hearing loss.

CV: Decreased exercise tolerance, occasional chest pain with SOB.

Respiratory: No cough or hemoptysis.

GI: Negative.

GU: Benign.

Skin/Skeletal: No rashes, pain, or joint stiffness.

PHYSICAL EXAMINATION:

Vitals: Stable.

General: NAD. Some anxiety about upcoming procedure.

HEENT: Normocephalic, atraumatic. Neck is supple with no lymphadenopathy. PERRL. EOMI.

Chest: CTA bilaterally.

CV: RRR. S1 and S2 normal.

Abd: No tenderness, guarding, or rigidity. Bowel sounds are present.

Ext: WNL.

GU/Rectal: Deferred.

Skin/Musculoskeletal: WNL.

Neuro: Alert and oriented. Cranial nerves intact. Gait is normal.

Patient was admitted for cardiac catheterization and possible PCI depending on the findings.

Final Report

CARDIOVASCULAR DIAGNOSTIC LABORATORY INVASIVE/INTERVENTIONAL CARDIOLOGY PROCEDURE REPORT:

Procedures performed:
1. Vascular access.
2. Coronary arteriography.
3. Percutaneous coronary intervention.
4. Iliofemoral arteriogram.

Pt height (in/em): 67.0/170.2.

Pt weight (lb/kg): 226.6/103.0.

Fluoro time (min): 24.4.

History: The patient is an 80-year-old man with known coronary artery disease s/p CABG (LAD and SVG to LADD). Thereafter, he underwent a balloon angioplasty procedure. Subsequently, he experienced an inferior MI. Cardiac catheterization then showed a totally occluded RCA and patent grafts. Two 3.0 ACS Duet stents were deployed in the proximal RCA. He recently developed recurrent angina. An adenosine myocardial perfusion SPECT study showed an LVEF of 38% and partially reversible defects of the inferolateral and anterolateral walls. His risk factors for CAD include remote tobacco use, dyslipidemia, and hypertension. He had a minor stroke 3 years ago and a left carotid endarterectomy.

Procedure description: After the usual sterile prep and drape, the site was locally anesthetized and vascular sheaths were inserted as described below. With use of the catheters described below, coronary angiography was performed in multiple projections. With the catheters and devices described below, percutaneous coronary intervention (PCI) with drug-eluting stent deployment in the RCA and LCX was performed with appropriate anticoagulation. The attending physician performed the procedure and interpreted the results.

Impression:

Coronary angiography: Mild coronary calcification. Right dominant circulation. Normal LM. Totally occluded proximal LAD distal to the first septal branch. The distal LAD was visualized by injection of LIMA graft. Large-caliber LCX with proximal 90% stenosis. The LCX gave origin to a medium-caliber bifurcating CXM that has a proximal 70% stenosis. Large-caliber dominant RCA with proximal 90% stenosis. Previously deployed RCA stents were patent with mild in-stent restenosis. The distal RCA gave origin to a large-caliber RPDA with mild proximal disease. The large-caliber RPLB has a proximal 70% stenosis.

Widely patent LIMA graft to the LAD. The distal LAD is a small-caliber vessel with a 60% stenosis. There is extensive retrograde perfusion to the LAD diagonal that has an ostial 90% stenosis. Totally occluded SVG to LADD. Successful proximal RCA PCI with drug-eluting stent deployment with a 3.5 × 18-mm Cypher stent converting the 90% stenosis to 0% residual.

Successful proximal LCX PCI with drug-eluting stent deployment with a 2.5 × 28-mm Cypher stent converting 90% stenosis to 0% residual.

Recommendations: Long-term ASA and Plavix × 1 year. Continued aggressive medical management. Will follow renal function post procedure.

Procedure Data

Contrast: Visipaque 270.0 cc, vascular.

Devices:

Stents:

Manufacturer	**Implanted**	**Implanted**
Manufacturer	Cordis	Cordis
Model	Cypher	Cypher
Model #	3.5 × 18	2.5 × 28
Serial #	AAAAA	BBBBB
Vessel	RCA	LCx

VASCULAR ACCESS:

Vessel art: Femoral

Access type: Percutaneous puncture

Sheath count: 1

Vessel side: Right

Sheath size: 6

Vascular closure: Angioseal device

CORONARY ARTERIOGRAPHY:

Indications: Primary indication: angina, stable.

Catheters:

	Obs #1	**Obs #2**	**Obs #3**
Vessel	LM	RCA	Other (see comment)
Catheter size	6	6	6 French
Catheter shape	JL4	JR4	JR4
Engagement	Good	Good	Good

Comment: SVG to LADD totally occluded.

	Obs #4
Vessel	LIMA
Catheter size	6 French
Catheter shape	IMA
Engagement	Good

CORONARY ANATOMY:

Dominance: Right
Territory supplied LAD system: Large
Territory supplied Cx system: Large
Territory size RCA system: Large

SUMMARY RESULTS:

Preliminary recommendation: Proceed with PCI.

PERCUTANEOUS CORONARY INTERVENTION:

Indications: Primary indication: angina, stable.

Target lesion:
Vessel type: Native coronary
Segment name: pRCA proximal RCA
Location in segment: Proximal
Percent stenosis, %: 90
Stenosis length, mm: 15

168

Reference vessel diameter, mm: 3.5
Lesion type: De novo
TIMI flow: 3
Territory distal to lesion: Large
Patent graft nearby: Stenosis of ungrafted vessel
Distal vessel graftability: Poor
Could patient withstand CAB? Poor candidate

PCI SEQUENCE:

	Obs #1	Obs #2	Obs #3
Device type	GC guide catheter	GW guidewire	BAL balloon
Description/model	Launcher JR4	Pilot 50	Voyager
Size	6 inches/French		
Intracoronary diameter, mm	2.5		
Intracoronary length, mm	9		
Successful	Yes	Yes	Yes

# 2 inflations/passes	
Maximum pressure	8 atm
Maximum duration, mm:ss	1.00

	Obs #4
Device type	DEST drug-eluting stent
Description/model	Cypher
Intracoronary diameter	3.5 mm
Intracoronary length, mm	18
Successful	Yes
#	1 inflation/pass
Maximum pressure	18 atm
Maximum duration	1.00 mm:ss

FINAL RESULT:

	Observation
Final (residual) stenosis, %	0
TIMI flow	3
Procedural antithrombotic Rx	Bivalirudin
Procedural antiplatelet Rx	Oral agents only
Procedural ACT sec	400
Final PCI result	Successful

PERCUTANEOUS INTERVENTION:

Indications: primary indication: angina, stable

Target lesion:
Vessel type: Native coronary
Segment name: pCIRC proximal circumflex
Location in segment: Proximal
Percent stenosis, %: 90
Stenosis length, mm: 20
Reference vessel diameter, mm: 2.5
Lesion type: De novo
TIMI flow: 3
Territory distal to lesion: Large
Patent graft nearby: Stenosis of ungrafted vessel
Distal vessel graftability: Poor
Could patient withstand CAB? Poor candidate

PCI sequence:

	Obs #1	Obs #2	Obs #3
Device type	GC guide catheter	GW guidewire	BAL balloon
Description/model	Launcher AL2	Pilot 50	Voyager
Size	6 inches/French		
Intracoronary diameter, mm	2.5		
Intracoronary length, mm	20		
Successful	Yes	Yes	Yes
#: 2 inflations/passes			
Maximum pressure	16 atm		
Maximum duration	1.00 mm:ss		

	Obs #4
Device type	DEST drug-eluting stent
Description/model	Cypher
Intracoronary diameter, mm	2.5
Intracoronary length, mm	28
Successful	Yes
#: 2 inflations/passes	
Maximum pressure	19 atm
Maximum duration	1.00 mm:ss

FINAL RESULT:

	Observation
Final (residual) stenosis, %	0
TIMI flow	3
Procedural antithrombotic Rx	Bivalirudin
Procedural antiplatelet Rx	Oral agents only
Procedural ACT, sec	400
Final PCI result	Successful

ILIOFEMORAL ARTERIOGRAM:

Indications: Primary indication: arterial stricture/stenosis. No right iliac disease. Angioseal deployed.

Discharge Summary

DIAGNOSES/PROBLEMS:

1. Coronary artery disease.
2. Stable angina pectoris.
3. Status post coronary artery bypass graft surgery many years ago with a left internal mammary artery graft to the left anterior descending and a saphenous vein graft to the left anterior descending diagonal coronary arteries.
4. Status post angioplasty of the right coronary artery left circumflex and right posterior descending coronary arteries.
5. Status post inferior wall myocardial infarction complicated by ventricular fibrillation.
6. Status post percutaneous transluminal coronary angioplasty with stent deployment in the right coronary artery.
7. Hypertension.
8. Hyperlipidemia.
9. Status post cerebrovascular accident.
10. Status post left carotid endarterectomy.
11. Gastroesophageal reflux disease.
12. Gout.
13. Left total knee replacement.
14. Left eye enucleation status post trauma.
15. Right eye cataract extraction.

PROCEDURES:

1. Left heart cardiac catheterization.
2. Percutaneous transluminal coronary angioplasty with drug-eluting stent deployment in the right coronary artery.
3. Percutaneous transluminal coronary angioplasty with drug-eluting stent deployment in the proximal left circumflex coronary artery.
4. Right iliac angiogram with application of an Angioseal closure device.

HISTORY, MAJOR FINDINGS, AND HOSPITAL COURSE:

Brief history: This 80-year-old man with known coronary artery disease who is status post bypass surgery and subsequent balloon angioplasty and angioplasty with stent procedures was referred for cardiac catheterization because of recurrent chest pain. His last coronary interventional procedure about 8 years ago involved the deployment of two 3.0-mm Duet stents in the proximal right coronary artery. Recently, he developed recurrent angina. An adenosine perfusion SPECT study showed a left ventricular ejection fraction of 38% and evidence of reversible ischemia in the inferolateral and anterolateral walls.

On the basis of these findings, he was referred for cardiac catheterization. He was admitted to the hospital and underwent coronary angiography on that same day.

Coronary angiography demonstrated the following: There was mild coronary calcification. The distribution was right dominant. The left main coronary artery was normal. The proximal LAD was totally occluded just distal to the first septal branch. The distal LAD was visualized by injection of the LIMA graft. The left circumflex was a large-caliber vessel with proximal 90% stenosis. The left circumflex gave origin to a medium-caliber bifurcating circumflex marginal that had a proximal 70% stenosis. The right coronary artery was a large-caliber dominant vessel with proximal 90% stenosis. Previously deployed RCA stents were patent with mild in-stent restenosis. The distal right coronary artery gave origin to a large-caliber right posterior descending artery that had mild proximal disease. The large-caliber right posterolateral branch had a proximal 70% stenosis.

The LIMA graft to the LAD was widely patent. The distal LAD was a small-caliber vessel with a 60% stenosis. There was also extensive retrograde perfusion to the more proximal LAD and a medium-caliber LAD diagonal that had an ostial 90% stenosis. The saphenous vein graft to the LAD diagonal was totally occluded.

On the basis of these findings, we elected to proceed with percutaneous intervention on both the right coronary artery and the left circumflex coronary artery. We first performed intervention on the proximal right coronary artery with drug-eluting stent deployment with a 3.5 × 18-mm Cypher stent that converted to 90% stenosis to 0% residual. We then proceeded with intervention on the proximal left circumflex with drug-eluting stent deployment with a 2.5 × 28-mm Cypher stent that converted to 90% stenosis to 0% residual.

His postangioplasty stent course was uncomplicated, and he was discharged home in stable condition.

Discharge condition: Stable.

DISCHARGE MEDICATIONS:

Aspirin 81 mg every day
Lipitor 10 mg nightly
Plavix 75 mg every day
Irbesartan 300 mg every evening
Nexium 40 mg every day
Probenecid/colchicine 500/0.5 mg 1 tablet by mouth 2 times a day
Nitroglycerin 0.4 mg sublingual as needed for chest pain
Fish oil 1000 mg a day
Metoprolol 75 mg every morning and 50 mg every evening

171

The patient will be seen in follow-up with the cardiologist.

Progress Note

Patient is recovering from PCI to the proximal RCA and circumflex. No evidence of groin hematoma. Patient can be discharged home later today.

CASE STUDY QUESTIONS

15-3a.   Admit diagnosis: _____

15-3b.   Discharge disposition: _____

15-3c.   Principal diagnosis: _____

15-3d.   Secondary diagnoses (indicate POA status for secondary diagnoses):

_____

_____

_____

_____

_____

_____

15-3e.   Principal procedure: _____

15-3f.   Secondary procedures: _____

_____

15-3g.   Assign MS-DRG: _____

15-3h.   Relative weight of MS-DRG: _____

15-3i.   Can this MS-DRG be optimized with the addition of a CC? Yes or No
         Can this MS-DRG be optimized with the addition of an MCC? Yes or No

15-3j.   Is there a main guideline pertinent to selection of the principal diagnosis in this case study?

_____

_____

15-3k.   Is there another diagnosis that meets the definition for principal diagnosis? Yes or No

15-3l.   If yes, what is the other diagnosis? _____

15-3m.   Is there any opportunity for physician query?

_____

_____

15-3n.   What is the drug Plavix used to treat? _____

172

16 Diseases of the Respiratory System (ICD-10-CM Chapter 10, Codes J00-J99)

ABBREVIATIONS/ACRONYMS

Without the use of reference materials, define the following abbreviations or acronyms.

1. RSV _____

2. O_2 _____

3. BAL _____

4. RAD _____

5. PCP _____

6. COPD _____

7. VATS _____

8. CAP _____

9. CHF _____

10. *H. flu* _____

GLOSSARY DEFINITIONS

Match the glossary term to the correct definition.

1. _____ Thoracentesis

2. _____ Pneumothorax

3. _____ Aspiration pneumonia

4. _____ Hemothorax

5. _____ Empyema

6. _____ Nosocomial pneumonia

7. _____ Tracheostomy

8. _____ Pleural effusion

9. _____ Bronchoscopy

10. _____ Community-acquired pneumonia

11. _____ Chronic bronchitis

12. _____ Asthma

13. _____ Influenza

14. _____ Pulmonary edema

15. _____ Chronic obstructive pulmonary disease

16. _____ Sinusitis

A. Blood that accumulates in the pleural space

B. Lung disease due to inhalation of coal dust

C. Disease that is defined by a mucus-producing cough most days of the month, 3 months of a year for 2 successive years with no other underlying disease to explain the cough

D. Air that accumulates in the pleural space

E. Procedure in which an artificial opening is made in the front of the trachea through the skin of the neck

F. Chronic disease that affects the airways that carry air into and out of the lungs

G. Lung disease due to inhalation of asbestos

H. Contagious viral infection of the respiratory tract that causes coughing, difficulty breathing, headache, muscle aches, and weakness

I. Broad term used to define pneumonias that are contracted outside of the hospital or nursing home setting

J. Condition in which fluid accumulates in the lungs

Continued

173

17. _____ Asbestosis

18. _____ Black lung

19. _____ Emphysema

20. _____ Mechanical ventilation

K. Condition where the linings of one or more sinuses become infected; usually due to viruses or bacteria

L. Puncture of the chest wall to remove fluid from the space between the pleura and the chest wall

M. Fluid that accumulated in the pleural space because of trauma or disease

N. Diagnostic endoscopic procedure in which a tube with a tiny camera on the end is inserted through the nose or mouth into the lungs

O. Inflammation of the lungs and bronchial tubes due to aspiration of foreign material into the lung

P. Chronic lung disease of gradual onset that can be attributed to chronic infection and inflammation or irritation from cigarette smoke

Q. Pneumonia that is acquired while a patient is in a hospital-type setting

R. General term used to describe lung disease in which the airways become obstructed, making it difficult for air to get into and out of the lungs

S. Accumulation of pus in the pleural space

T. The use of a machine to induce alternating inflation and deflation of the lungs, to regulate the exchange rate of gases in the blood

CODING

Using the code book, code the following.

1. Emphysematous bleb _____

2. Influenza with *Streptococcus pneumoniae* pneumonia _____

3. Steroid-dependent asthma (systemic steroids) _____

4. Right middle lobe syndrome _____

5. Acute on chronic respiratory failure due to end-stage COPD. Patient is on home oxygen. _____

6. Acute bronchiolitis due to RSV _____

7. Tension pneumothorax, right _____

8. Patient admitted for change of tracheostomy tube _____

9. Aspiration pneumonia in a patient who has dysphagia due to previous CVA _____

10. Chronic lung disease _____

11. Right malignant pleural effusion due to cancer of the right lung _____

12. Mediastinitis _____

13. Paralysis of diaphragm _____

14. Edema of larynx _____

15. Acute bronchospasm due to exercise

CASE SCENARIOS

Using the code book, code the following cases.

1. Patient is a 67-year-old female who presented to the ER with shortness of breath. She was in her usual state of health until 1 week ago, when she began to have chills, fever, and a cough. Patient was admitted and started on IV antibiotics for pneumonia. Her COPD exacerbation was treated with albuterol treatments and oxygen by nasal cannula. Sputum cultures grew *Klebsiella pneumoniae*. Coumadin was continued for treatment of the patient's chronic atrial fibrillation.

   Final Diagnoses: Pneumonia due to *Klebsiella*.
   Chronic obstructive pulmonary disease with acute decompensation.
   Atrial fibrillation.

   _____

   _____

2. Patient was admitted with acute respiratory distress syndrome due to hantavirus. The patient was intubated and was placed on mechanical ventilation. After admission to ICU, the patient continued to deteriorate and expired within a few hours.

   Cause of Death: Hantavirus.

   _____

   _____

3. Patient is admitted with shortness of breath and fever that has been present for 2 to 3 weeks and has gotten progressively worse. Patient has a history of rheumatoid arthritis. CT scan showed evidence of bronchiolitis obliterans organizing pneumonia (BOOP). Patient was started on prednisone and discharged when symptoms had resolved.

   Final Diagnoses: BOOP.
   Rheumatoid arthritis.

   _____

   _____

4. Patient was admitted with acute bronchitis that is exacerbating the patient's COPD. Patient quit smoking 5 years ago. X-ray was negative for any pneumonia. Patient takes medications for CAD, stable angina, and hypertension.

   Final Diagnoses: Exacerbation of COPD.
   Acute bronchitis.
   Angina.
   Coronary artery disease.
   Hypertension.

   _____

   _____

5. Patient is admitted with acute on chronic respiratory failure due to emphysema. Patient has depression with anxiety, is dependent on oxygen, and has had numerous admissions for pneumonia, history of kidney stones, and pulmonary hypertension. Patient was treated with BIPAP for 48 hours and is a DNR/DNI. Blood gases show evidence of acidosis. No infection is identified, and deterioration in respiratory status is thought to be a progression of his emphysema. Patient is discharged to at home hospice care.

   Final Diagnoses: End-stage emphysema.

                  Chronic respiratory failure with hypercapnia.

                  Pulmonary hypertension.

   Procedure: BIPAP.

   _____

   _____

6. Patient was admitted with acute pulmonary edema due to chemical reaction. She was doing some housecleaning and mixed products containing bleach with an acid-containing toilet bowl cleaner. This resulted in the inhalation of chlorine gas. Patient was treated in the ICU and made an uneventful recovery.

   Discharge Diagnosis: Noncardiogenic pulmonary edema.

   _____

   _____

7. This 1-year-old male child was admitted with barking cough, stridor, and hoarseness. The patient was up-to-date on all vaccinations and had achieved normal developmental milestones. Patient was treated for laryngotracheobronchitis and recovered.

   Discharge Diagnosis: Laryngotracheobronchitis.

   _____

   _____

8. Patient is an alcoholic who may have aspirated while having a seizure because of withdrawal. Patient's seizure is stabilized in the ER, and patient is admitted for treatment of possible aspiration pneumonia. Social history reveals that the patient is homeless and drinks 1 quart of whiskey each day. Additional investigations reveal that the patient has cirrhosis of the liver likely due to alcohol. Ultrasound also reveals ascites. The patient is emaciated. Nutrition and social work consults are obtained.

   Final Diagnoses: Seizure due to alcohol withdrawal.

                  Aspiration pneumonia.

                  Cirrhosis due to alcoholism.

   _____

   _____

9. Patient is admitted for treatment of pneumonia. She has had a cough and fever for the past 3 days. Patient is currently being treated for metastasis to the lung and is dehydrated. Patient has a history of breast cancer and takes medications for rheumatoid arthritis, eczema, and benign hypertension. Patient has mild COPD with emphysema. She is treated with IV fluids and antibiotics.

   Final Diagnoses: Fever due to pneumonia.

                  Dehydration.

                  Metastatic breast cancer.

                  COPD.

   _____

   _____

10. Patient was treated for pneumonia as an outpatient but continued to cough and to have fever and pleuritic chest pain. A chest tube was inserted for drainage in the right pleural cavity. Cultures of the drainage and sputum grew *Haemophilus influenzae*. IV antibiotics were administered, and the patient started to improve. Patient has the following medical conditions: chronic alcohol-induced pancreatitis, alcoholism with daily use, and tobacco abuse.

Final Diagnosis: *Haemophilus influenzae* pneumonia with empyema.

_____

_____

CASE STUDIES

Using the code book, code and answer questions about the following case studies.

16-1. CASE STUDY

Admission History and Physical

Reason for admission: The patient is admitted because of worsening shortness of breath and cough.

History of present illness: The patient is a 53-year-old female. She has a history of non–small cell lung cancer. She is status post right lower lobe lobectomy. She has had a recurrence and has been treated with chemotherapy, including Taxotere. She had induction chemotherapy prior to her surgery. She was also on Tarceva. She also received radiation therapy this year.

She comes in reporting a couple of days of nasal congestion, sore throat, cough, and shortness of breath. On initial chest x-ray in the Emergency Room, no pneumonia was found. On CT scan, there was no evidence of pulmonary embolism. The patient was treated with nebulizers, antibiotics, and steroids; however, she did not significantly improve and in fact desaturated when she was mobilized. She was then brought to our service. She has not noted any improvement in the past 48 hours. Her main complaint is shortness of breath with any exertion. She has pain throughout the chest, which is an old problem. She continues to have nasal congestion and sore throat. She has not had any fevers. She did have green sputum for a couple of days.

Past medical history:
1. Rheumatoid arthritis.
2. GERD.
3. History of bronchitis.

Medications:
1. OxyContin.
2. Oxycodone.
3. Advair.
4. ATRA.
5. Prednisone.
6. Nexium.

Social history: Continues to smoke.

Allergies: NKDA.

Physical examination: On examination this morning, she was sitting up in bed. She was awake and alert. Her vital signs were stable. She was afebrile. O_2 saturation was 94% on room air. Her mouth and pharynx were clear. Her neck was supple. There was no JVD. The heart was regular rate and rhythm. The abdomen was soft. There was wheezing throughout both lung fields. No peripheral edema.

Diagnostic studies: Laboratory studies from late yesterday show a hematocrit of 35.1, white count of 7600, and platelet count of 297,000. Chemistry panel is unremarkable.

Imaging studies: CT scan of the chest again shows no evidence of pneumonia or pulmonary embolism. There is a growing mass in the right lung. This is in the right hilum and compresses the right main stem bronchus and bronchus intermedius. It also may extend into the mediastinum and subcarinal region. This has been a clear progression from previous scan.

Impression and plan: The patient is a 53-year-old female with local/regionally recurrent non–small cell lung cancer who has been through several therapies. It is not clear now whether her symptoms are related to just an exacerbation of COPD plus/minus a viral infection, or whether her symptoms are related to the progression of her disease and compression of the right main stem bronchus. At this point, she does not seem to be improving much with conservative measures.

We will continue on our current course of antibiotics, steroids, and nebulizers. If she has not improved, we will need to have Pulmonary see her regarding bronchoscopy and possible stent placement.

The patient was seen and was discussed with the medical house staff and Pulmonary Medicine. Everyone agrees with the above plan.

Thoracic with Contrast CT

RESULT:

Clinical history: Shortness of breath, cough, non–small cell lung carcinoma.
Comparison: CT chest from October.

Technique: Axial CT of the chest was obtained after administration of intravenous contrast without adverse reaction.

CT chest: No evidence of PE seen. The patient is status post right lower lobectomy. Surgical clips again seen in the right hilar region. Round soft tissue density around the surgical suture material in the right hilum posterior to the right main bronchus and bronchus intermedius, increasing in size. It measures approximately 4 × 3 cm on current examination and previously measured 3 × 2 cm. This mass causes significant compression of the bronchus intermedius/proximal right middle lobe bronchi, which appear patent distally. Mass appears to be invading the adjacent mediastinum in the subcarinal region. Right infrahilar lymph node adjacent to the mass has increased by 1.7 × 1.1 cm, previously 1.0 × 0.8 cm.

Mild subpleural atelectasis or scarring and adjacent pleural thickening medial aspect of the adjacent right lung slightly worsened. Diffuse pulmonary emphysema. Minimal subpleural nodule or nodular scarring measuring up to 3 mm in the right upper lobe unchanged.

Minimal scarring in the right lung base unchanged. Small calcified nodule in the left thyroid unchanged. Atherosclerosis of the thoracic aorta. Subcentimeter mediastinal lymph nodes unchanged. Calcified right hilar and subcarinal lymph nodes unchanged. Coronary artery calcifications. Atherosclerosis of the thoracic aorta.

Impression: Increasing size of right hilar soft tissue mass consistent with recurrent non–small cell lung carcinoma. This mass causes significant compression of the bronchus intermedius/proximal right middle lobe bronchus and may be possibly extending into the subcarinal portion of the mediastinum. Increased size of adjacent right infrahilar lymph node noted. Slight worsening of atelectasis right upper lobe.

Discharge Summary

DIAGNOSES/PROBLEMS:

1. Non–small cell lung cancer.
2. Exacerbation of COPD.

178

History, Major Findings, and Hospital Course:

The patient is a 53-year-old African American female with a history of recurrent non–small cell lung cancer status post radiation and chemotherapy.

The patient was treated with chemotherapy, including Taxotere and carboplatin. She was also on Tarceva. Radiation was done this year.

The patient reported nasal congestion, sore throat, cough, and shortness of breath. Chest x-ray in the ER shows no pneumonia. CT scan shows no evidence of pulmonary embolism. However, increasing size of right hilar soft tissue mass is consistent with recurrent non–small cell lung carcinoma, which caused significant compression of the bronchus intermedius/proximal right middle lobe bronchus and may be possibly extending into the subcarinal portion of the mediastinum. There is also increased size of adjacent right infrahilar lymph node, and slight worsening of atelectasis of the right upper lobe is noted. Therefore, the patient's respiratory symptoms seem to be caused by an exacerbation of her COPD and/or the worsening of local recurrence of the tumor. Sputum cultures show little normal upper respiratory flora with few polymorphonuclear cells; blood culture is negative. The patient was treated symptomatically with albuterol and Atrovent nebulizers and Advair inhaler, as well as Robitussin and Mucomyst.

The patient was afebrile with a white count of 10.3. She was treated with azithromycin 250 mg daily. Initially, she required oxygenation with nasal cannula of 2 L of oxygen for hypoxemia. Her symptoms improved significantly after she also received intravenous methylprednisolone of 12.5 mg 3 times a day.

Eventually, the patient did not require any oxygenation even though she had mild expiratory wheezing during the examination. Her steroid was tapered and was changed to prednisone 40 mg daily. She was continued on nebulizers and inhalers. The patient also reported pain, which was controlled with OxyContin 20 mg 2 times a day and oxycodone 10 mg every 6 hours as needed. She was encouraged to ambulate, which she tolerated without taking oxygen.

The patient's systolic blood pressure was running between 150 and 180. Therefore, she was started on Norvasc 5 mg daily on the day of discharge.

Discharge Medications:

Azithromycin 250 mg by mouth daily for 7 days
OxyContin 20 mg by mouth 2 times a day
Oxycodone 10 mg by mouth every 6 hours as needed
Albuterol and Atrovent nebulizers every 6 hours
Advair 250/50 mcg two puffs 2 times a day
Prednisone 40 mg daily for 2 days, then 20 mg daily for 2 days, then 10 mg daily for 2 days, and then 5 mg daily
Nexium 40 mg daily
Colace
Senna
Norvasc 5 mg daily

Discharge Instructions:

Diet: The patient can resume a low-salt diet.

Activity: As she tolerates.

Other: She should call us if she has increasing shortness of breath, chest pain, fever, or chills.

The patient should make an appointment with her oncologist to discuss further treatment for her cancer.

Progress Notes

DAY 1

Widespread inspiratory wheeze. Ongoing chest and abd discomfort.

D/C oral prednisone and start Solu-Medrol IV 125 mg q8h.

Nebs q4h.

Continue antibiotic, not febrile; no increase in WBC, sating well.

DAY 2

Still wheezy. Unable to expectorate. Stable WBC.

Continue IV steroids. Follow hyperglycemic protocol.

Await C&S.

Monitor BP.

DAY 3

Wheezing much improved with less SOB.

Change to oral steroids.

Blood pressure elevated, ? due to pain. Add Norvasc.

Discharge home.

Oncology Consultation

The patient is a 53-year-old woman with recurrent non–small cell lung carcinoma. She finished radiation therapy to her right chest. She has progressed. She had five cycles of Taxotere. She had progressed, then was status post four cycles of Tarceva, with progression. She then was given radiation therapy earlier this year, but this was complicated by serious esophagitis. Earlier, she also received Taxol with carboplatinum and had a good response but did not tolerate the treatment at all. She was hospitalized for significant shortness of breath and wheezing over the weekend and was found to have progression of disease in her right lung and subcarina. This is compressing her bronchus intermedius and right upper lobe; however, most of her symptoms were believed by Pulmonary to be due to a COPD exacerbation. Her symptoms are improving. She is not requiring oxygen at this point, and she is due to go home today.

Again, scans show evidence of progression. We did discuss her case in Tumor Board, and it was believed that photodynamic therapy may be palliative. In the meantime, I think we should treat her with Alimta. We went over Alimta given IV once every 3 weeks. I would start this in the first part of January, see how she tolerates this, and then discuss photodynamic therapy, particularly if her disease progresses. Otherwise, her options are limited. Because she has not tolerated therapy that well in the past, it is unclear whether or not she will tolerate Alimta. We went over the fact that she needs to start folic acid. We will give her a B_{12} shot when she comes in next week, and then consider starting Alimta the first week of January, depending on how she feels. I will arrange for follow-up with her as an outpatient.

CASE STUDY QUESTIONS

16-1a.   Admit diagnosis: _____

16-1b.   Discharge disposition: _____

16-1c.   Principal diagnosis:_____

16-1d.   Secondary diagnoses (indicate POA status for secondary diagnoses):

_____

_____

_____

_____

_____

16-1e.   Principal procedure: _____

16-1f.   Secondary procedures: _____

_____

16-1g.   Assign MS-DRG: _____

16-1h.   Relative weight of MS-DRG: _____

16-1i.   Can this MS-DRG be optimized with the addition of a CC? Yes or No
         Can this MS-DRG be optimized with the addition of an MCC? Yes or No

16-1j.   What main guideline is pertinent to selection of the principal diagnosis in this case study?

_____

_____

16-1k.   Is there another diagnosis that meets the definition for principal diagnosis? Yes or No

16-1l.   If yes, what is the other diagnosis? _____

16-1m.   Is there any opportunity for physician query?

_____

_____

16-1n.   What is the drug Alimta used to treat? _____

Chapter **16 Diseases of the Respiratory System**

CC: SOB.

HPI: The patient is an 87-year-old gentleman who presents with shortness of breath and dyspnea on exertion. He was feeling short of breath with walking for the past 2 or 3 weeks. He had an exercise tolerance of 2 miles prior to the last few weeks and says he can walk less than half a block now before becoming dyspneic. He says his symptoms have been stable over the course of 2 to 3 weeks. His cough initially was productive of green sputum; now it is dry with no fever or chills, no chest pain, no orthopnea, and no PND. His wife was sick with URI symptoms about 3 weeks ago and was treated with antibiotics for about 10 days. No recent travel. He has had the flu vaccine but has not had the pneumococcal vaccine.

Past medical history: A leg fracture, status post internal reduction and fixation. Bilateral cataracts, hypertension, hypothyroidism, hypercholesterolemia, and arthritis.

Medications:
Avalox 400 mg daily
Synthroid 75 mcg daily
Lipitor 10 mg nightly
Aspirin 81 mg daily
Hydrochlorothiazide 5 mg by mouth daily
Lotrel

Social history: Former smoker, not currently. No alcohol. No illicits. Lives with his wife.

Retired plumber, has one daughter.

Family history: Sister with arthritis. Does not know about the parents' status.

Allergies: Percocet.

PHYSICAL EXAMINATION:

Vitals: T 97.2, HR 75, BP 164/77, RR 20, saturating at 95% on 3 L of oxygen. Weight is 73 kg.

General: A pleasant elderly gentleman in no acute distress.

HEENT: Mucous membranes were moist. Normocephalic and atraumatic.

Neck: No masses or enlarged nodes.

Chest: Mild crackles half way up bilaterally. No wheezes and no rhonchi.

Heart: Irregularly irregular. No murmurs, rubs, or gallops.

Abd: Soft and nontender. Bowel sounds were present.

Rectal: Deferred.

Extremities: Calf tenderness bilaterally with no edema. Dorsalis pedis pulses 2 plus bilaterally.

Neurologic: Grossly nonfocal.

A/P: Patient is admitted for treatment of pneumonia. IV antibiotics will be started. Doppler examination of the lower extremities will be ordered.

DIAGNOSES/PROBLEMS:

1. Community-acquired pneumonia this admission.
2. Deep venous thrombosis.
3. Hypertension.
4. Hypothyroidism.
5. Arthritis.

PROCEDURES:

1. Chest CT shows bilateral interstitial fibrosis and possible pneumonia.
2. Lower extremity ultrasound shows nearly occlusive thrombosis of the right femoral vein and nearly occlusive thrombosis of the left common femoral vein.
3. Renal ultrasound shows multiple renal cysts and nonobstructive renal calculi.
4. Pulmonary function studies show a moderately obstructive ventilatory defect and a possible moderately restrictive ventilatory defect.

HISTORY, MAJOR FINDINGS, AND HOSPITAL COURSE:

The patient is an 87-year-old gentleman with the above past medical history who presents with shortness of breath and dyspnea on exertion. He was feeling short of breath with walking for the last 2 or 3 weeks. He had an exercise tolerance of 2 miles prior to the last few weeks and says he can walk less than half a block now before becoming dyspneic. He says his symptoms have been stable over the course of 2 to 3 weeks. His cough initially was productive of green sputum; now it is dry with no fever or chills, no chest pain, no orthopnea, and no PND. His wife was sick with URI symptoms about 3 weeks ago and was treated with antibiotics for about 10 days. No recent travel. He has had the flu vaccine but has not had the pneumococcal vaccine.

Past medical history: As per above, in addition to a leg fracture status post repair and bilateral cataracts.

Medications:
Avalox 400 mg daily
Synthroid 75 mcg daily
Lipitor 10 mg nightly
Aspirin 81 mg daily
Hydrochlorothiazide 5 mg by mouth daily
Lotrel

Social history: Former smoker, not currently. No alcohol. No illicits. Lives with his wife. Retired plumber, has one daughter.

Family history: Sister with arthritis. Does not know about the parents' status.

Allergies: Percocet.

Review of systems: See HPI. Otherwise negative.

Physical examination: Temperature is 97.2°, heart rate is 75, blood pressure 164/77, respiratory rate 20, saturating 95% on 3 L, and weight is 73 kg.

General: A pleasant elderly gentleman in no acute distress.

HEENT: Mucous membranes were moist. Normocephalic and atraumatic.

Neck: No masses or enlarged nodes.

Chest: Mild crackles halfway up bilaterally. No wheezes and no rhonchi. Heart was irregularly irregular. No murmurs, rubs, or gallops.

Abd: Abdomen was soft and nontender. Bowel sounds were present.

Extremities: Calf tenderness bilaterally with no edema. Dorsalis pedis pulses 2 plus bilaterally. Neurologic examination is grossly nonfocal.

Lab work: White count was 7.2 and hematocrit was 40. Creatinine was 1.6. INR was 1.3.

Summary: This is an 87-year-old gentleman with likely pneumonia who presents with dyspnea on exertion and shortness of breath for several weeks. The patient has presumptive pneumonia with an oxygen requirement, potentially also with some underlying diffuse interstitial lung disease.

Pulmonary: The patient requires oxygen on admission. However, the patient's oxygenation eventually improved on antibiotics and other supportive care. The pulmonary team was consulted and was not overtly impressed; team recommended checking a V/Q scan and echocardiogram and having the patient follow up in the Pulmonary Clinic later. The patient continued to improve and eventually was discharged without requiring home oxygen. To further evaluate the possibility of an underlying interstitial process, rheumatologic workup was begun. ANA was positive, 1:40 nucleolar pattern. Rheumatoid factor was 28, which is negative. HIV was negative. ANCA was negative. Glomerular membrane was negative. ACE levels were normal. The patient continued to improve on antibiotics.

DVT: The patient was initiated on anticoagulation therapy; this will continue on an outpatient basis.

Endocrine: The patient has a slightly elevated TSH of 5.18 and was maintained on levothyroxine dosing at 75 mcg daily.

Platelets: Platelets have been falling some during this admission but stabilized and did not continue to fall. Antiplatelet antibodies were ordered.

DISCHARGE MEDICATIONS:

Lovenox 60 mg subcutaneous daily
Levothyroxine 75 mcg orally daily
Coumadin 5 mg orally daily
Hydrochlorothiazide 12.5 mg daily
Moxifloxacin 400 mg orally daily for 5 days
Lipitor 10 mg nightly
Combivent 2 puffs every 6 hours as needed for shortness of breath

FOLLOW-UP CARE:

1. The patient is to follow up at the Coumadin clinic.
2. Pulmonary will call the patient for an appointment.

The patient is to follow up with PMD. The patient will have home physical therapy arranged.

Progress Notes

DAY 1

The patient was seen and examined by the resident, and the history and physical findings were reviewed. The patient is an 87-year-old man admitted with pneumonia and hypoxia. Per his wife, the patient is otherwise functional at home. The patient is making general clinical improvement. We will continue him on a fluoroquinolone for community-acquired pneumonia and will follow him closely. Initiate anticoagulation therapy for incidental DVT finding.

Day 2

The patient was seen and examined by the resident, and the history and physical findings were reviewed. The patient is an 87-year-old man who was admitted with pneumonia. He has been treated with antibiotics. He is improving and has a lower oxygen requirement than yesterday. Continue anticoagulant therapy for DVT.

Day 3

The patient was seen and examined by the resident, and the history and physical findings were reviewed. The patient is an 87-year-old man admitted with community-acquired pneumonia. He is doing great today. He is on room air and has been up and ambulating. We have discussed this case with his family, who are looking forward to taking care of him and bringing him home. He will be discharged accordingly today. Arrangements have been made for home physical therapy.

CASE STUDY QUESTIONS

16-2a. Admit diagnosis: _____

16-2b. Discharge disposition: _____

16-2c. Principal diagnosis: _____

16-2d. Secondary diagnoses (indicate POA status for secondary diagnoses):

_____

_____

_____

_____

_____

_____

16-2e. Principal procedure: _____

16-2f. Secondary procedures: _____

_____

16-2g. Assign MS-DRG: _____

16-2h. Relative weight of MS-DRG: _____

16-2i. Can this MS-DRG be optimized with the addition of a CC? Yes or No
        Can this MS-DRG be optimized with the addition of an MCC? Yes or No

16-2j. Is there a main guideline pertinent to selection of the principal diagnosis in this case study?

_____

_____

16-2k. Is there another diagnosis that meets the definition for principal diagnosis? Yes or No

16-2l.   If yes, what is the other diagnosis? _____

16-2m. Is there any opportunity for physician query?

_____

_____

16-2n. What is the drug Lovenox used to treat? _____

16-3. CASE STUDY

History and Physical

CC: Acute respiratory failure.

HPI: The patient is a 70-year-old female who presented from her nursing home with severe shortness of breath. The patient was emergently intubated in the ER and was admitted to the critical care unit. The patient received Lasix in the ER. ABGs were drawn.

Past medical history: Obtained from previous records. Hypertension, aortic stenosis, DM type II on insulin, CVA ×3, bilateral carotid stenosis, CAD, OSA, tardive dyskinesia, and hyperlipidemia.

Social history: History of 40 pack-years of cigs, none now. No alcohol. Lives in a nursing home. Family is involved.

Allergies: Penicillin, Haldol, Primidone.

Review of systems: Unable to obtain from the patient because of intubation. Notes from the nursing home indicate the following:

Constitutional: No fevers. Patient has been fatigued for the past week.

Neuro: Weakness. No headache or syncope.

HEENT: Patient had cataract surgery 2 weeks ago.

CV: Decreased exercise tolerance.

Resp: Increasing SOB.

GI: No complaints.

GU: No complaints.

Musculoskeletal: Right shoulder pain.

Physical examination:

General: Patient is intubated.

HEENT: Recent cataract surgery. Neck is supple without bruit. No JVD, but neck is obese, so unreliable. Tongue midline.

Chest: Crackles. Diminished breath sounds at the bases.

Heart: RRR. 3/6 SEM.

Abd: Soft. Obese.

Ext: 2+ lower extremity edema. Varicose veins.

GU/Rectal: Not done.

Skin: WNL.

Neuro: Cranial nerves WNL.

186

Chest x-ray shows pulmonary vascular congestion and edema since previous examination compatible with congestive heart failure. Cardiomegaly with CTR: 20/30. Minimal tortuosity of thoracic aorta. Moderate degenerative arthritis right shoulder. Marked obesity limits detail examination.

A/P: Admit to critical care unit for monitoring and treatment of acute respiratory failure due to congestive heart failure. Patient will be diuresed and maintained on mechanical ventilation. Check BNP.

Discharge Summary

DIAGNOSES/PROBLEMS:

1. Acute respiratory failure due to CHF exacerbation (diastolic dysfunction).
2. HTN.
3. DM type II.
4. Morbid obesity.
5. CVA ×3.
6. Bilateral carotid stenosis.
7. CAD.
8. Obstructive sleep apnea.
9. Anxiety.
10. Hx tardive dyskinesia—treated and controlled with Clonopin.
11. Hyperlipidemia.
12. Iron deficiency anemia.

PROCEDURES:

1. Chest x-ray—vascular congestion compatible with CHF.
2. VQ scan—low probability for PE; high resolution.
3. CT scan—no interstitial lung process; resolving pulmonary edema.
4. Echocardiogram—mild valvular aortic stenosis. Mean aortic gradient 18 mm Hg. Trace aortic regurgitation. The left ventricle is not well visualized. Left ventricular systolic function is normal. Technically challenging study; however, available images suggest normal LV systolic function with estimated LVEF of 60% to 65%.
5. Mechanical ventilation.

HISTORY, MAJOR FINDINGS, AND HOSPITAL COURSE:

The patient is a 70-year-old female who presented from her nursing facility with severe shortness of breath and low saturations on RA. Patient was intubated in the ER for acute respiratory failure and was admitted for further treatment. The patient's CXR and presentation were consistent with CHF exacerbation. She was started on IV Lasix with good diuresis and improved oxygenation over the next 2 to 3 days. We were able to wean her from the ventilator on hospital day 2. She had an echocardiogram with results as described above. Patient developed acute on chronic renal failure with creatinine elevated up to 2.8 from her baseline but returned to 1.2 with decreased Lasix dosing. After good initial response, patient did not improve much over the next 2 to 3 days despite adequate diuresis, and we investigated for acute pulmonary process. We obtained a VQ scan that ruled out a PE, and high-resolution CT scan was negative for pneumonia and interstitial lung disease that had been suggested by an earlier PFT. Her PFTs did not show a restrictive pattern either. At this point, patient had reached her baseline status, at 4 L of oxygen. During her stay, her iron studies showed an Fe of 36 and percent saturation of 12% with normal transferring and iron-binding capacity. She was started on iron supplements. No records of colonoscopy are available, and this case may be pursued on an outpatient basis. An incidental finding on the patient's high-resolution CT scan was a foreign body in her GE junction, likely a pill. This could be followed up with further imaging as an outpatient. Patient's blood glucose levels were mostly in the 70 to 150 range over the past 2 days in the hospital, with no episodes of hypoglycemia reported. We have decreased her Lantus, and her blood sugars will need further monitoring. We are switching the patient to 40 mg Lasix oral on the day of discharge, and further need for Lasix should be assessed 1 to 2 weeks from now. On the day of discharge, patient felt she had returned to her baseline respiratory status and had no new complaints. Her examination findings were as follows:

Vitals: HR 68, temp 36.5°C, BP 142/66, respiratory rate 20.

HEENT: Oral mucosa moist, no JVD.

Chest: CTAP; CVS; RRR.

Abd: Obese, nontender ext 1 + edema.

Labs: WBC 7420, Hb 9.2, Plt 34.4, Na 137, K 4.9, BUN/Cr 49/1.2.

DISCHARGE MEDICATIONS:

Lisinopril enteral 10 mg PO daily routine
Clopidogrel enteral 75 mg PO daily routine
Simvastatin enteral 20 mg PO daily routine
   Nurse: Please notify the Nutrition Department (via computer) to exclude grapefruit juice from the diet. Grapefruit juice increases bioavailability and may lead to toxicity.
Insulin glargine human inj 16 unit subQ prn routine
Escitalopram oxalate enteral 10 mg PO daily routine
Milk of Magnesia 30 mL PO at bedtime, prn constipation, routine
Ferrous sulfate enteral 300 mg PO tid routine
   Food/drug interaction: At discharge, instruct patient to take dose 1 hour before or 2 hours after meals to increase absorption.
Trazodone HCl enteral 50 mg PO at bedtime routine prn insomnia
Regular human insulin sliding scale before meals and at bedtime. One amp 050; notify MD if BS <60 0 unit, if BS 61 to 200 6 unit, if BS 201 to 250 8 unit, if BS 251 to 300 10 unit, if BS 301 to 350 12 unit, if BS 351 to 400 NHO, if BS >400; subQ routine
Brimonidine tartrate ophth soln 0.2%; 1 drop both eyes q8h, routine
Clonazepam enteral 1 mg PO tid, routine
Travoprost ophthalmic soln 0.004% NF; 2 drops both eyes daily, routine
Lasix 40 mg PO daily for 2 weeks

DISCHARGE INSTRUCTIONS:

Discharge to nursing home, activity as tolerated, diabetic and low-salt diet.

FOLLOW-UP CARE:

Treatments/follow-up:
1. Please have blood work drawn for primary care physician in 1 week (reason: electrolyte monitoring while on Lasix).
2. Follow-up imaging for foreign body in distal esophagus per primary care physician.
3. Outpatient colonoscopy to evaluate for iron deficiency anemia; follow-up.

Progress Notes

DAY 1

Patient was admitted to the CCU yesterday from the nursing home in respiratory failure. Intubated and on ventilation. She has been on the heart monitor and has been treated with IV Lasix for the past 24 hours. Monitor daily weights. Keep accurate I/Os. Continue Lantus 24 units qhs for her DM. Monitor Accu-Chek. Nutrition consult for morbid obesity. HTN is stable.

Day 2

Patient is much improved and was extubated early this morning. Patient's creatinine is elevated at 2.8, indicating acute renal failure, likely from aggressive diuresis. If it continues to go higher, will consider holding Lasix. Ordered CPAP for OSA. Will investigate patient's anemia by sending iron studies.

Day 3

No acute events overnight. Still has some SOB. Chest x-ray is improved. Dietary indiscretions are likely the cause of this exacerbation. MI was ruled out. Increased Lasix to 60 IV bid. Per TTE, patient meets the criteria for moderate aortic stenosis. Continue CPAP.

Day 4

Patient is getting closer to baseline. She is able to walk in the corridor. Patient is continuing to diurese nicely. Her diabetes has been well controlled during her stay. CT scan did not show any interstitial process. Her renal function is stabilizing with the current Lasix dose. Patient will be discharged back to the nursing home. Her family has been notified of these plans.

CASE STUDY QUESTIONS

16-3a.   Admit diagnosis: _____

16-3b.   Discharge disposition: _____

16-3c.   Principal diagnosis: _____

16-3d.   Secondary diagnoses (indicate POA status for secondary diagnoses):

_____

_____

_____

_____

_____

_____

16-3e.   Principal procedure: _____

16-3f.   Secondary procedures: _____

_____

16-3g. Assign MS-DRG: _____

16-3h. Relative weight of MS-DRG: _____

16-3i.   Can this MS-DRG be optimized with the addition of a CC? Yes or No
         Can this MS-DRG be optimized with the addition of an MCC? Yes or No

_____

16-3j.   Is there a main guideline pertinent to selection of the principal diagnosis in this case study?

_____

_____

16-3k.   Is there another diagnosis that meets the definition for principal diagnosis? Yes or No

16-3l.   If yes, what is the other diagnosis? _____

16-3m.   Is there any opportunity for physician query?

_____

_____

16-3n.   What is the drug Clopidogrel used to treat? _____

17 Diseases of the Digestive System (ICD-10-CM Chapter 11, Codes K00-K94)

ABBREVIATIONS/ACRONYMS

Without the use of reference materials, define the following abbreviations or acronyms.

1. EGD _____
2. UGI _____
3. PEG _____
4. GERD _____
5. ERCP _____
6. PUD _____
7. ESWL _____
8. UC _____
9. SBO _____
10. GI _____

GLOSSARY DEFINITIONS

Match the glossary term to the correct definition.

1. _____ Ileus
2. _____ Mastication
3. _____ Necrotic
4. _____ Peristalsis
5. _____ Anorexia
6. _____ Lysis
7. _____ Intussusception
8. _____ Adhesion
9. _____ Impaction
10. _____ Anastomosis

A. Hard stool in rectum that does not allow normal passage of feces

B. Rhythmic muscle contractions that move food down the digestive tract

C. Loss of appetite

D. Portion of the intestine that telescopes into another portion, causing bowel obstruction

E. Scar tissue that forms an abnormal connection between body parts

F. Dead tissue that blocks the blood supply

G. Surgically formed connection between two structures

H. Chewing of food

I. Destruction of adhesions

J. Absence of normal movement within the intestine

CODING

Using the code book, code the following.

1. Aphthous stomatitis _____

2. Acute and chronic gingivitis _____

3. Osteomyelitis of the jaw _____

4. Tracheoesophageal fistula _____

5. Black hairy tongue _____

6. Ulcer of the esophagus due to aspirin ingestion _____

7. Acute peptic ulcer with perforation and hemorrhage _____

8. Chronic ulcerative ileocolitis _____

9. Fecalith of the appendix _____

10. Umbilical hernia _____

11. Crohn's disease _____

12. Pseudopolyposis of the colon _____

13. Enterocolitis due to radiation _____

14. Rectal polyp _____

15. Portal hypertension due to cirrhosis from chronic hepatitis C _____

CASE SCENARIOS

Using the code book, code the following cases.

1. Patient is admitted with the diagnosis of incarcerated incisional hernia. A repair is performed with the use of mesh.

_____

_____

2. The patient has a diagnosis of esophageal stricture and a history of COPD. An EGD with dilatation of the stricture is performed.

_____

_____

3. Patient presents to the ER with severe abdominal pain and a long history of alcohol abuse. Patient is currently drinking a fifth of liquor a day. Patient is admitted to the hospital with a diagnosis of acute pancreatitis secondary to alcoholism.

_____

_____

4. Patient is admitted to the hospital with abdominal pain. After testing, it is determined that the patient has impaction of the colon. Prior to surgery, the anesthesiologist documents that the patient also has MVP and requires preop antibiotics. The patient is taken to the OR for disimpaction of feces from the rectum and descending colon.

_____

_____

5. A patient is taken to the hospital by ambulance after collapsing at home. Upon arrival to the ER, it is determined that this patient has a history of HTN, DM, chronic constipation, and hypercholesterolemia. The patient is admitted for syncope. After workup, it is determined that the patient collapsed from a volvulus. The patient is taken immediately to the OR for repair. A reduction of the left descending colon is performed.

_____

_____

6. Patient with vomiting and abdominal pain is admitted to the hospital. After workup, it is determined that the patient has appendicitis. The patient is taken to the OR for a laparoscopic appendectomy. The pathology report shows that the patient suffered from acute appendicitis with an abscess, which is confirmed by the attending in the discharge summary.

_____

_____

7. The ER physician documents that the patient is being admitted for hematemesis. The patient has a Hct of 24.3. A transfusion of unit PRBCs is administered, and the patient is taken to the OR for an EGD. The EGD reveals that the patient has an acute perforated duodenal ulcer that is causing the bleed. The patient is treated with IV antibiotics, antiulcer meds, and NG tube.

_____

_____

8. The patient presents to the ER with facial swelling in the area of the jaw. After workup, it is determined that the patient has sialolithiasis. He is taken to the OR for removal of the stone by incision.

_____

_____

9. Patient is admitted with abdominal pain. It is determined that the patient is dehydrated because of an exacerbation of Crohn's disease.

_____

_____

10. Patient has severe abdominal pain with known DM. She is diagnosed and treated for diabetic gastroparesis.

_____

_____

Using the code book, code and answer questions about the following case studies.

17-1. CASE STUDY

History and Physical

CC: "My stomach is hurting."

HPI: This is a 60-year-old man with a past history of prostate cancer and hernia repair (twice) who comes in reporting abdominal pain since yesterday at 3 PM. It began on the left side, more in the lower quadrants, and did not radiate. The pain felt different from prior pain resulting from kidney stones. He has not felt like eating; he has been nauseous and has thrown up. Last night, he could not sleep, and it hurt if he tossed and turned. This morning, he had fever and chills and came to the ED. He has had one bowel movement (this AM) since this all began. The patient denies any change in his stool and reports no HA, no SOB, and no chest pain. He has felt better since he was given morphine in the ED.

Past medical history: Prostate cancer, hypercholesterolemia, and kidney stones.

Past surgical history: Resection of prostate with left inguinal hernia repair at the same time. Two years later, he underwent bilateral inguinal hernia repair, both with mesh.

Social history: Tobacco: PPD for 40 years. Alcohol: Rare wine. Illicits: None. Business owner. Married with two kids.

Family history: No family history of colon cancer. Positive for CAD.

Allergies: NKDA.

Medications: None.

Review of systems:

Constitutional: Fever and chills; fatigue.

Neuro: No headache, syncope, or weakness.

HEENT: Negative.

CV: No chest pain, palpitations, PND, or orthopnea.

Respiratory: No SOB, pleuritic pain, or cough.

GI: See HPI.

GU: No dysuria.

Skin/Skeletal: No rashes.

Physical examination:

General: No acute distress, but mildly uncomfortable.

HEENT: Patient has an NG tube. MMM. PERRL. Oropharynx is clear. Neck is supple with no masses.

Chest: Clear to auscultation.

CV: Regular S1 and S2. No murmur or gallop.

Abd: Mildly distended with guarding. No bowel sounds. Tender to palpation in epigastrium and LLQ. No CVAT.

Ext: Normal.

Skin: Normal.

Neuro: Alert and oriented. CN III to XII intact.

194

Chest x-ray: Chest clear. Air-fluid levels. CT shows partial SBO. No masses.

EKG: Sinus rhythm with nl axis and intervals. TWI 3, F with slight ST depression.

Assessment/Plan: This 60-year-old man is admitted with a partial small-bowel obstruction, likely from prior abdominal surgeries and adhesions. Will attempt to manage conservatively. Continue NG suction and IV fluids. At this point, he is nontoxic. Other issues include polycythemia and EKG changes.

Discharge Summary

DIAGNOSES/PROBLEMS:

1. Small-bowel obstruction.
2. Nausea, vomiting.
3. History of kidney stones.
4. Tobacco use.

PROCEDURES:

CT of the abdomen and chest x-ray. Repeat CT of abdomen.

HISTORY, MAJOR FINDINGS, AND HOSPITAL COURSE:

This is a 60-year-old patient with a history of prostate cancer and hernia repair ×2 who comes in with a 1-day history of abdominal pain that began on the left side, more in the lower quadrant, and did not radiate, but it is different from prior kidney stone pains. The patient did not feel like eating, felt nauseated, and also has thrown up. The patient denies any headache, shortness of breath, or chest pain.

Past medical history: Prostate cancer, bilateral inguinal hernia repairs, kidney stones, hypercholesterolemia.

Social history: The patient is a smoker with occasional alcohol use and no drugs.

Allergies: No known drug allergies.

Medications: None according to the patient.

Physical examination:

Vital signs: Stable.

Abdomen: Mildly distended without guarding, not tympanic. No bowel sounds.

Hospital course: The patient was hospitalized. CAT scan showed partial small-bowel obstruction but no mass. Intravenous fluids were started, antiemetics were started, and pain control was instituted. NG tube was put to low intermittent suction. The patient improved during his admission and started eating, and he was discharged home.

Condition on discharge: Improved.

Discharge medications: Protonix 40 mg daily.

Discharge instructions: Soft diet; advance as tolerated.

Follow-up care: Follow up with the patient's primary care physician.

Progress Notes

DAY 1

Patient is feeling better. Abdomen is soft, nontender, and no longer distended. Patient has normal bowel sounds. Had a BM this morning. Passing gas. NG tube can be removed.

Patient is doing great. Tolerating regular diet. No abdominal pain. EKG is similar to one from a couple of years ago. Had a negative stress test. His polycythemia was most likely due to dehydration. Will recheck prior to discharge. Patient can be discharged home after lunch.

CASE STUDY QUESTION

17-1a.   Admit diagnosis: _____

17-1b.   Discharge disposition: _____

17-1c.   Principal diagnosis: _____

17-1d.   Secondary diagnoses (indicate POA status for secondary diagnoses):

_____

_____

_____

_____

_____

_____

17-1e.   Principal procedure: _____

17-1f.   Secondary procedures: _____

_____

17-1g.   Assign MS-DRG: _____

17-1h.   Relative weight of MS-DRG: _____

17-1i.   Can this MS-DRG be optimized with the addition of a CC? Yes or No
Can this MS-DRG be optimized with the addition of an MCC? Yes or No

17-1j.   Is there a main guideline pertinent to selection of the principal diagnosis in this case study?

_____

_____

17-1k.   Is there another diagnosis that meets the definition for principal diagnosis? Yes or No

17-1l.   If yes, what is the other diagnosis? _____

17-1m. Is there any opportunity for physician query?

_____

_____

17-1n. What are antiemetics used to treat? _____

17-2. CASE STUDY

History and Physical

CC: Vomiting and FTT.

HPI: This 11-week ex-full-term male infant was born via induced vaginal delivery to mother who reported that the only complication during pregnancy was gestational diabetes. The patient was growing initially with occasional spitting up immediately with or within 12 to 20 minutes of feeds. Birth weight was 7 pounds 5 ounces, weight at 1 month was 9 pounds 10 oz, and weight at 2 months was 9 pounds 15 ounces. At that time, Mom noted that the infant was arching and was looking uncomfortable with feeds. PMD recommended starting Zantac. Per Mom, vomiting/arching initially improved after start of Zantac 1 week ago, but then worsened again. Mom now reports nonbilious, nonbloody vomiting within 15 minutes of feeding, estimated close to full feed.

Past medical history: Pregnancy complicated by GDM. Induced 1 week early—vaginal delivery without complication. GERD. Physiologic jaundice treated with bili blanket at home ×5 days.

Development: Tracks, turns to sounds, smiles, holds head up.

Social history: Lives with Mom and Dad, 2 dogs, no smoking.

Family history: Noncontributory. No history of pyloric stenosis.

Allergies: NKDA.

Review of systems:

Constitutional: No fevers. Slight increase in fussiness.

Neuro: No lethargy.

GI: No diarrhea. Slight decrease in number of stools.

GU: Normal number of wet diapers.

All other systems were reviewed and are negative.

Physical examination:

Vitals: Afebrile. HR 123, RR 32, BP 90/55, length 59 cm.

General: NAD.

HEENT: NCAT. PERRL. Full range EOM. TMs are clear. Neck is supple without masses.

Chest: CTA. No wheezing or rhonchi.

CV: RRR.

Abd: Normal bowel sounds. Soft. Not distended. No organomegaly.

Ext: WNL.

Skin/Musculoskeletal: Benign.

Assessment/Plan: Will continue with Zantac with PO ad lib breastfeeding. Will check daily weight and monitor strict I/Os. Follow up with official ultrasound results.

Consider further imaging to determine etiology. Plan to check labs to assess lytes. May need IVs for extra fluids.

Discharge Summary

DIAGNOSES/PROBLEMS:

Gastroesophageal reflux.

PROCEDURES:

Ultrasound of abdomen UGI.

HISTORY, MAJOR FINDINGS, AND HOSPITAL COURSE:

39-wk GA, now 11-week-old male born via vaginal delivery to a mother with gestational diabetes was noted to have increased spitting up with feeds, fussiness, and arching behavior at his 2-month well child check. He was prescribed Zantac but did not start taking until about 1 week prior to admit. On the day of admit, he was seen by his PMD, who was concerned about inadequate weight gain and recommended further evaluation. His birth weight was 3.3 kg, and admit weight was 4.5 kg. Abdominal US showed a slightly elongated pylorus but adequate passing of feeds. A UGI study showed a large amount of gastroesophageal reflux. While in the hospital, the infant was observed to breastfeed well, about every 2 hours, without further significant emesis. The Zantac dose was maximized; addition of a PPI was recommended, and the patient was discharged to home.

Discharge medications: Zantac.

Discharge instructions: Call PMD if emesis becomes more forceful or more frequent, or if poor feeding develops.

Follow-up care: Schedule follow-up appointment with pediatrician.

Stomach/Pylorus

Indication: Vomiting. Evaluate for pyloric stenosis. Sonographic evaluation of the pylorus was performed.

Findings: The pylorus was identified and is normal in appearance. The muscular walls are normal in thickness measuring 2 mm each in the sagittal and coronal planes. The pyloric channel is minimally elongated, measuring 16 mm. Fluid is seen passing freely through the pyloric channel.

Impression: Minimally elongated pyloric channel measuring 16 mm in length. Otherwise unremarkable pylorus without evidence of obstruction or hypertrophy at this time. Given minimal elongation, it is possible that pyloric stenosis is developing. If symptoms persist, please repeat the ultrasound test.

Upper GI Series

Indication: Vomiting, question of gastric outlet obstruction.

Procedure: The patient swallowed 15 cc of thin barium without an adverse reaction. Multiple spot films were taken of the esophagus and stomach. An overhead film was taken.

Interpretation: Preliminary film of the abdomen shows air within distended stomach, small bowel, and colon. Multiple episodes of GE reflux were reported to the mid portion of the esophagus just above the carina. The stomach is horizontal in orientation, with the fundus lower in position than the body of the stomach. Prompt emptying from the stomach into the duodenum and the proximal jejunum was noted.

198

Minimal redundancy of the second and third portions of the duodenum was seen. The duodenum crosses the midline to the left side and reaches the level of the duodenal bulb. No dilatation of the proximal small bowel is noted.

Impression:

1. Marked GE reflux to the level of the carina.
2. Slight redundancy of the second and the third portions of the duodenum with no evidence of obstruction.

Progress Notes

DAY 1

The patient was admitted with FTT and vomiting. The infant is lying quietly asleep with IV in L arm. US shows minimally elongated pylorus. No obstruction. Physical examination is benign. Will get upper GI. Monitor VS, I/Os, weights, emesis, reflux precautions, and nutrition consult. GERD versus pyloric stenosis is most likely.

DAY 2

Infant admitted with history of vomiting and poor weight gain. Patient taking adequate PO overnight. Cause of FTT in this patient is likely extreme GERD. Afebrile with no acute issues.

DAY 3

Upper GI showed significant GERD. Otherwise normal anatomy. Infant has had some weight gain during hospital stay. Maximize Zantac dose, add Reglan. Discussed reflux precautions with Mom. Infant to be discharged home to care of parents.

CASE STUDY QUESTION

17-2a.   Admit diagnosis: _____

17-2b.   Discharge disposition: _____

17-2c.   Principal diagnosis: _____

17-2d.   Secondary diagnoses (indicate POA status for secondary diagnoses):

_____

_____

_____

_____

_____

_____

17-2e.   Principal procedure: _____

17-2f.   Secondary procedures: _____

_____

17-2g.   Assign MS-DRG: _____

17-2h.   Relative weight of MS-DRG: _____

17-2i.   Can this MS-DRG be optimized with the addition of a CC? Yes or No
          Can this MS-DRG be optimized with the addition of an MCC? Yes or No

17-2j.   Is there a main guideline pertinent to selection of the principal diagnosis in this case study?

_____

_____

17-2k.   Is there another diagnosis that meets the definition for principal diagnosis? Yes or No

17-2l.   If yes, what is the other diagnosis? _____

17-2m.   Is there any opportunity for physician query?

_____

_____

17-2n.   What is the drug Reglan used to treat? _____

17-3. CASE STUDY

History and Physical

CC: Abdominal pain.

HPI: The patient is a 48-year-old male with HIV (CD4 949 a couple of months ago) who was recently admitted with pancreatitis of unknown etiology. He was discharged home this afternoon. He states that when he got home, he started to experience severe abdominal pain that was much worse than the pain that he had experienced on initial presentation. He stated that he had not taken anything by mouth yet. He was instructed to proceed to the Emergency Room. The ED physician was notified of his arrival.

The patient states that he was feeling well when he left the hospital, and that about 90 minutes later, he started to have severe abdominal pain that responded poorly to PO pain meds. The pain is epigastric in location with some back pain, but no clear radiation. The pain is 7/10 in intensity. He also had some nausea, not vomiting, and gagging since the pain started. CT of the abdomen was done in the ER.

Past medical history includes the following:

1. History of HIV with CD4 count of 949 during his recent stay here. Of note, he has a history of splenectomy; thus, his CD4 count must be interpreted judiciously in that setting.
2. History of GERD.
3. Renal stone 15 years ago.
4. Hepatitis B S/P blood transfusion.
5. Status post splenectomy secondary to motor vehicle accident.
6. Depression.
7. Obstructive sleep apnea.
8. History of diabetes mellitus, well controlled.
9. History of recurrent candidiasis in the setting of earlier, poorly controlled diabetes.
10. Peripheral neuropathy.

11. Hypertension.
12. Hypercholesterolemia.

Allergies: The patient reports a history of an allergy to Augmentin and amoxicillin, both of which cause hives.

Medications: After his recent discharge, his medications included fluoxetine 40 mg by mouth every day, nystatin swish and swallow 500,000 units every 6 hours, lisinopril 40 mg by mouth every day, senna and Colace, amitriptyline 50 mg by mouth every day, Nexium 40 mg by mouth 2 times a day, metformin 1 g by mouth 2 times a day, Flexeril 10 mg by mouth 3 times a day as needed for pain, Dilaudid 2 mg by mouth every 4 hours as needed for pain, Phenergan 12.5 mg by mouth every 4 hours as needed for nausea, Reglan 10 mg by mouth as needed for pain, and Pravachol 10 mg by mouth every day.

His social history is notable for his being a one-pack-a-day smoker for the past 40 years. He rarely drinks alcohol. He reports that he was drinking a minimal amount prior to his most recent admission here. He occasionally uses marijuana.

REVIEW OF SYSTEMS:

Constitutional: No fever or chills.

Neuro: Positive for headache, light-headedness, and dizziness.

HEENT: No diplopia, sore throat, or lymphadenopathy.

CV: No chest pain.

Respiratory: No SOB.

GI: Abdominal pain with nausea. No vomiting, diarrhea, constipation, melena, BRBPR, reflux, or hematemesis.

GU: No dysuria or frequency.

Skin/Skeletal: No rashes or myalgias.

Physical examination:

Vitals: T 36.0, HR 98, BP 128/85.

General: NAD, resting comfortably. Received pain meds in the ER.

HEENT: NCAT, no oral thrush, EOMI. Erythematous macular rash on both cheeks. No adenopathy.

Chest: CTA bilaterally.

CV: RRR. 2/6 murmur right upper sternal border radiating to bilateral carotids.

Abd: Decreased BS. TTP mid upper abdomen. No rebound or guarding, no peritoneal signs.

Ext: No edema.

GU/Rectal: Deferred.

Neuro: A&O. CN II through XII intact. Gait normal.

Assessment/Plan: Clinically and by labs, presentation is consistent with pancreatitis. Imaging is worrisome for abscess formation. NPO for now with IVF. PPN tomorrow. Cover broadly with antibiotics. Elevated WBC—do blood cultures. Concern for development of possible SIRS/septic picture.

Discharge Summary

DIAGNOSES/PROBLEMS:

1. Pancreatitis.
2. Human immunodeficiency virus.

PROCEDURES:

None.

HISTORY, MAJOR FINDINGS, AND HOSPITAL COURSE:

This is a 48-year-old male with a history of HIV and CD4 count of 949 in the setting of a history of splenectomy, who was recently admitted to our service with a diagnosis of pancreatitis of unclear origin and was discharged home earlier on the day of admission, only to return with abdominal pain. Regarding his prior history, the patient reported that approximately 2 weeks prior to this admission, he had begun developing some intermittent sharp epigastric pain that was nonradiating and was not affected by meals. The patient was seen in multiple Emergency Rooms and by his primary care physician, as well as by a GI physician, and was given a diagnosis of potential gastritis in the setting of negative imaging, including CT scans and right upper quadrant ultrasound. On admission, he again presented with abdominal pain that was most severe; CT scan of the abdomen and pelvis revealed findings consistent with acute pancreatitis. His stay here was notable for an initially maintained NPO and for resolution of or improvement in his abdominal pain. He was also evaluated by the GI service, including by an EGD, and was noted to have some mild gastritis. At the time of his discharge, the patient was tolerating oral with minimal amount of discomfort. After returning home, he stated that he began to experience severe abdominal pain that was much worse than the pain he had experienced on initial presentation. He reported that he had not yet taken anything by mouth after the time of his discharge. He attempted to take oral pain medications without relief of the pain, which he graded as 7 out of 10 in intensity. It was associated with nausea, but not vomiting.

Past medical history includes the following:

1. History of HIV with CD4 count of 949 during his recent stay here. Of note, he has a history of splenectomy; thus, his CD4 count must be interpreted judiciously in that setting.
2. History of GERD.
3. Renal stone 15 years ago.
4. Hepatitis B.
5. Status post splenectomy secondary to motor vehicle accident.
6. Depression.
7. Obstructive sleep apnea.
8. History of diabetes mellitus, well controlled.
9. History of recurrent candidiasis in the setting of earlier, poorly controlled diabetes.
10. Peripheral neuropathy.
11. Hypertension.
12. Hypercholesterolemia.

Allergies: The patient reports a history of an allergy to Augmentin and amoxicillin, both of which cause hives.

Medications: After his recent discharge, medications included fluoxetine 40 mg by mouth every day, nystatin swish and swallow 500,000 units every 6 hours, lisinopril 40 mg by mouth every day, senna and Colace, amitriptyline 50 mg by mouth every day, Nexium 40 mg by mouth 2 times a day, metformin 1 g by mouth 2 times a day, Flexeril 10 mg by mouth 3 times a day as needed for pain, Dilaudid 2 mg by mouth every 4 hours as needed for pain, Phenergan 12.5 mg by mouth every 4 hours as needed for nausea, Reglan 10 mg by mouth as needed for pain, and Pravachol 10 mg by mouth every day.

His social history is notable for his being a one-pack-a-day smoker for the past 40 years. He rarely drinks alcohol. The patient reports that he was drinking a minimal amount prior to his most recent admission here. He occasionally uses marijuana.

Physical examination: On presentation here, the patient was afebrile at 36°. His heart rate was 98 and blood pressure 128/85; he was breathing comfortably and

202

saturating 96% on room air. He appeared initially comfortable on examination. His HEENT examination was notable for no oral lesions. JVP was flat. Lungs were clear to auscultation. Cardiovascular examination revealed 2 out of 6 systolic murmurs at the right upper sternal border that radiated to the carotid. His abdomen revealed decreased bowel sounds. The patient was tender to palpation in the mid upper abdomen, but with no rebound, guarding, or peritoneal signs. Extremities revealed no edema, and no skin lesions or joint involvement was noted.

Admission labs were notable for white count of 13.7, up from 9.7 on the morning of discharge; hemoglobin was 13.8 and platelets 446. His panel was notable for a bicarbonate of 20 and normal renal function with creatinine of 0.7. LFTs were within normal limits, but amylase was elevated at 93, lipase was 167, and lactate was 3.4.

CT of the abdomen and pelvis, performed on readmission here, revealed inflammation around the pancreas compatible with pancreatitis. Multiple, small, loculated-appearing fluid collections around the head and neck of the pancreas were ill-defined from the prior examination and were compatible with pseudocyst or abscess formation.

Hospital course: This is a 48-year-old gentleman with a history of HIV, who was recently admitted to our service in the setting of pancreatitis. He returns with a relapse in his symptoms and an increased white count, and CT scan shows progression of his pancreatitis findings.

1. GI. Admission lab data and clinical picture are consistent with finding of pancreatitis. Imaging reveals better definition of cyst formation, and potential abscess formation is a matter of concern. Given his history of pancreatitis, the patient was maintained strictly NPO, and supplemental parenteral nutrition was started. Additionally, given his prior diagnosis of mild gastritis, the patient was maintained on his 2 times a day PPI. With an elevated white count and findings on CT, the patient was initially maintained on Cipro and Flagyl in the setting of his penicillin allergy. Given rare reports of ACE-I–related pancreatitis, his lisinopril was held, and later his statin was held as well. When abdominal pain persisted and appeared refractory to initial conservative measurements, a GI consultation was called. At the request of consultants, an MRCP was performed that revealed normal proximal and distal pancreatic ducts with evidence of inflammatory collection measuring approximately 5 × 4 cm. The patient was given total bowel rest and after several days, he reported improvement in pain on the PCA. His narcotic needs were slowly weaned away. Repeat imaging revealed changes consistent with pancreatitis that had decreased in severity without evidence of necrosis. PCA was weaned, and diet was advanced. The patient was discharged to home on a full diet with instructions to return, should his pain reemerge. He was maintained off his ACE-I and statin on discharge, given no other clear precipitant for the pancreatitis, despite the rarity of these reactions. Reinitiation can be considered on an outpatient basis.
2. HIV. On his recent visit here, the patient was noted to have a CD4 count of 949 and a viral load of 52,000. He is currently off antiretroviral and has no clear indication for any prophylaxis at this time. His initiation of HMRT in this settlement is likely to be a function of alternative measure, rather than his CD4 count, given his history of splenectomy.

Discharge medications: Promethazine 25 mg PO q6h PRN nausea, amitriptyline 50 mg PO at bedtime, Fluoxetine 40 mg PO at bedtime, Flexeril 10 mg PO TID PRN pain; Dilaudid 2 mg PO every 4 to 6 hours as needed for pain, Metformin 1 g by mouth twice daily, and Nexium 40 mg by mouth daily.

DISCHARGE INSTRUCTIONS:

The patient was instructed to maintain a low-fat, low-residue, low-sugar, low-salt diet and to call his physician if he has any of the following problems: fevers, chills, abdominal pain, nausea, or vomiting.

Please follow up with your physician.

CT Abd with and Without Contrast with Pelvis

Clinical history: The patient has abdominal pain, and the study is done for evaluation. The study consists of dural phase imaging. On lung windows, no evidence of infiltrate is seen. The patient has evidence of multiple accessory spleens. The patient has acute pancreatitis and inflammation, particularly in the body and neck of the pancreas; peripancreatic inflammation is seen. Pseudocysts may be developing in the region of the body of the pancreas, where several zones are a bit small, but they do not enhance to any degree. However, they are present in the rest of the gland.

Very early pancreatic necrosis based on lack of glandular enhancement may be present. On venous phase imaging, a dilated pancreatic duct with glandular inflammation is again seen. No venous thrombosis is noted.

Impression: Acute pancreatitis is seen with what appears to be developing pseudocyst in the neck of the pancreas. Portal vein and SMV appear patent. SMA and celiac axis are unremarkable. No other findings of note were gathered in this study.

Progress Notes

DAY 1

Patient was discharged yesterday but returned shortly thereafter with severe epigastric pain and nausea. Repeat CT shows findings consistent with pseudocyst/abscess and pancreatitis. Lipase is elevated.

Impression: Pancreatitis with pseudocyst. Continue NPO, PPN, fluids, pain meds, and empiric antibiotic coverage. Check daily amylase/lipase.

DAY 2

Patient still complains of abdominal pain. States he is hungry. Abdomen is TTP in epigastrium on deep palpation. In setting of elevated WBC and lactic acidosis, we will continue antibiotic. DM is in good control. Uses CPAP for OSA. Cr is stable.

DAY 3

Abdominal pain has improved. Blood cultures are negative. PPN. May repeat CT. Consult GI.

DAY 4

Patient with signs and symptoms of acute pancreatitis. Patient had MRCP, which showed peripancreatic edema with a 5 × 4–cm area of body necrosis. Blood cultures are negative to date.

Impression: Acute necrotizing pancreatitis. HIV. Continue conservative management.

DAY 5

Patient has been pain-free for 24 hours. Will discontinue antibiotics. Advance diet.

DAY 6

Patient has tolerated feeds. Remains pain-free. Discharge today.

CASE STUDY QUESTIONS

17-3a. Admit diagnosis: _____

17-3b. Discharge disposition: _____

17-3c. Principal diagnosis: _____

17-3d. Secondary diagnoses (indicate POA status for secondary diagnoses):

_____

_____

_____

_____

_____

_____

17-3e. Principal procedure: _____

17-3f. Secondary procedures: _____

_____

17-3g. Assign MS-DRG: _____

17-3h. Relative weight of MS-DRG: _____

17-3i. Can this MS-DRG be optimized with the addition of a CC? Yes or No
Can this MS-DRG be optimized with the addition of an MCC? Yes or No

17-3j. Is there a main guideline pertinent to selection of the principal diagnosis in this case study?

_____

_____

17-3k. Is there another diagnosis that meets the definition for principal diagnosis? Yes or No

17-3l. If yes, what is the other diagnosis? _____

17-3m. Is there any opportunity for physician query?

_____

_____

17-3n. What is the drug Dilaudid used to treat? _____

Diseases of the Skin and Subcutaneous Tissue (ICD-10-CM Chapter 12, Codes L00-L99)

18

ABBREVIATIONS/ACRONYMS

Without the use of reference materials, define the following abbreviations or acronyms.

1. I&D _____

2. CEA _____

3. STSG _____

4. MS-DRG _____

5. FTSG _____

GLOSSARY DEFINITIONS

Match the glossary term to the correct definition.

1. _____ Stasis ulcer   A. Itching

2. _____ Furuncle   B. Hives

3. _____ Heterograft   C. Another name for skin

4. _____ Allograft   D. Graft from another species

5. _____ Decubitus ulcer   E. Dermatitis caused by something taken internally

6. _____ Integumentary   F. Bed sore

7. _____ Endogenous   G. A boil

8. _____ Urticaria   H. Ulcer associated with varicose veins

9. _____ Pruritus   I. Graft between individuals of the same species

10. _____ Homograft   J. Same as an allograft

CODING

Using the code book, code the following.

1. Malignant pemphigus   _____

2. Dermatitis due to jewelry, patient is allergic to metal   _____

3. Severe sunburn of the face   _____

4. Infected pilonidal cyst   _____

5. Pityriasis rosea   _____

6. Toxic epidermal necrolysis   _____

7. Lichen urticatus   _____

8. Hirsutism   _____

9. Vitiligo   _____

10. Cicatrix   _____

11. Comedo   _____

12. Stage III decubitus ulcer of the sacrum with   _____
    osteomyelitis

13. Rosacea   _____

14. Felon of the right finger   _____

15. Staph cellulitis of the left hand   _____

CASE SCENARIOS

Using the code book, code the following cases.

1. Patient presents to the ER with severe dermatitis. History reveals that patient was being treated for scabies. The patient had been treated with Elimite, which is the cause of dermatitis.

   _____

   _____

2. A child presents to the pediatrician with a crusty, itchy rash. The diagnosis is impetigo of the legs.

   _____

   _____

3. A heroin addict presents with cellulitis to the right toe caused by needlesticks.

   _____

   _____

4. A patient presents to the hospital for removal of keloid of right forearm.

   _____

   _____

5. A patient is admitted to the hospital for hidradenitis suppurativa in the right axillary area. The surgeon removes the sweat glands.

   _____

   _____

6. Patient was admitted because of the development of blistering and erosion of skin and mucous membranes. About 5 days ago, the patient had fever, sore throat, and headache and was thought to have influenza. The patient was diagnosed with Stevens-Johnson syndrome.

   _____

   _____

7. Patient was admitted for colostomy because of stage II sacral and stage III buttock pressure ulcer. A temporary percutaneous colostomy of the sigmoid colon is performed to allow better healing of the ulcers. Patient is paraplegic due to previous spinal cord injury as a result of a MUA.

_____

_____

8. Patient was admitted for further testing and investigation of an autoimmune condition. Results of various tests indicate that this patient most likely has scleroderma.

_____

_____

9. A 10-month-old infant was admitted with swelling of the glands in the neck. Siblings have recently been treated for strep throat. The child has not been eating well and has been running a fever.

Impression: Acute lymphadenitis likely due to strep.

_____

_____

CASE STUDIES

Using the code book, code and answer questions about the following case studies.

18-1. CASE STUDY

History and Physical

CC: Erythema legs.

HPI: The patient is a 51-year-old gentleman with medical history notable for severe eczema for the past 30 years, as well as prior superinfection of his eczema, presented to the hospital with 3 days of bilateral lower extremity pain. During the 3 days prior to admission, his eczema had flared up per his report, with redness extending bilaterally to the shin and excessive drainage and fissuring of the skin. He denied fevers and chills but noted severe pain that limited his ability to ambulate. He also had swelling of his right eye, such that he could not open it any longer. He has had eczema in this area of his face as well in the past. He presented to the clinic prior to hospitalization and was treated with prednisone. He reported that his eye swelling improved, but his legs worsened, at which point he presented to the Emergency Room. He was admitted for further evaluation and treatment with antibiotics.

Past medical history: As noted above, including severe eczema for the past 30 years. He has had prior superinfection of the affected region. He also has a history of scoliosis, tinnitus, head trauma, splenectomy, and alcoholism.

Past surgical history: Splenectomy.

Social history: Notable for active tobacco abuse. He smokes one-half to one pack per day and has done so for the past 40 years. He is a prior alcoholic but reports now that he drinks only occasionally; he had his last drink 1 day prior to admission. He also has a history of prior cocaine and heroin abuse, but his urine tox screen was negative on admission. He is homeless and has lived in a halfway shelter before. His family includes 3 children and 1 nephew. He usually works doing home improvements when he can find work.

Family history: Notable for heart disease in his parents, asthma in his mother, and an unspecified type of cancer in his father.

Medications: Prednisone 10 mg daily, Benadryl as needed, and a daily multivitamin.

Allergies: He has an allergy to penicillin but is able to tolerate Keflex.

REVIEW OF SYSTEMS:

Constitutional: No fever or chills.

Neuro: No headache or seizures. No dizziness.

HEENT: Denies any visual changes.

CV: No chest pain.

Respiratory: No SOB or cough.

GI: No GI symptoms.

GU: Benign.

Skin/Skeletal: See HPI.

PHYSICAL EXAMINATION:

Vitals: T 98.7, HR 75, BP 113/62, RR 16, and SaO_2 99%.

General: Lying in bed. NAD.

HEENT: Mild conjunctival erythema. Right eyelid is swollen. MMM. Oropharynx clear. No pain with eye movement. No photophobia. Neck is supple without masses.

Chest: CTA bilaterally.

CV: RRR.

Abd: Normal BS, soft. No masses or organomegaly.

Ext: Prominent bilateral inguinal node lymphadenopathy.

GU/Rectal: Deferred.

Skin/Musculoskeletal: Both legs with cracks, scabbing, erythema, and edema of feet. The skin is peeling with a blister on the right foot.

Neuro: A&O ×3.

Orbital CT with contrast showed mild inflammation around the right orbit compatible with periorbital cellulitis and no evidence of abscess. Mucoperiosteal thickening of the ethmoid air cell compatible with chronic sinusitis was also noted.

Assessment/Plan: Patient with likely superficial infection of lower extremities. Appears more like impetigo on top of eczema. Hydration and Dermatology consult ordered.

Inpatient Dermatology Consultation Note

Chief complaint: Bad eczema.

History of present illness: A 51-year-old Caucasian male with a long-standing history of eczema without recent treatments who is having a severe flare with superinfection. Gram-positive cocci were noted in the bloodstream, and he had been started on ceftriaxone and vancomycin. The patient stated that his eczema is usually confined to the hands, feet, and face, but over the past week, he also developed a flare in areas of the back, arms, legs, and around the belly button, which was extremely pruritic.

Family history was positive for atopy. He received a recent prednisone taper and had some mild improvement. He is currently homeless.

Past medical history: Rhinitis, eczema, and splenectomy.

Family history: Atopy.

Social history: As above.

Medications: Benadryl, ceftriaxone, vancomycin, and oxazepam.

Allergies: Penicillin.

Laboratory results: White count of 11.9 and platelets of 471.

Review of systems: Itch; otherwise benign.

Major findings: A well-developed, well-nourished Caucasian male who is thin, awake, alert, and oriented ×3 in a pleasant, calm mood. Temperature 36.8°.

Complete skin examination, including scalp, face, neck, chest, back, abdomen, buttocks, and bilateral upper and lower extremities, including palms, toes, and nails, was significant for the following: erythematous lichenified plaques in the periorbital region, right greater than left, with mild bulbar injection; evidence of deep-seated old palmar vesicles; denuded plaques at dorsal feet and shins with overlying scaling and crust; discrete pinpoint excoriated erythematous papules around the umbilicus, on the arms and the back, and on the thighs.

Assessment: Atopic dermatitis with impetiginization; scabies.

Plan: The patient had superinfected atopic dermatitis. However, the new rash described last week in the web space of the fingers and umbilicus suggested concurrent scabies infection. We recommend Alomide cream from the neck down nightly and washing of the clothes and sheets in the morning with repetition in 1 week. Also, recommend treating his bedmate. After the first treatment, he can begin triamcinolone 0.1% cream 2 times a day as needed to the face, arms, and legs, transitioning to plain moisturizers. We suggested Atarax 25 mg by mouth nightly as needed to help sleep through the night. In addition, he can perform general wash to debride some of the crusted areas on the feet, along with continued oral antibiotics to treat his superinfection and appropriate foot care. I asked the patient to follow up in the Dermatology Clinic in 1 month for reassessment.

Discharge Summary

DIAGNOSES/PROBLEMS:

1. Impetigo this admission.
2. Eczema.
3. Preseptal cellulitis.
4. Scoliosis.
5. History of head trauma.
6. History of splenectomy due to traumatic injury.
7. History of tinnitus.

PROCEDURES:

1. PA and lateral chest x-ray showed minimal hyperinflation and minimal spondylosis of the thoracic spine with no other abnormalities and a normal cardiac silhouette.
2. Orbital CT with contrast showed mild inflammation around the right orbit compatible with periorbital cellulitis and no evidence of abscess. Mucoperiosteal thickening of the ethmoid air cell compatible with chronic sinusitis was also noted.

HISTORY, MAJOR FINDINGS, AND HOSPITAL COURSE:

The patient is a 51-year-old gentleman with medical history notable for severe eczema for the past 30 years, as well as prior superinfection of his eczema; he presented to the hospital with 3 days of bilateral lower extremity pain. During the 3 days prior to admission, his eczema had flared up per his report, with redness extending bilaterally to the shin and excessive drainage and fissuring of the skin. He denied fevers and chills but noted severe pain that limited his ability to ambulate. He also had swelling of his right eye, such that he could not open it any longer. He has had eczema in this area of his face in the past. He presented to the clinic prior to hospitalization and was treated with prednisone. He reported that his eye swelling improved, but his legs worsened, at which point he presented to the Emergency Room. His triage vital signs were as follows: Temperature 98.2 degrees, pulse 118 beats per minute, pressure 142/86 mm Hg, and respiratory rate 18. He received clindamycin 600 mg intravenous, as well as Tylenol and Benadryl, and was admitted for further evaluation.

Past medical history is as noted above, including severe eczema for the past 30 years. He has had prior superinfection of the affected region. He also has a history of scoliosis, tinnitus, head trauma, splenectomy, and alcoholism. He has an allergy to penicillin but is able to tolerate Keflex. On admission, the medication he was taking included prednisone 10 mg daily, as well as Benadryl as needed, and a daily multivitamin.

Social history is notable for active tobacco abuse. He smokes one-half to one pack per day and has done so for the past 40 years. He is a prior alcoholic but reports now that he drinks only occasionally; he had his last drink 1 day prior to admission. He also has a history of prior cocaine and heroin abuse, but his urine tox screen was negative on admission. He is homeless and has lived in a halfway shelter before. His family includes 3 children and 1 nephew. He usually worked doing home improvements when he could find work.

Family history is notable for heart disease in his parents, asthma in his mother, and an unspecified type of cancer in his father.

On admission physical examination, his temperature was 98.7° with heart rate 79, blood pressure 113/62 mm Hg, respiratory rate 16, and oxygen saturation 99% on room air. He appeared comfortable but did have prominent swelling around his right eye. Examination of his eye was otherwise unremarkable. No purulent discharge, no scleral abnormalities, and no difficulty with extraocular movement were noted. Neck examination was unremarkable. On auscultation of his chest, the lungs were clear to auscultation bilaterally, and heart rate and rhythm were regular. No murmurs, rubs, or gallops were detected. Abdominal examination was normal. Examination of his extremities revealed bilateral erythema with the demarcation just below his knees and significant fissuring and cracking consistent with eczema. Severe tenderness to palpation was observed over his extremities. Neurologic examination was nonfocal.

Admission laboratory results were notable for a white blood cell count of 19.6 with differential showing 77% neutrophils. For the rest of his laboratory results, please see EPR. EKG on admission showed normal sinus rhythm with left ventricular hypertrophy and nonspecific T-wave inversions in V1 and V2. Chest x-ray on admission is reported earlier.

Summary of hospitalization: The patient had superinfection of his eczema. His cellulitis was treated with ciprofloxacin and clindamycin intravenous. His antibiotics were continued until day 3 of hospitalization, at which time ciprofloxacin was discontinued and clindamycin was changed from intravenous to oral. Given the severity of his disease, Dermatology was consulted. They gave him a diagnosis of atopic dermatitis with impetiginization, as well as scabies. They recommended treatment with Elimite cream for scabies. They also recommended triamcinolone 0.1% cream 2 times daily as needed to the face, arms, and legs. Atarax was added to help with itching as needed.

Given that the patient was unable to ambulate because of pain produced by the severe atopic dermatitis, Social Work was consulted and made arrangements for the patient to stay at a center for the homeless. He was discharged to this facility and received an influenza vaccination prior to discharge.

Discharge medications: Clindamycin 300 mg by mouth 3 times a day, Atarax 25 mg at bedtime as needed for itching, triamcinolone cream 0.1% 2 times a day, Benadryl

25 mg every 4 to 6 hours as needed for itching, and vitamin A and D ointment to be applied to the affected areas.

DISCHARGE INSTRUCTIONS:

The patient was discharged to a center for the homeless with instructions to resume normal activity as tolerated and a normal diet.

FOLLOW-UP CARE:

The patient is going to follow up with Dermatology.

WOUND CARE SPECIALIST:

Asked to see patient for superinfected eczema. Patient was evaluated by Dermatology yesterday and was given a diagnosis of scabies. The patient's care is complicated by homelessness. His feet and lower legs have erythema and dry flaking skin. No necrotic or debrideable tissue is evident; therefore, no wound care modalities other than whirlpool are appropriate. He should continue the creams and ointments prescribed by Dermatology. He may use a petrolatum preparation like vitamin A and D ointment to the feet and legs to soften the flaking skin.

Progress Notes

DAY 1

The patient has no complaints. Lesions on lower extremities and right face are erythematous and weepy. Continue Vanco. Not orbital but preseptal cellulitis. Watch for alcohol withdrawal. Patient is being treated with Serax.

DAY 2

Still has some pain in legs from superinfected eczema with impetigo and preseptal cellulitis. Edema is slightly better. Appreciate Dermatology consult and recommendations. Taper Serax.

DAY 3

Homeless man with bad eczema and superinfection. Was also treated for dehydration. Still has some itching, otherwise no complaints. Patient also has scabies infestation, which is being treated.

DAY 4

Patient's preseptal cellulitis and lower extremity eczema and impetigo are much improved. Patient is being discharged to a center for the homeless to facilitate better care of skin condition.

CASE STUDY QUESTIONS

18-1a. Admit diagnosis: _____

18-1b. Discharge disposition: _____

18-1c. Principal diagnosis: _____

18-1d. Secondary diagnoses (indicate POA status for secondary diagnoses):

_____

_____

_____

_____

_____

_____

18-1e. Principal procedure: _____

18-1f. Secondary procedures: _____

_____

18-1g. Assign MS-DRG: _____

18-1h. Relative weight of MS-DRG: _____

18-1i. Can this MS-DRG be optimized with the addition of a CC? Yes or No
       Can this MS-DRG be optimized with the addition of an MCC? Yes or No

18-1j. Is there a main guideline pertinent to selection of the principal diagnosis in this case study?

_____

_____

18-1k. Is there another diagnosis that meets the definition for principal diagnosis? Yes or No

18-1l. If yes, what is the other diagnosis? _____

18-1m. Is there any opportunity for physician query?

_____

_____

18-1n. What is the drug Serax used to treat? _____

18-2. CASE STUDY

History and Physical

CC: Chronic foot ulcer.

HPI: The patient is a 69-year-old male who presents with a small right foot ulcer just below the large right metatarsal. There is no history of trauma. Denies fever or chills.

Past medical history: Hypercholesterolemia and hypertension.

Social history: The patient does not smoke, drink, or use drugs. The patient lives with his wife.

Family history: Both parents died of old age.

Medications: Lipitor 10 mg by mouth at bedtime, aspirin 81 mg by mouth every day, lisinopril 10 mg by mouth every day, and gemfibrozil 600 mg by mouth 2 times a day.

Allergies: No known drug allergies.

Review of systems:

Constitutional: No fevers, chills, or night sweats. No heat or cold intolerance.

Neuro: No headache, seizures, light-headedness, dizziness, or weakness.

HEENT: No visual changes. No sore throat.

CV: No chest pain or palpitations.

Respiratory: No SOB, wheezing, sputum production, or hemoptysis. Has a dry cough.

GI: No reflux, hematemesis, abdominal pain, N/V/D/C.

GU: No dysuria or frequency.

Skin/Skeletal: Chronic ulcer. Denies severe foot pain.

Physical examination:

Vitals: T 37.5, HR 90, BP 135/74, RR 20.

General: NAD.

HEENT: NC/AT. PERRL. EOMI. Sclera anicteric. MMM. Oropharynx clear.

Chest: CTA. No crackles, rales, or rhonchi.

CV: RRR.

Abd: Normal bowel sounds. Soft. Nontender, nondistended. No organomegaly.

Ext: No calf tenderness. 2 × 2–cm ulcer of right foot with surrounding cellulitis.

GU/Rectal: Not done.

Neuro: Alert and oriented ×3. Gait is normal.

X-ray of foot shows a small amount of air in the soft tissues medial to the proximal phalanx of the great toe, consistent with abscess. No radiographic evidence of osteomyelitis.

Assessment/Plan: Admit patient for treatment of ulcer and associated cellulitis of right foot. Check UA for proteinuria. Continue lisinopril for HTN. Regular diet. Investigate microcytic anemia.

Discharge Summary

1. Foot ulcer.
2. Mixed hypercholesterolemia (total cholesterol 199, triglycerides 403, HDL 42).
3. Erythromicrocytosis likely secondary to beta- or alpha-thalassemia minor.
4. Possible vitamin B_{12} deficiency.
5. Hypertension.

PROCEDURES:

1. Chest x-ray.
2. Electrocardiogram.
3. Excisional wound debridement and culture.

History, Major Findings, and Hospital Course:

The patient is a 69-year-old male who presents with a small right foot ulcer just below the large right metatarsal. The patient was afebrile on admission. The patient underwent bedside debridement by general surgery. The patient was seen by the wound care specialist, who recommended daily soap and water cleansing in the shower, as well as a gauze and Hydrogel dressing during the day.

Social history: The patient does not smoke, drink, or use drugs. The patient lives with his wife.

Family history: Both parents died of old age.

Medications: Lipitor 10 mg by mouth at bedtime, aspirin 81 mg by mouth every day, lisinopril 10 mg by mouth every day, and gemfibrozil 600 mg by mouth 2 times a day.

Allergies: No known drug allergies.

Physical examination: The patient's temperature on admission was 37.5 degrees, heart rate was 90 beats per minute, blood pressure was 146/84, and respiratory rate was 20.

Pertinent physical examination findings: A 2×2–cm ulcer on the right plantar aspect of the first metatarsal with surrounding erythema. No evidence of heat or erythema more proximally.

Laboratory data: WBC was 5.5, hematocrit was 42.8, MCV was 72, and platelets were 237,000. Vitamin B_{12} was 243. Ferritin was 372. Blood cultures, 3 times, were negative.

Hospital Course by Symptoms:

Infectious disease: Right foot ulcer. The patient was started on Zosyn and was discharged on ciprofloxacin to complete a 14-day course of antibiotic therapy. In addition, the patient was told how to clean the wound and to use Hydrogel dressing. The patient will follow up with Podiatry in 1 week.

The patient was found to have significant hypertriglyceridemia of 403. His LDL could not be calculated, but he reports hypercholesterolemia in the past. The patient's Lipitor was increased to 40 mg daily, and he was started on gemfibrozil 600 mg by mouth 2 times a day.

Cardiovascular: The patient has a history of hypertension and was normotensive on this admission with lisinopril 10 mg by mouth daily.

Hematology: The patient has erythromicrocytosis without anemia. Thalassemia screen was ordered. The patient was found to have a borderline low vitamin B_{12} level and thus was started on supplementation.

Discharge medications: Aspirin 81 mg by mouth every day, lisinopril 10 mg by mouth every day, Lipitor 40 mg by mouth at bedtime, gemfibrozil 600 mg by mouth 2 times a day, vitamin B_{12} 2000 mcg by mouth every day ×7 days followed by 1000 mcg by mouth every day thereafter, and ciprofloxacin 500 mg by mouth 2 times a day to complete a 14-day course.

Follow-up Care:

The patient has a follow-up appointment with a podiatrist.

Wound Care Specialist:

Appreciate consult to evaluate patient with right great toe wounds. Patient was debrided by surgery at the bedside (unroofed), but he required further debridement today because purulent drainage was evident under the loose callus. I unroofed the entire plantar toe to reveal two more broken areas with necrotic bases. I was unable to probe to bone. The patient had a medial toe wound measuring 1.2 × 1.5 × 0 cm with a clean pink base. The medial aspect of the plantar surface had a 0.5 × 0.7 × 0.2 cm wound, and the plantar aspect had a wound that measured 0.7 × 1.4 × 0.2 cm at both necrotic bases. Periwound skin was macerated. The patient will need close follow-up with Podiatry.

Recommendations:

1. Right foot: Patient may shower and clean toe with soap and water, dry well. Apply Vaseline to skin around the open areas, apply gauze strip that has been "mushed up" with Hydrogel to open areas, cover all with dry gauze, and secure to foot with wrap or tape daily.
2. Follow up with Podiatry. Need toe off-loading device in foot.

Final Report

Ankle brachial indices:

History: Right great toe ulcer.

Procedure description: ABI.

Impression: Bilateral ABI testing reveals normal arterial perfusion at rest based on ankle pressure criteria and Doppler waveform analysis.

Procedure data: Ankle brachial indices:

Indications: Athero w/ulceration.

ABI/TBI

Brach	Right	Left
PTA	126	106
DPA	120	130
ABI	1.03	1.05

Progress Notes

DAY 1

Patient presented with ulcer/cellulitis of right foot. MRI may be needed to rule out osteo. Continue medications for HTN and hypercholesterolemia. Blood cultures are pending.

DAY 2

Patient admitted for ulcer care and antibiotics. Right foot ulcer was debrided at bedside. Patient feels well. No fevers. ABI done, report pending.

DAY 3

Patient is much improved and is ready for discharge.

CASE STUDY QUESTIONS

18-2a. Admit diagnosis: _____

18-2b. Discharge disposition: _____

18-2c. Principal diagnosis: _____

217

18-2d. Secondary diagnoses (indicate POA status for secondary diagnoses):

_____

_____

_____

_____

_____

_____

18-2e. Principal procedure: _____

18-2f. Secondary procedures: _____

_____

18-2g. Assign MS-DRG: _____

18-2h. Relative weight of MS-DRG: _____

18-2i. Can this MS-DRG be optimized with the addition of a CC? Yes or No
        Can this MS-DRG be optimized with the addition of an MCC? Yes or No

18-2j. Is there a main guideline pertinent to selection of the principal diagnosis in this
case study?

_____

_____

18-2k. Is there another diagnosis that meets the definition for principal diagnosis? Yes or No

18-2l. If yes, what is the other diagnosis? _____

18-2m. Is there any opportunity for physician query?

_____

_____

18-2n. What is the drug gemfibrozil used to treat? _____

Diseases of the Musculoskeletal System and Connective Tissue (ICD-10-CM Chapter 13, Codes M00-M99)

19

ABBREVIATIONS/ACRONYMS

Without the use of reference materials, define the following abbreviations or acronyms.

1. SLE _____
2. MRI _____
3. OA _____
4. JRA _____
5. NSAIDs _____
6. RA _____
7. DJD _____
8. DEXA _____
9. PMR _____
10. PV _____

GLOSSARY DEFINITIONS

Match the glossary term to the correct definition.

1. _____ Scoliosis
2. _____ Anterior
3. _____ Fibromyalgia
4. _____ Pathologic fracture
5. _____ Myelopathy
6. _____ Radiculopathy
7. _____ Distal
8. _____ Spondylosis
9. _____ Spinal fusion
10. _____ Kyphosis
11. _____ Osteoarthritis
12. _____ Proximal
13. _____ Percutaneous vertebroplasty
14. _____ Arthropathy

A. Break in a bone that occurs because of underlying disorders that weaken the bone, including malignancy, benign bone tumors, metabolic disorders, infection, and osteoporosis

B. Compression of the spinal cord

C. Disease that affects the joints

D. Farther from the median plane; often is used to describe a location in the limbs

E. Metabolic bone disorder that results in decreased bone mass and density

F. Type of arthritis that develops as the result of wear and tear on the joints

G. Lateral or sideways curvature of the spine

H. Compression of a nerve root

I. Another term for spinal osteoarthritis

J. Describes the front of the body or an organ

Continued

15. _____ Spinal stenosis

16. _____ Necrotizing fasciitis

17. _____ Rheumatoid arthritis

18. _____ Osteoporosis

19. _____ Posterior

K. Technique by which an acrylic cement is injected into a collapsed or weakened vertebra under x-ray guidance to reduce pain caused by compression fractures

L. One of the most common diseases affecting the muscles; characterized by widespread muscle pain associated with chronic fatigue

M. Relates to the back of the body or an organ

N. Excessive posterior curvature of the thoracic spine that may not be detected until a hump in the upper back is noticeable

O. Rare but serious condition in which an infection occurs in the tissues below the skin, or "flesh-eating disease"

P. Closer to the median plane

Q. Chronic, inflammatory, systemic disease that affects the joints, often causing deformity

R. Narrowing of the central spinal canal or the areas of the spine where the nerve roots exit

S. Creation of a solid bone bridge between two or more adjacent vertebrae to provide stability between levels of the spine

CODING

Using the code book, code the following.

1. Septic left knee joint due to *Staphylococcus aureus*   _____

2. Hunchback   _____

3. Recurrent dislocation of right shoulder; reduction of dislocation   _____

4. Chronic osteomyelitis of the sacrum; closed biopsy of sacrum   _____

5. Healing pathologic fracture of right hip   _____

6. Patient admitted for rod-lengthening procedure; patient has progressive infantile idiopathic scoliosis of the thoracic spine   _____

7. Sciatica due to herniated disc at L5-S1   _____

8. Avascular necrosis of right shoulder joint due to long-term steroid use for rheumatoid arthritis   _____

9. Chondrocalcinosis of right knee   _____

10. Acute osteomyelitis of the left calcaneus in a patient with a decubitus ulcer left heel and a diabetic foot due to peripheral vascular disease   _____

11. Lumbar radiculitis   _____

12. Steroid-induced osteoporosis; patient takes prednisone for polymyalgia rheumatica   _____

13. Loose body elbow joint, right   _____

14. Pathologic fracture of right rib due to metastatic breast _____
carcinoma; this female patient is continuing to undergo
chemotherapy treatment

15. Osteoarthritis of right knee; total knee replacement _____

CASE SCENARIOS

Using the code book, code the following cases.

1. A pediatric patient was admitted with a pathologic fracture of the proximal right humerus. Radiographic evidence suggests that the fracture was caused by a unicameral bone cyst. An orthopedic consult was obtained to see whether this should be treated surgically. It was decided to treat conservatively and monitor healing with serial x-rays.
Final Diagnosis: Unicameral bone cyst proximal right humerus with pathologic fracture.

_____

_____

2. This 54-year-old gentleman with chronic arm and neck pain was admitted for spinal fusion. The patient's preoperative and postoperative diagnosis is cervical spondylosis with cervical radiculopathy of C6-7. A herniated disc is noted at C6-7. The patient takes medications for hypertension, hypercholesterolemia, and anxiety. The patient underwent anterior cervical discectomy and fusion with allograft bone and anterior cervical locking plates and screws.
Discharge Diagnoses: Cervical spondylosis with C6-7 radiculopathy.
               Herniated disc.
               Hypertension.
               Hypercholesterolemia.
               Anxiety.
Procedures: Anterior cervical discectomy with C6-7 spinal fusion.

_____

_____

3. The patient was admitted with disc herniation at L4-5. The patient has failed conservative treatments such as physical therapy. NSAIDs and even steroid injections did not provide much relief. The patient was taken to surgery, and a discectomy was performed. The patient recovered uneventfully and was discharged. Instructions were given to avoid lifting anything over 10 pounds until after the postoperative clinic visit.
Final Diagnosis: Herniated disc.
Procedure: Discectomy.

_____

_____

4. The patient has a history of ESRD due to diabetic nephropathy and is on dialysis M-W-F. She has been having increased back pain. There is extreme tenderness to palpation over the low back. X-rays were suspicious for osteomyelitis, and a bone scan confirmed acute osteomyelitis of the lumbar vertebra. A percutaneous bone biopsy was done, and cultures were taken. The patient will have to be treated with 6 to 8 weeks of IV antibiotics. Prior to discharge, the patient had a PICC line inserted. The patient was continued on medications for hypertension and takes insulin for her diabetes, renal osteodystrophy, and secondary hyperparathyroidism.
Final Diagnosis: Acute osteomyelitis of lumbar vertebra due to *Staphylococcus aureus*.
Procedures: Percutaneous needle biopsy of lumbar vertebra.
               Hemodialysis.

_____

_____

221

5. The patient has been bothered with shoulder pain for a long time and was diagnosed with a rotator cuff tear. Physical therapy worked for a while, but recently the patient has experienced weakness and limited motion in his right arm. The patient has a medical history of an embolic stroke 3 years ago and an ablation procedure for atrial fibrillation that initially resulted in resolution, but the atrial fibrillation has recurred. He has diabetic retinopathy.
   Final Diagnoses: Weakness of right arm due to rotator cuff tear.
                 Atrial fibrillation.
                 Diabetic retinopathy, type II.
                 History of stroke.
   Procedure: Repair of right rotator cuff tear.

   _____

   _____

6. The patient was admitted for a knee replacement. He was in an MVA many years ago with dislocation/fracture of the right knee joint. His condition has worsened because of the corticosteroids that he takes for his Crohn's disease. The patient's only complication during his stay was hyperglycemia due to steroid use. The patient had a total knee replacement. He was seen by the physical therapist prior to discharge to inpatient rehabilitation.
   Final Diagnoses: Traumatic arthritis of right knee.
                 Crohn's disease (ileocolitis).
                 Hyperglycemia.
   Procedure: Total right knee arthroplasty.

   _____

   _____

7. This elderly woman has been bothered by chronic back pain that has been getting progressively worse. X-rays confirmed the presence of compression fractures from T8-T10. The patient has steroid-dependent asthma and has developed severe osteoporosis caused by the steroids. She also complains of constipation, most likely related to her pain medications (narcotics). The patient was seen by the interventional radiologist, and a percutaneous vertebroplasty was performed. She recovered with no complications.
   Final Diagnoses: Compression fractures T8-T10 due to steroid-induced osteoporosis.
                 Constipation.
                 Steroid-dependent asthma, inhaled steroids.
   Procedure: Percutaneous vertebroplasty.

   _____

   _____

8. The patient was admitted to the hospital because of severe left hip pain that is often worse during the night. X-rays of the hip were taken in the ER. A preliminary report showed that the patient possibly had Paget's disease, which was responsible for the patient's pain. Alkaline phosphatase was elevated, and a bone scan was done to determine the extent of the disease. The patient's other medical conditions include stable angina, coronary artery disease with stent placement, and a history of kidney stones.

Final Diagnoses: Severe hip pain due to Paget's disease.
　　　　　　　 Stable angina.
　　　　　　　 Coronary artery disease.
　　　　　　　 History of kidney stones.

_____

_____

9. The patient was admitted from the ER for chest pain, to rule out MI. The patient also had some difficulty breathing and pain when taking a deep breath. The patient does have a family history of ischemic heart disease and is positive for the following cardiac risk factors: male gender, over age 65, hypertension, smoker, and overweight. After evaluation and monitoring, an MI was ruled out. Cardiology thought the most likely cause for his chest pain was costochondritis.

Final Diagnoses: Chest pain due to costochondritis.
　　　　　　　 Hypertension.
　　　　　　　 Smoker, current nicotine dependence on cigarettes.
　　　　　　　 Overweight.
　　　　　　　 Family history of ischemic heart disease.

_____

_____

CASE STUDIES

Using the code book, code and answer questions about the following case studies.

19-1. CASE STUDY

History and Physical

CC: Ulceration of left foot.

HPI: The patient has a history of peripheral neuropathy and has had previous surgical intervention applied to the foot bilaterally, including transmetatarsal amputation on the right and previous first and second toe amputations on the left. The patient states that he noticed an ulceration in the region over 3 weeks ago and has tried to treat it conservatively with local ulcer care. The patient was admitted to the Emergency Room with an infected ulceration to the region. X-ray shows changes to the third metatarsal head that are suspicious for osteomyelitis. The patient will be admitted for IV antibiotics.

Past medical history: See HPI. The patient has CRI and HTN. The patient has a history of asthma in childhood but has had no attacks for many years.

Past surgical history: Right metatarsal amputation and left first and second metatarsal amputations.

Allergies: NKDA.

Social history: The patient works as a forklift operator. Married with two kids. Drinks 6 beers on the weekends. No tobacco. No drugs.

ROS: The patient denies any fevers, chills, or night sweats. No change in weight. Good appetite. No headaches, seizures, or dizziness. He has no visual changes or hearing loss. No chest pain, palpitations, orthopnea, PND, or edema. No cough, wheezing, or sputum production. The patient reports occasional heartburn, but no nausea, vomiting, or diarrhea. No dysuria, nocturia, or frequency. No skin rashes.

PHYSICAL EXAMINATION:

General: NAD. Has some pain in the left foot.

HEENT: PERRLA. EOMI. Moist mucous membranes. Neck is supple. Trachea is midline.

Chest: Clear to auscultation bilaterally.

CV: RRR, S1 and S2 normal. No murmurs, rubs, or gallops.

Abd: Positive bowel sounds. No hepatosplenomegaly.

Ext: Large ulcer on the left foot. Metatarsal amputation on left and right feet.

Neuro: Intact.

A/P: Patient will be admitted for IV antibiotics for possible osteomyelitis. Podiatry consult will be obtained. MRI will be obtained.

Podiatry Consult

Reason for consultation: Ulceration of left foot.

History of present illness: The patient has a history of peripheral neuropathy and has undergone previous surgical intervention to the foot bilaterally, including transmetatarsal amputation on the right and previous first and second right amputations on the left. The patient states that he noticed an ulceration to the region over 3 weeks ago and has tried to treat it conservatively with local ulcer care. The patient was admitted to the Emergency Room with an infected ulceration to the region. X-ray shows changes to the third metatarsal head that are suspicious for osteomyelitis. The patient at this time has no acute fevers, chills, or night sweats and has been started on intravenous antibiotics.

Past family and social history: See record.

Past medical problems: See record.

Review of systems: See record.

Physical examination: The patient's vascular status shows weakly palpable pulses. The patient underwent vascular testing, which shows adequate flow to the extremities bilaterally. The patient has no acute ischemia to the remaining digits of the left forefoot. The patient's neurologic evaluation shows decreased sharp, dull, and light touch sensation. The patient has reduced plantar sensation bilaterally with a monofilament. The patient's reflexes are diminished, and the patient does have occasional paresthesias distally bilaterally. The patient's range of motion shows adequate ankle and subtalar joint motion on the right. The patient has adequate ankle, subtalar joint, and midfoot range of motion on the left. The patient has a previous transmetatarsal amputation on the right and a previous first and second ray amputation on the left with prominent metatarsal heads three through five and obvious hammertoe contractures of the lesser digits of the left foot. The patient's dermatologic evaluation shows that the patient has a Wagner grade 2 ulceration measuring approximately 3 × 3.5 cm. The patient has a fibrotic and necrotic base to the area with slightly devitalized tissue and some malodor. The patient at this time has no acute cellulitis. No purulence is seen coming from the wound, and it is most likely that he has underlying osteomyelitis in the region. The right foot appears to be stable at this time, and no acute ulceration is noted in the left heel.

DIAGNOSIS:

1. Ulceration of the left forefoot with osteomyelitis of third metatarsal.
2. Previous transmetatarsal amputation of right foot.
3. Peripheral neuropathy.
4. Hypertension.
5. Chronic renal insufficiency.

Treatment plan: The patient had an initial consultation. The ulcer site was cleaned, and an excisional debridement was performed. The area was repacked with a dry sterile dressing. The patient was advised that he would probably need surgical intervention in the future. We are awaiting MRI results to confirm the diagnosis of osteomyelitis of the third metatarsal. The patient was advised of his surgical versus conservative treatment options. At this time, we recommend additional surgical intervention, including transmetatarsal amputation to the area. The patient was given a detailed explanation of the surgical procedure, as well as details on complications of pain, scar, swelling/infection, neurovascular damage/RSD/DVT, AVN, poor healing, dehiscence of the wound, continued infection, and the possible need for additional surgery, including more proximal amputation of the foot or leg. At this time, if the patient's white blood cell count remains stable, and the patient relates no fevers, chills, or systemic signs of infection, it is possible that the patient may be discharged from the hospital and may undergo surgery on an outpatient basis. The patient will have to continue with local wound care and will be using crutches to keep weight off the area. Oral antibiotics will be continued until the time of surgery. We will discuss his continued treatment with the medical team. At this time, we will continue to provide conservative care.

X-ray: Foot, Left

Indication: Infection.

Impression: Amputation through proximal first metatarsal and mid second metatarsal. Dislocation and medial angulation third phalanx. Cortical disruption and lucency of third metatarsal head/suspicious for osteomyelitis. Advise MRI or nuclear medicine bone scan for further evaluation. Soft tissue swelling over dorsal and lateral foot and toes. Small dense fragment adjacent to fourth distal phalanx, possibly small bony fragment.

MRI Left Lower Extremity

History: History of right foot pain with elevated CRP and ESR suspicious for osteomyelitis.

Technique: Axial T1 and T2 images. T1 and STIR coronal images. The patient received 0.1 mmol/kg gadolinium for postcontrast T1 images.

Comparison: Plain film radiograph of the left foot from 9/23/06.

Findings: The patient is status post amputations at the mid second metatarsal and base of the first metatarsal. Within the shaft of the third metatarsal are increased T2 and STIR signal, as well as decreased T1 signal with enhancement within the bone and surrounding soft tissues compatible with osteomyelitis. Marked dislocation of the proximal third phalanx is noted at the MTP joint. Views of the third phalanges are limited, and osteomyelitis cannot be excluded. A large ulcer is seen along the plantar surface of the left foot, extending within the fascial layers.

Impression:

1. Osteomyelitis of the left third metatarsal. Marked dislocation of the third MTP; cannot exclude osteomyelitis in the third phalanges.
2. Large left plantar fascial ulcer.
3. Status post amputations at the mid second metatarsal and base of the first metatarsal.

225

DIAGNOSES/PROBLEMS:

Left foot ulcer.

PROCEDURES:

1. MRI.
2. Excisional debridement.

HISTORY, MAJOR FINDINGS, AND HOSPITAL COURSE:

This is a 43 y/o man with a PMHx of HTN and peripheral neuropathy who presented to the ED complaining of left foot ulcer. He was noted to have a large ulcer on the left foot and was admitted for IV antibiotics and possible operative management. He was started on Zosyn. The ulcer was debrided at the bedside; wound cultures and blood cultures were sent. The patient had no event overnight. To examine the patient's circulation, ABI from the vascular laboratory was ordered. To rule out osteomyelitis, MRI of the L lower extremity was also ordered. The patient underwent the vascular study, which showed abnormal arterial flow on ABI. Because of the patient's culture results and infectious disease recommendations, the patient was switched from Zosyn to clindamycin. Wound cultures grew out light *Strep viridans*.

Podiatry was consulted, and the patient underwent MRI. The patient continued to have dressing changes to his wound. It was recommended that the patient may be a candidate for a transmetatarsal amputation as an outpatient. The patient's MRI revealed osteomyelitis of the third metatarsal. The patient experienced no additional events, and his blood cultures are negative to date. The patient agreed that he will follow up with his physician as an outpatient, and he was deemed satisfactory to go home.

PMHx: HTN and peripheral vascular disease.

PSHx: R metatarsal amputation.

L 1st and 2nd metatarsal amputations.

Allergies: NKDA.

Discharge medications: Tylenol 650 mg, clindamycin 650 mg.

DISCHARGE INSTRUCTIONS:

Wound: Please apply wet to dry dressing twice a day.

Activity: Partial weight bearing LLE, heel touch 50%.

When to call doctor: If bleeding from wound, if severe pain arises, if pus emerges from wound.

FOLLOW-UP CARE:

Follow up with orthopedics as needed.

DAY 1

MRI was done. Appreciate podiatry's consult and recommendations. The patient's pain has improved. Continue IV antibiotics. Blood and wound cultures are still pending. May need amputation.

Day 2

MRI confirms osteomyelitis of the left third metatarsal. Continue IV antibiotics. Wet to dry dressing twice daily. Ulceration looks better. Partial weight bearing for left lower extremity.

Day 3

Blood cultures are negative. The patient was switched from Zosyn to clindamycin because wound cultures grew *Strep viridans*. The patient is ready for discharge. Will follow up with Podiatry regarding possible amputation.

CASE STUDY QUESTIONS

19-1a. Admit diagnosis: _____

19-1b. Discharge disposition: _____

19-1c. Principal diagnosis:_____

19-1d. Secondary diagnoses (indicate POA status for secondary diagnoses):

_____

_____

_____

_____

_____

_____

19-1e. Principal procedure: _____

19-1f. Secondary procedures: _____

_____

19-1g. Assign MS-DRG: _____

19-1h. Relative weight of MS-DRG: _____

19-1i. Can this MS-DRG be optimized with the addition of a CC? Yes or No
       Can this MS-DRG be optimized with the addition of an MCC? Yes or No

19-1j. Is there a main guideline pertinent to selection of the principal diagnosis in this case study?

_____

_____

19-1k. Is there another diagnosis that meets the definition for principal diagnosis? Yes or No

19-1l. If yes, what is the other diagnosis? _____

19-1m. Is there any opportunity for physician query?

_____

_____

19-1n. What is the drug Zosyn used to treat? _____

19-2. CASE STUDY

Clinic Note/Preop Evaluation

History of present illness: The patient returns today for reevaluation of his right shoulder in consideration of right total shoulder arthroplasty. He is here with his wife today. His shoulder continues to be significantly sore and painful with limitations of activity. On his left side, he has had it replaced. He is very happy with the result and has no complaints.

Past medical history is significant for diabetes mellitus type II, hypercholesterolemia.

Past surgical history is significant for left shoulder replacement.

Social history is significant for previous tobacco use. Occasional alcohol.

Medications: Lipitor and Glucotrol. Patient has been taking NSAIDs for shoulder pain.

Allergies: None.

Major findings: He is a very pleasant gentleman in no acute distress at the time of examination.

Vital signs: Stable.

HEENT: PERRLA. Neck is supple. Trachea is midline. Thyroid is normal. No lymphadenopathy is reported.

Chest: CTA bilaterally.

Heart: RRR.

Abd: Soft. Bowel sounds present. No tenderness, guarding, or rigidity. No hepatosplenomegaly.

GI/GU: Rectal exam deferred.

Extremities: He elevates his right shoulder only to about 50 to 60 degrees. His rotations are also significantly limited. He has no weakness in abduction or external rotation. He does not appear to have an incompetent subscapularis, but he cannot internally rotate enough to test it.

X-rays show significant degenerative arthritis and a slightly high-riding humeral head.

Assessments: The patient would benefit from a total shoulder arthroplasty. He has some thinning of his rotator cuff, so we should be available to do a reverse, if possible. I gave him reading material about this. I told him I thought there was a 95% chance he would need a standard total shoulder replacement. I told him I could not rule out a reverse prosthesis, however. I did discuss with him getting an MRI of his shoulder prior to surgery. We need to see the results of that scan.

Plans: We discussed with the patient the complications of surgery, including but not exclusive of infection, nerve or artery damage, stiffness, loss of range of motion, incomplete relief of pain, incomplete return of function, incomplete return of motion, medical complications, surgical complications, anesthesia complications, and long-term loosening. The patient has been through this before and understands all of the risks. We did review the consent forms with him line by line, even though it has been done before. He and his wife understand that there are no guarantees. We will see him back for his surgery and asked him to call us if he has any questions or problems.

Discharge Summary

DIAGNOSES/PROBLEMS:

1. Right shoulder osteoarthritis.
2. Diabetes mellitus type II.
3. Hypertension.

PROCEDURES:

Right total shoulder arthroplasty.

HISTORY, MAJOR FINDINGS, AND HOSPITAL COURSE:

The patient is a pleasant 76-year-old gentleman with a history of diabetes and hypertension, as stated above. The patient has a long-standing history of osteoarthritis of both shoulders. The left shoulder was replaced previously. The patient has been evaluated for replacement of the right shoulder and was determined to be a candidate. The patient was brought to the operating theater, where a right total shoulder arthroplasty was performed without complication. For details of the operative procedure, please refer to the dictated operative note.

Postoperatively, the patient was transferred to the floor for recovery and pain management. His peripheral nerve catheter was deemed not to be working on postoperative day 1 and was therefore discontinued by the pain service. The patient throughout this hospitalization had the Iceman cooling device applied to the right shoulder. Pain was controlled with Tylox solely, and the patient's diet was advanced as tolerated. The patient was discharged on postoperative day 2 without complication. He will receive home health physical therapy services.

Discharge medications: Tylox 1 to 2 tablets by mouth every 4 to 6 hours as needed for pain. The patient is to resume home medications.

DISCHARGE INSTRUCTIONS:

Activity: The patient is to avoid any lifting over the shoulder level until he is seen in clinic. The patient is to avoid physical therapy until he is seen in clinic.

Other: The patient is to follow instructions as per the handout that has been given. The patient is to remain in the ice band for as close to 24 hours a day as he can tolerate. The patient is instructed to call the office if he has a fever of 101.5 degrees, drainage from the wound, or change in motor or sensory function of the right upper extremity.

Operative Report

Title of operation: Total shoulder arthroplasty right shoulder (Stryker solar system; uncemented plasma sprayed humeral stem size 12; cemented keeled glenoid component size 7; 45 × 12 mm concentric head). Biceps tenodesis, right shoulder.

Indications for surgery: The patient has been seen multiple times preoperatively. He was found to have intractable arthritis of the shoulder. Risks and benefits of the procedure have been discussed at length inclusive but not exclusive of infection, nerve or artery damage, stiffness, loss of range of motion, incomplete relief of pain, incomplete return of function, long-term loosening, medical complications, surgical complications, and anesthesia complications. The patient underwent prerotator cuff repair, and concerns were expressed that he might have a consistent or repeat tears; whether reverse prosthesis was available if necessary was also discussed at length.

Preoperative diagnosis: Degenerative arthritis, right shoulder.

Postoperative diagnosis: Degenerative arthritis, right shoulder; biceps tenosynovitis, right shoulder.

Surgeon's Narrative

The patient was placed in supine position. A Foley catheter was placed in his bladder. He was then placed in a beach-chair position. All bony prominences were padded, and the patient was brought in on the side of the table and secured with towels and tape. His head was placed in the neutral position with no lateral bending or extension. His head was secured with paper tape, with assurance that no tape was placed on his orbits or his auricular cartilages. His right upper extremity was then prepped and draped in usual sterile fashion. He was given antibiotics well before the start of the procedure to decrease the risk of infection. Once he had been prepped and draped, the patient was prepped the second time with a DuraPrep. This allowed the Loban bandages to be placed more closely to the skin, thereby decreasing the risk of infection.

A deltopectoral incision was made. Mediolateral skin flaps were developed. The cephalic vein was identified and protected throughout the procedure. The deltopectoral ala was developed down to the clavipectoral fascia. The patient had a significant number of adhesions between the deltoid and the underlying rotator cuff. These were very carefully and tediously released until the proximal humerus could be completely exposed.

The shaft was also exposed, and the deltoid insertion was released by approximately half its width because the patient was very tight. The nerve was also taken all the way to the clavicle. The upper one half of the pectoralis insertion was released to increase his external rotation. The biceps tendon was then identified. The transverse ligament was split over the top of the tendon but sounded as though it was somewhat partially torn with tenosynovitis. As a result, it was released with a level of the joint and was tagged with a 0 Vicryl suture; it was later tenodesed to the #2 Ti-Cron sutures, which were placed at the calcar region for the subscapularis.

The capsule and subscapularis muscles were then released off the lesser tuberosity as a unit. This was kept on the bone the entire time to protect the axillary nerve. Retractors were placed inferiorly so as to increase exposure to protect the axillary nerve. Dissection was taken off of the proximal humerus in the upper one half of the latissimus dorsi tendon, which was also released. This was done with an increase in external rotation until the edge could be dislocated. The patient had a moderate number of spurs, which were easily removed.

The arm was then dislocated, and the arm was brought to the side. The patient was found to have an entirely intact supraspinatus tendon, so it was elected to proceed with the standard total shoulder arthroplasty and not a reverse prosthesis. The humeral head cut was then made in the usual manner. The retractor was placed superiorly to protect the rotator cuff. The retractor was then placed inferiorly to protect the axillary nerve. The retractor was placed medially to protect the glenoid and the brachial plexus. The humeral head cut then was made in the usual manner with the use of a guide and 30 degrees of retroversion. The patient's proximal bone was fairly sturdy. The shaft itself was identified with a rongeur. Sequential reamers were then placed distally up to a size 12. Proximal rotators were placed at 30 degrees in retroversion at size 12. Axial with counter sink a little bit into the proximal humerus. As a result, it was elected to use a plasma spray prosthesis, which provided increasing stability proximally.

Attention was then directed to the glenoid. The biceps tendon was removed along with the labrum circumferentially. The confines of the glenoid were carefully evaluated at size 9 and would have been entirely too large, so a size 7 was believed to be the best fit. The patient did have some scalping of the glenoid, but no particular anterior or posterior erosions were noted. As a result, an anchoring hole was made in the mid portion of the glenoid. A size 7 reamer was then used to smooth down the edges as much as possible.

The keyhole was anchored in the usual manner with curettes and a handheld bur. The size 7 component was easily fitted into the keyhole with no difficulty. The glenoid was then drilled with multiple small drill holes to enhance cement fixation. Excess blood was removed with the use of irrigation and sponges. Hemostasis was obtained with Gelfoam. When the cement was mixed, it was removed, along with excess blood. The keyhole and the glenoid were then finger packed with cement in the usual manner. The component was then placed with no difficulty, and excess cement was removed. It was felt digitally to be in position, with no toddling until the cement had hardened. It was found to be very secure once this had been completed.

The proximal humerus was thoroughly irrigated. The real component was placed in 30 degrees of retroversion. It should be noted that a plasma spray component with hydroxyapatite was used rather than a cementing component. This occurred primarily because it was believed that the mismatch measured only approximately 0.5 mm; therefore, we did not believe that it was necessary to cement the smaller component. Once the component had been packed, it had excellent position and good bone fixation.

Sequential reductions were then made with different head sizes; it was found that a 45 × 15 mm concentric head gave the best stability with the greatest external rotation. The rear head was then inserted after the fluid had been moved from the Morse taper; it was packed in position and was very sturdy. Reduction was performed again, and stability was quite good. The subscapularis was closed back with the proximal humerus with placement of a #2 Ti-Cron. Prior to insertion of the glenoid component, approximately 4 to 5 #2 Ti-Cron sutures were placed in the calcar region. Also, rotator cuff intervals were closed with multiple #2 Ti-Cron sutures. Once this had been completed, the patient had excellent anterior and posterior stability with no subluxation. External rotation width, before tension was placed on the repair, was 15 degrees with arm at the side and 15 degrees with arm abducted 90 degrees. The wound was thoroughly irrigated throughout with antibiotic-impregnated solution. Two Hemovac drains were placed inferiorly to the wound. The biceps tendon was then tenodesed back to the calcar region with #2 Ti-Cron sutures and was placed under good tension, so it would have good form later. This was reinforced with multiple 0-Vicryl sutures, as was the subscapularis repair. The deltopectoral was then closed with interrupted 0-Vicryl sutures. The deep and superficial subcutaneous tissues were closed with interrupted 2-0 Vicryl sutures. The skin was closed with staples. A sterile bandage was applied, along with a cold device and a shoulder immobilizer. The patient was sent to the recovery room in stable and satisfactory condition.

Shoulder X-ray

Result: Right shoulder AP portable.

Clinical information: Postop.

Result: Normal postop right humeral head replacement with soft tissue drain in place.

for addressograph plate

Date	Time	
12/12	1000	Ortho Brief op note
		pre-op dx: (R) shoulder arthritis
		post-op dx: same
		procedure: (R) Total shoulder arthroplasty
		surgeon: _____ Brock.
		GETA
		IVF: 2200 cc EBL: 250 cc UOP: 200 cc
		Implant: #12 stem (plasma) 45x12 mm head # 7 glenoid
		Specimen: humeral head
		Drains: x2
		Comp: ø
		Dispo: PACU

for addressograph plate

Date	Time	
12/13	0810	AAHO
		37⁴ 90-110 105-142/59-87 94% RA i: 2950 o. 715
		Drsn 115/20 ⁷ᵗ/10
		MAD, pain controlled
		wnd dvcky C1&1 I
		Kerman in place
		Sensation slightly ↓ C5-T1
		mdr ↓ D ⁴/5 B/T ³/5 INT/APB ³/5
		A/P pt dg well
		① PT ndy
		② await d/c PNC to eval strength/function

Date	Time	
12/14	0545	C/Ano
		37⁷ 86~60 122~135 /65~78 93% RA (757/3610
		NAD Hx cur rected
		Pt uncooperative c̄ exam
		Mecy c̄ID/F und intact
		Sensation intact c5-T1
		motor D/B/T/IWT/APB 4/5 - 2012 pt cooperation/poor
		Atp Pt RUP A 2 c/p ® TSA, dry well
		① D/C name
12/16		o su Attend
	0650	As above.
		M intact - Incision A ~ or signs sepsis
		Stable, DC truly
		PMiRPT
12/14	11²⁵	Attempted PT follow up — pt received amb
		in unit mod I c̄ shoulder immobilization.
		Pt v. preoccupied c̄ discharge — no one can
		pick him up despite being told of discharge
		today—looking into option. Will follow up later this

CASE STUDY QUESTIONS

19-2a. Admit diagnosis: _____

19-2b. Discharge disposition: _____

19-2c. Principal diagnosis: _____

19-2d. Secondary diagnoses (indicate POA status for secondary diagnoses):

_____

_____

_____

_____

_____

_____

19-2e. Principal procedure: _____

19-2f. Secondary procedures: _____

_____

19-2g. Assign MS-DRG: _____

19-2h. Relative weight of MS-DRG: _____

19-2i. Can this MS-DRG be optimized with the addition of a CC? Yes or No
Can this MS-DRG be optimized with the addition of an MCC? Yes or No

19-2j. Is there a main guideline pertinent to selection of the principal diagnosis in this case study?

_____

_____

19-2k. Is there another diagnosis that meets the definition for principal diagnosis? Yes or No

19-2l. If yes, what is the other diagnosis? _____

19-2m. Is there any opportunity for physician query?

_____

_____

19-2n. What is the drug Tylox used to treat? _____

Clinic Note/Preop Evaluation

Reason for visit: Preop evaluation.

History of present illness: A 56-year-old with low back pain and left lower extremity weakness. She is otherwise healthy.

Past medical history includes migraine, mitral valve prolapse confirmed by echocardiogram, obesity, and multiple drug allergies and sensitivities. The patient underwent hysterectomy without anesthetic complications. No airway difficulties were noted. The patient has no significant family problems with anesthesia.

ROS: The patient denies chest pain, shortness of breath, orthopnea, PND, or fatigue. She claims she is able to climb three flights of stairs without stopping, except that she does get pain in her legs and back.

Medications: Premarin 0.0625 mg daily, Verapamil 240 mg SR, Mobic 7.5 mg (last dose 12/3/06), Clarinex 5 mg daily, amitriptyline, Flonase, Darvocet 100 mg prn, Percocet 5 mg prn (3 doses over past few weeks), Skelaxin 800 mg, Maxalt prn, Calcium, MVI, Fibercon Stool Softener, and flaxseed oil.

Allergies: Demerol, Dilantin, Dilaudid, codeine, sulfa, latex, lidocaine, and surgical steel.

Physical Examination:

Vital signs: Stable.

General: NAD. Pleasant female patient with chronic back pain.

HEENT: PERRLA. Trachea is central. JVP not raised. No carotid bruit.

Chest: Clear.

Heart: RRR.

Abd: Obese. No tenderness.

Extremities: Weakness on the left.

Assessments: This 56-year-old female is scheduled for an L2-L5 spinal fusion. The patient has chronic back pain and is currently taking several pain medications. The patient has a history of mitral valve prolapse, confirmed by ECHO per patient. She was told that the ECHO was otherwise normal. She has no other cardiac history. She experiences chronic migraines; typically, one occurs each month. She normally takes Maxalt when she realizes they are starting.

Plans: We sent this patient for Heme 8, CMP, and T&C for two units PCs. We also sent her for an ECG. Provided there are no significant findings, we need no further testing.

Medication changes: The patient was instructed to take her normal medications on the evening prior to surgery, but to take only Premarin and verapamil on the morning of surgery. She was told to bring her Maxalt with her to the hospital, in case she begins to develop a migraine headache. She was also instructed that she could take one Darvocet on the morning of surgery.

Discharge Summary

DIAGNOSES/PROBLEMS:

1. Lumbar stenosis and spondylolisthesis at L3-4.
2. Scoliosis and spondylosis.

PROCEDURES:

1. L3-4 laminectomy with bilateral facetectomy.
2. Resection of pars.
3. Decompression of L3-4 nerve root bilateral.
4. Pedicle screw instrumentation L2 through L5.
5. Reduction of scoliotic deformity.
6. Arthrodesis L2 to L5 with autograft, allograft, and demineralized bone matrix.

HISTORY, MAJOR FINDINGS, AND HOSPITAL COURSE:

This is a 56-year-old female with complaints of weakness and pain in the left lower extremity and back pain. An MRI and x-rays of the lumbosacral spine showed L3-4 spondylolisthesis with degenerative scoliosis and bilateral foraminal stenosis L3-4, L4-5 bilateral. In addition to this, the patient had central canal stenosis. She underwent the above surgical procedures. She tolerated the procedures well and was transferred to the neuro intensive care unit. The patient was stable and was then transferred to the floor. Her wound was clean, dry, and intact with no fluid collection. She was seen by the Department of Rehabilitation Medicine for mobilization. The patient was doing well. She had a mild headache that eventually stopped. This headache was positional. No leakage from the drain sites was noted. The wound continued to be clean, dry, and intact. The patient had done extremely well. She denied any further headache, was ambulating, and continued to be neurologically stable. Her pain was well controlled. The patient was ready for discharge to her home.

Reportable diseases: None.

Adverse drug reactions: None.

Allergies: None.

Complications of the procedure: None.

Condition on discharge: Good.

Discharge medications: Resume her prior preop medications. Flexeril 5 mg 3 times a day as needed.

DISCHARGE INSTRUCTIONS:

Diet: Regular.

Activity: As tolerated.

FOLLOW-UP CARE:

To have staples removed in approximately 10 days and to see surgeon in 4 to 6 weeks for follow-up.

Operative Report

Title of operation: L3-L4 laminectomy. L3-L4 bilateral facetectomy and resection of pars (Smith Peterson Osteotomy). Decompression of the L3-L4 nerve roots bilaterally. Pedicle screw instrumentation from L2 through L5. Reduction of scoliotic deformity and L3-L4 dislocation from L2 to L5. Arthrodesis from L2 to L5 with locally obtained autograft, allograft, and demineralized bone matrix.

Indications for surgery: This 56-year-old female initially presented to the Neurosurgery Service with complaints of weakness and pain going down her left lower extremity and significant back pain. She underwent MRI scan and x-ray examination of her lumbosacral spine, which revealed L3-L4 spondylolisthesis with degenerative scoliosis, as well as bilateral foraminal stenosis at L3-L4 and L4-L5 bilaterally. In addition, she had central canal stenosis. Given her constellation of symptoms of radiculopathy and neurogenic claudication, as well as the scoliosis and deformity, we discussed with her various treatment options. One option would be conservative therapy, and the other would be surgical intervention. Surgical intervention would involve an L2 to L5 instrumented fusion with correction of the scoliotic deformity and L3-L4 decompression. She understood the risks and benefits of the procedure. The risks included but were not limited to bleeding, infection, injury to nerves, pain, paralysis, need for another operation, failure of instrumentation, failure to fuse, and death. Despite these risks, the patient decided to undergo the operation.

Preoperative diagnosis: Lumbar stenosis, L3-L4. Spondylolisthesis at L3-L4. Scoliosis. Spondylosis. Back pain.

Postoperative diagnosis: Lumbar stenosis, L3-L4. Spondylolisthesis at L3-L4. Scoliosis. Spondylosis. Back pain.

Surgeon's Narrative

Description of operation in detail: The patient was taken to the Operating Room and was placed supine on the operating table. After general endotracheal anesthesia was provided, the patient was taken from the supine position and was placed prone on the Jackson table. Areas of pressure were carefully padded. Then, the lumbosacral region was cleaned in a normal fashion. The first time out was performed, and it was verified that indeed we were performing the correct operation on the correct patient in the correct location, and that preoperative antibiotics had been given. We then prepped and draped the spine in the usual sterile fashion. A midline incision was made from approximately L2 through L5 with a #15 blade scalpel carried down through the subcutaneous tissue and fascia with the Bovie cautery.

After the fascia had been incised with a Bovie cautery, we carefully dissected between the paraspinous muscle and the fascia out laterally on both sides. We opened the plane between the multifidus and the paraspinous muscle bilaterally through the Wiltse approach, by identifying the transverse processes of L2, L3, L4, and L5. Using this approach, we carefully exposed the lateral aspect of the facet, the mamillary process, and the transverse processes of L2, L3, L4, and L5 bilaterally. After the exposure had been completed, self-retaining retractors were placed, thereby maintaining our exposure. We then proceeded to place our instrumentation in the pedicles of L2 and L3 and L5. We used the Click'X pedicle screw instrumentation from Synthes for instrumentation. At L4, we used the Click'X spondylolisthesis reduction instrumentation for instrumentation at that level. Using normal anatomic landmarks for entry points and trajectories, we placed our pedicle screw instrumentation. Intraoperative x-ray was obtained in the AP and lateral projections, verifying that indeed the instrumentation was in good position. After instrumentation was confirmed to be in good position, we proceeded with our midline exposure.

Self-retaining retractors were removed, and we then proceeded at the midline in a subperiosteal dissection, exposing the spinous process of the lamina and the medial facets of L3 and L4. Self-retaining retractors were placed, thereby maintaining our exposure. We then resected the spinous processes of L3 and L4 and, using the high-speed cutting bur followed by Kerrison punches, removed the laminae of L3 and L4. During the laminectomy of L3, a durotomy was encountered, and this was carefully controlled by gentle suction and cottonoids. We worked around the durotomy, decompressing the lateral gutters and resecting the hypertrophied ligamentum flavum. We exposed the L3 and L4 nerve roots bilaterally and carefully traced these out laterally. After the thecal sac had been completely decompressed, we then turned our attention to the durotomy. The durotomy was closed with a running 6-0 Prolene suture, and this closure was reinforced with fibrin glue.

After the durotomy had been completed and the thecal sac had been completely decompressed, and the L3 and L4 nerve roots had been completely decompressed, we then turned our attention to the spondylolisthesis correction.

238

Given the degree of dislocation in this region, we felt that it would be beneficial to reduce the spondylolisthesis. In addition, the spine was rotated in this region, causing the scoliosis as well; we therefore believed that correcting the spondylolisthesis and correcting the rotation of the spine in this region would correct the deformity. We performed complete facetectomies of L3-L4 bilaterally, further exposing these nerve roots and also further freeing the spine at this level by completing the facetectomies and resection of pars at this level. We performed Smith-Peterson osteotomies, which later allowed us to achieve further lordosis of the spine. After the Smith-Peterson osteotomies had been performed and the spine was made mobile, we contoured two rods such that they would span from L2 to L5 on both sides. The rod on the righthand side was positioned first and then was locked into place on the L2 and L3 screw heads. After it had been locked into place, we used the spondylolisthesis reduction instrumentation on the right-hand L4 screw and carefully reduced L4 onto L3, thus reducing the dislocation and the spondylolisthesis, and derotating the spine in this fashion. After the L4 screw had been reduced onto the rod, this was locked into position. Then, a locking screw was positioned onto the L5 screw. By performing the spondylolisthesis reduction and using a precontoured rod, we were able to achieve greater lordosis from the Smith-Peterson osteotomy, and we were able to derotate the L4 vertebral body and reduce the dislocation and scoliosis. After this rod was in position, we selected a separate contoured rod to place on the left-hand side; this was placed from L2 to L5 and was locked into position again.

We then decorticated the transverse processes of L2, L3, L4, and L5, with the Leksell rongeur, and we decorticated the facet joints of L2-L3 and L4-L5. This was done with a high-speed cutting burr. The facet joints were packed with locally obtained allograft and autograft and demineralized bone matrix. We placed the locally obtained allograft, autograft, and demineralized bone matrix from L2 to L5 on the transverse processes, producing an arthrodesis. After the graft material and instrumentation were in good position, we placed two subfascial drains over the instrumentation and carried these out through two separate stab incisions. The lumbosacral fascia was then reapproximated with interrupted 0-Vicryl sutures. The Scarpa layer was reapproximated with interrupted 0-Vicryl sutures. The subcuticular layer was reapproximated with interrupted 3-0-Vicryl sutures, and the skin was closed with a running 3-0 nylon suture.

All instrument, sponge, and needle counts were correct at the end of the procedure. Estimated blood loss was less than 650 cubic centimeters. No complications were associated with the procedure. No transfusions were needed.

Lumbar Spine Port in OR

Lumbosacral and lower thoracic spine operative lateral.

Results: Posteriorly placed drill tips in anterior portions of L2, L3, and vertebral bodies and at anterior cortex L4 vertebral body. Hook retractors posterior to L2-3, L3-4, and L4-5.

CT Left Spine Without Contrast Complex

Indication: Status post lumbar spine fusion.

Technique: Axial CT scans were performed through the lumbar spine with sagittal reconstructions without contrast administration.

Findings: Posterior fusion with bilateral rods, screws, and bone graft was seen from L2-5. L3 and L4 laminectomy was performed. Lumbar spine alignment is normal. Evidence of severe degenerative disc disease was noted at the L3-4 level with end-plate sclerosis, Schmorl's nodes, and vacuum cleft deformity. Small anterior osteophytes are present throughout the lumbar spine, most pronounced at L3-4. Expected postoperative changes are present, including soft tissue emphysema and swelling. At the T12-L1 level, the central canal and neural foramina are widely patent. At the L1-2 level, the central canal and neural foramina are widely patent. At the L2-3 level, a diffuse broad-based disc bulge minimally effaces the ventral thecal sac and narrows the central canal in combination with ligamentum flavum and facet joint hypertrophy. A small focus of air, likely postoperative, is present posterior and lateral to the cord at this level. Mild to moderate bilateral neural foramina stenosis is apparent.

At the L3-4 level, evidence suggests severe degenerative disc disease. A few small foci of air are present in the region of the central canal, likely postoperative in nature. The central canal/cord is not well delineated at this level secondary to extensive soft tissue swelling/inflammatory change and is likely postoperative in nature. Mild left neural foraminal stenosis with disc material appears to extend into the left neural foramen. The right neural foramen remains widely patent.

At the L4-5 level, a mild diffuse disc bulge is seen. A tiny calcification is present to the left of the central canal at table position 1718—probably a small bone fragment. Facet joint hypertrophic changes cause mild right neural foraminal stenosis. The left neural foramen is widely patent.

At the L5-S1 level, a mild disc bulge is present. The central canal and neural foramina are widely patent. Spina bifida occulta is present on the left side. Visualized intra-abdominal structures are unremarkable except for atherosclerosis of the aorta and a normal variant retroaortic left renal vein.

Impression: Postoperative changes status post L2-5 posterior fusion and L3/L4 laminectomy. Multilevel degenerative changes, most pronounced at L2-3.

Progress Notes

POSTOP NOTE

Preop diagnosis: L3-4 spondylolisthesis; scoliosis.

Postop diagnosis: Same.

Proc: L3-4 laminectomy; L2-L5 spinal fusion.

Anes: General.

IVF: 7000 cc crystalloid; EBL: 600 cc; UO: 1000 cc; drains: 2 JP.

Complication: Durotomy.

Dispo: To NCCU.

Vitals: T 36.4, P 109, RR 22, BP 101/55.

Neuro status stable. Pain is controlled. At risk for hemorrhage, radiculopathy, myelopathy, and CSF leak.

S/P L2-L5 fusion with scoliosis correction. Surgical bandages dry. Pain well controlled on PCA; 5/5 bilateral LE.

Plan: PT/OT; D/C Foley; continue PCA; CT scan of hardware.

DAY 1

Afebrile; urine output good.

Alert and oriented ×3.

5/5 bilateral LE.

Incision/wound: C/D/I no collection.

Day 2

Pain well controlled. Mild headache.

Neuro is stable. Inc C/D/I.

Doing well. Mild tachycardia. Continue PT/OT.

Day 3

No headache. Urinary function is good.

Tolerating regular diet. Ready for discharge.

CASE STUDY QUESTIONS

19-3a. Admit diagnosis: _____

19-3b. Discharge disposition: _____

19-3c. Principal diagnosis: _____

19-3d. Secondary diagnoses (indicate POA status for secondary diagnoses):

_____

_____

_____

_____

_____

_____

19-3e. Principal procedure: _____

19-3f. Secondary procedures: _____

_____

19-3g. Assign MS-DRG: _____

19-3h. Relative weight of MS-DRG: _____

19-3i. Can this MS-DRG be optimized with the addition of a CC? Yes or No
Can this MS-DRG be optimized with the addition of an MCC? Yes or No

19-3j. Is there a main guideline pertinent to selection of the principal diagnosis in this case study?

_____

_____

19-3k. Is there another diagnosis that meets the definition for principal diagnosis? Yes or No

19-3l.   If yes, what is the other diagnosis? _____

19-3m. Is there any opportunity for physician query?

_____

_____

19-3n. What is the drug Flexeril used to treat? _____

20 Diseases of the Genitourinary System (ICD-10-CM Chapter 14, Codes N00-N99)

ABBREVIATIONS/ACRONYMS

Without the use of reference materials, define the following abbreviations or acronyms.

1. DIEP _____
2. VUR _____
3. TURP _____
4. CKD _____
5. LUTS _____
6. PID _____
7. FSG _____
8. ESRD _____
9. ARF _____
10. LAVH _____

GLOSSARY DEFINITIONS

Match the glossary term to the correct definition.

1. _____ Hydronephrosis
2. _____ Urolithiasis
3. _____ Prostatitis
4. _____ Mixed incontinence
5. _____ Hematuria
6. _____ Acute renal failure
7. _____ Pedicle flap
8. _____ Salpingitis
9. _____ Pelvic inflammatory disease
10. _____ Benign prostatic hypertrophy
11. _____ Rectocele
12. _____ Stress incontinence
13. _____ Pyelonephritis
14. _____ Cystitis
15. _____ Free flap
16. _____ Fistula

A. Inflammation of the prostate that can be acute and/or chronic in nature

B. Describes a stone in the urinary tract

C. Abnormal passage or communication between two internal organs or leading from an organ to the surface of the body

D. Lower urinary tract infection that affects the bladder

E. Inflammation of the uterus

F. Condition that results in enlargement of the prostate gland and usually occurs in men older than 50 years of age

G. Approach to many procedures of the urinary tract

H. Abnormal dilatation of the renal pelvis caused by pressure from urine that cannot cannot flow past an obstruction in the urinary tract

I. Upper tract infection that involves the kidneys

J. Involuntary loss of small amounts of urine due to increased pressure from coughing, sneezing, or laughing

Continued

243

17. _____ Endometritis

18. _____ Cystoscopy

19. _____ Extracorporeal shockwave lithotripsy

20. _____ Calculi

K. Sudden and severe impairment of renal function characterized by oliguria, increased serum urea, and acidosis

L. Term for a stone

M. The presence of blood in the urine

N. Vaginal and cervical infections that spread and involve the uterus, fallopian tubes, ovaries, and surrounding tissues

O. Flap that remains attached to its original blood supply and tunnels it under the skin to a particular area such as the breast

P. Combination of stress and urge incontinence

Q. Descent of the rectum and pressing of the rectum against the vaginal wall

R. Inflammation of the fallopian tubes

S. The cutting of skin, fat, blood vessels, and muscle free from its location and movement of it to another area such as the chest

T. Procedure performed to break kidney stones up into small particles that can then pass through the urinary tract in the urine

CODING

Using the code book, code the following.

1. Hemorrhagic cystitis _____

2. BPH with postvoid dribbling _____

3. Vesicoureteral reflux _____

4. Acute on chronic renal insufficiency _____

5. Overactive bladder _____

6. Pyuria due to perinephric abscess _____

7. Renal osteodystrophy _____

8. Adhesions of right ureter _____

9. Mass of left kidney _____

10. Acute epididymitis due to *Streptococcus* _____

11. Prostatic intraepithelial neoplasia II _____

12. Torsion of testis _____

13. Diverticulum bladder _____

14. Solitary right renal cyst _____

15. Acute on chronic interstitial nephritis _____

CASE SCENARIOS

Using the code book, code the following cases.

1. This 60-year-old female patient was admitted for repair of a large cystocele and a small rectocele. The patient underwent surgery, and both were repaired. The patient has a medical history of previous kidney cancer with right nephrectomy, depression treated with Wellbutrin, and atrial fibrillation that is treated with Coumadin.
Final Diagnosis: Cystocele and rectocele.
Procedure: Repair of cystocele/rectocele.

   _____

   _____

2. A patient was admitted to the hospital for further evaluation of stage IV kidney disease. The patient is known to have been born with only one kidney and on routine check-up, it was found that the patient's kidney function was markedly abnormal. One year ago, the patient's laboratory tests were relatively normal. The patient's blood pressure was monitored, and it was decided that medications would be necessary to treat the patient's hypertension. The patient was advised about fluid intake and restriction and dietary considerations regarding protein and potassium. Referral was made to a nephrologist because the CKD appears to be progressing rapidly, and arrangements may be necessary for dialysis.
Final Diagnoses: Chronic progressive renal failure, stage IV.
                    Hypertension.

   _____

   _____

3. This 10-year-old female developed fatigue, fevers, and joint swelling and pain. Her symptoms were treated by her family practice physician with no improvement, so she was referred to a pediatric rheumatologist. The patient was admitted to the hospital for further testing. On hospital day 3, it was determined that a kidney biopsy was necessary to rule out lupus nephritis. After the percutaneous needle biopsy was performed, the patient was discharged. Pathology results confirmed lupus nephritis, which was suspected.
Final Diagnosis: Lupus nephritis.
Procedure: Kidney biopsy, right.

   _____

   _____

4. A patient is admitted to the hospital with fever and chills, flank pain, and burning on urination with increased frequency. CT scan shows stranding around the right kidney consistent with pyelonephritis. Urine culture is positive for proteus mirabilis. The patient has a long history of obstructive uropathy due to BPH. The patient is on medications for hypertension, osteoarthritis, and glaucoma.
Final Diagnoses: Fever due to acute pyelonephritis due to proteus mirabilis.
                    Obstructive uropathy due to benign prostatic hypertrophy.
                    Hypertension.

   _____

   _____

5. A patient was admitted for investigation of microscopic hematuria. The patient plans to donate a kidney to a family member, and any renal disease must be ruled out. The patient had a percutaneous needle biopsy of the left kidney. The patient has a past medical history of GERD, which is treated with Nexium, and had a pneumothorax caused by an MVA several years ago.
Final Diagnosis: Kidney donor with microscopic hematuria.
Procedure: Diagnostic kidney biopsy.

_____

_____

6. A patient was admitted for surgery to repair a hydrocele of the spermatic cord on the left side. This was accomplished with no problem.
Final Diagnosis: Hydrocele.
Procedure: Hydrocelectomy.

_____

_____

7. This 28-year-old female presented to the emergency department with nausea and vomiting, fever, lower abdominal pain, and vaginal discharge with foul odor. The patient was started on IV antibiotics and was transferred to the medical unit. Per social history, the patient has engaged in some high-risk heterosexual practices and was advised regarding safer sex practices. She was discharged with a prescription of oral antibiotics and will follow up with her regular GYN practitioner.
Final Diagnosis: Lower abdominal pain due to pelvic inflammatory disease.

_____

_____

8. This 32-year-old female patient has severe, debilitating endometriosis with very painful and heavy periods, chronic pelvic pain, and pain during sex. Conservative treatment with pain medications and hormonal therapy has failed. The patient was taken to the OR for a total hysterectomy with bilateral salpingo-oophorectomy. While in recovery, the patient developed symptoms of anaphylactic shock, most likely caused by the preoperative antibiotic cefotetan. The patient was reintubated (endotracheal) and was transferred to the surgical intensive care unit. She was mechanically ventilated for only a few hours, recovered with no additional complications, and was discharged home.
Final Diagnosis: Endometriosis uterus and ovaries.
Procedure: Total hysterectomy with bilateral salpingo-oophorectomy.

_____

_____

9. The patient was admitted for treatment of BPH with urinary retention and a history of frequent urinary tract infections. The patient's PSA was normal. Past medical history revealed that the patient has a shunt for normal pressure hydrocephalus, peripheral vascular disease, and a history of peptic ulcer disease. A TURP was performed. The patient recovered uneventfully with only minimal hematuria, which had resolved by the time of discharge.
Final Diagnosis: Benign prostatic hypertrophy.
Procedure: Transurethral resection of prostate.

_____

_____

10. A patient was admitted with renal colic due to kidney stone. Pain medications were administered with IV fluids. Urology staff was consulted and performed a percutaneous nephrostomy with fragmentation to remove the obstructing stone. Hydronephrosis was evident on ultrasound and hematuria per urinalysis.

Final Diagnoses: Renal colic and hematuria due to kidney stone on the right.
Hydronephrosis.

Procedure: Percutaneous nephrostomy with fragmentation for removal of stone.

_____

_____

CASE STUDIES

Using the code book, code and answer questions about the following case studies.

20-1. CASE STUDY

Clinic Note/Preop Evaluation

Reason for visit: Kidney donor evaluation.

History of present illness: The patient is a 59-year-old Caucasian male who wishes to donate a kidney to his son. His son has ESRD from an unclear hereditary condition that appears to have been transmitted through the mother's side of the family. The patient denies any history of renal disease, hematuria, kidney stones, foaminess to the urine, edema, or diabetes. Of note, he has been given a diagnosis of prehypertension. He states that he was begun on the antihypertensives lisinopril/HCTZ 1½ years ago for systolic blood pressures around 138. He has completed a 24-hour blood pressure reading for us, which shows a mean blood pressure of 114/70 while on his medication. Past history is also notable for prostate cancer, for which he underwent seed implantation 7 years ago. Tumor Registry has reported three cases of prostate cancer transmitted from a donor to a kidney transplant recipient. One of these was known to be metastatic, and the other two were noted at an unclear stage. It is emphasized that the risk is therefore non-zero. The patient has no evidence of lymph node involvement, and his PSA, which was 16 in 1998, prior to seed implantation, has been undetectable (<0.1) over the last 7 years.

Family history: Father deceased at age 45 from alcoholism, Mother deceased at age 92 with insulin resistance but not frank diabetes. Siblings include four sisters and two brothers, all healthy. No family history of renal disease, kidney stones, or malignancy is reported.

Social history: Works as a computer programmer. Denies use of tobacco, illicits, or alcohol at this time. The patient has a history of previous alcohol abuse but has been abstinent for a few years. The patient does not have a defined exercise program.

Review of systems: Denies fever, chills, night sweats, and exertional symptoms. Review is otherwise negative.

Medications: Lisinopril/HCTZ 20/12.5 QD, aspirin 81 mg QD

Allergies: Codeine causes pruritus.

Major findings: On examination, the patient appears well. Weight 72.5 kg for body mass index 27.3. Blood pressure 130/82, pulse 80, and temperature 36.5. HEENT unremarkable and without retinopathy. Neck without JVD, lymphadenopathy, thyromegaly, or bruit. Lungs clear to auscultation and without distress. CV regular rate and rhythm, without gallops, murmurs, or rub. Abdomen is soft without organomegaly or bruit. Extremities are without cyanosis or edema and have full pulses. Neurologic examination is intact to light touch and motor strength.

Labs: Urinalysis without heme or protein. 24-hour urine creatinine clearance 105 mL/min/1.73 m^2, and protein too low to calculate. Microalbumin 3 mg/g creatinine. Na 144, K 4.0, Cl1 04, CO_2 28, BUN 14, and creatinine 0.8 mg/dL. WBC 6.1, Hct 45.6%, and platelets 171. Liver function test results normal. Occult blood negative ×3. Colonoscopy with hemorrhoids in 7/02: PSA 0.1. Cholesterol 200, HDL 39, LDL 126, and triglyceride 177. Thallium cardiac stress test EF 65% with no ischemia, no left ventricular dilatation.

Assessments: The patient is a 59-year-old male who wishes to donate a kidney to his son.

PROBLEMS/DIAGNOSES:

1. Prehypertension on medication.

2. Prostate cancer 1999 with seed implantation; PSA 0.1.

3. Cervical neck fusion.

4. Right ulnar nerve repair.

PLANS:

Donor status: The patient appears to be a good kidney donor candidate. We will need a note from his urologist confirming resolution of his prior prostate cancer and the absence of lymphadenopathy or evidence of metastasis on prior imaging. The patient likely does not have true hypertension but meets criteria for donation even if he does, according to the Caucasian hypertensive donor protocol. He has well-controlled blood pressure, with no evidence of end-organ damage and low cardiac risk. I have recommended that he discontinue his ACE inhibitor 1 week prior to surgery to help avoid ATN. His blood pressure can be followed closely in the hospital to assess the need for antihypertensives. He would probably best benefit from short-term beta blockers and then a change back to an ACE inhibitor a few weeks after donation, if he is indeed hypertensive.

Discharge Summary

DIAGNOSES/PROBLEMS:

1. Living kidney donor.

2. Hypertensive donor protocol.

PROCEDURES:

Laparoscopic donor nephrectomy, 11/6/06.

HISTORY, MAJOR FINDINGS, AND HOSPITAL COURSE:

This 59-year-old male was admitted to donate a kidney to his son. Patient has an h/o prehypertension and was taking lisinopril/HCTZ prior to admission. Tolerated operative procedure well but had problems with nausea/vomiting after surgery. N/V improved after patient was changed from dolasetron to Zofran. Cr 1.4 mg/dL and Hct 29.4%. The patient has three port sites and a Pfannenstiel incision, which are steri-stripped. No purulent drainage from wound or erythema is noted. The patient has ecchymosis across the lower abdomen. BP range during this admission 123-156/72-87. Will be followed by nephrology as an outpatient because he is in the hypertensive donor protocol. Discharged to home, ambulatory and in good condition.

DISCHARGE MEDICATIONS:

Colace 100 mg PO bid

Lisinopril 20/HCTZ 12.5 mg PO 1/2 tablet qd

DISCHARGE INSTRUCTIONS:

Call for increased T, decreased UOP, N/V/D, constipation, wound infection, or any other unusual symptoms. No driving ×2 weeks or while on narcotics. No heavy lifting ×2 months. May shower. No soaps or lotions over incision.

FOLLOW-UP CARE:

Return in 2 weeks.

Operative Report

Title of operation: Laparoscopic left donor nephrectomy.

Indications for surgery: This is a middle-aged gentleman who is donating his kidney to his son. The patient has no particular prior medical history, other than prostate cancer. He has a history of a cervical fusion, and he has a history of alcohol abuse. The patient has been compliant with his alcohol abstinence program over the past few years and currently is in an excellent state of health. He underwent a complete workup prior to being cleared to become a donor; that workup did not elucidate any medical problems. All inherent risks of this operation were explained in great detail, and the patient signed the consents after I had explained all of these risks to him and to his family.

Preoperative diagnosis: Healthy kidney donor.

Postoperative diagnosis: Healthy kidney donor.

Anesthesia: General endotracheal anesthesia.

Complications: None.

Estimated blood loss: Minimal.

Surgeon's Narrative

The patient was brought to the Operating Room and was placed supine on the operating table. General endotracheal anesthesia was induced. Sequential compression devices were placed and Foley catheter was placed. Abdomen was prepped and draped on a standard, surgical protocol. Ports were placed at the umbilicus and subxiphoid region and left anterior axillary line. A Pfannenstiel incision was made, and a port was placed through this defect as well. The patient was placed in right lateral decubitus position, right side down, left side elevated. We began the operation by medially reflecting his left colon from the splenic flexure all the way down into the pelvis, exposing the retroperitoneum. We then began dissection in and about the retroperitoneum. We isolated retroperitoneal structures, including the gonadal vein and the ureter. We traced the gonadal vein superiorly to its junction with the left renal vein. We circumferentially dissected about the left renal vein and artery. We then circumferentially dissected about the kidney, taking down all of its retroperitoneal attachments. The patient had a very adherent adrenal gland; the dissection above the left adrenal gland was difficult, and there was some amount of hemorrhage, but this was eventually easily controlled. After we had isolated the vascular pedicle, we were ready to remove the kidney. We ligated the gonadal vein in the pelvis and cut through the ureter after ligating the distal aspect of the ureter with staples. Free, aggressive urine was afforded to occur inside the abdomen. The patient did receive induction antibiotics, as well as systemic heparinization and systemic diuretic medications. Good diuresis occurred at this point. We then proceeded to take down all retroperitoneal attachments for the kidney, and only the vascular pedicle held the kidney in place. Using the GIA linear stapling and the dividing device, we then stapled across the renal artery and vein and removed the kidney with the use of the endoscopic bag retrieval system through the Pfannenstiel incision; we handed the kidney off in good condition, as a specimen. Our attention then returned to the abdomen. We reconstituted the carbon dioxide pneumoperitoneum up to 50 mm Hg. We looked for any hemorrhage or intra-abdominal injury. None was seen. There was some hemorrhage—a small amount at the adrenal gland—that was easily controlled with the endoscopic argon beam coagulator. We then proceeded to close all port sites with the Carter-Thomason suture passing device. We closed the Pfannenstiel incision in layers; interrupted number 1 Maxon sutures were used to close the fascial layer. Skin incisions were all closed with 4-0 Biosyn, and sterile dressings were applied. The patient tolerated the procedure well. No complications were reported. The needle, instrument, and sponge count were correct at the end of the case. The patient was awakened, extubated, and transported to the postanesthesia care unit in stable condition.

Progress Notes

TRANSPLANT SURGERY NOTE

Preop diagnosis: Elective donor nephrectomy.

Postop diagnosis: Same.

Procedure: Elective left donor nephrectomy.

Anesth: General.

EBL: 400 cc.

UOP: 1600 cc.

Fluids: 4900 cc.

To PACU in stable condition.

DAY 1

Vital signs stable. UOP is good.

Nausea and vomiting.

Change to Zofran.

Wounds look good.

DAY 2

Vital signs are stable. Blood pressure is good. UOP remains good.

N/V has resolved.

Wounds have no drainage or erythema.

Continue antihypertensive medication.

Ready for discharge.

CASE STUDY QUESTIONS

20-1a. Admit diagnosis: _____

20-1b. Discharge disposition: _____

20-1c. Principal diagnosis: _____

20-1d. Secondary diagnoses (indicate POA status for secondary diagnoses):

_____

_____

_____

_____

_____

_____

20-1e. Principal procedure: _____

20-1f. Secondary procedures: _____

20-1g. Assign MS-DRG: _____

20-1h. Relative weight of MS-DRG: _____

20-1i. Can this MS-DRG be optimized with the addition of a CC? Yes or No
Can this MS-DRG be optimized with the addition of an MCC? Yes or No

20-1j. Is there a main guideline pertinent to selection of the principal diagnosis in this case study?

_____

_____

20-1k. Is there another diagnosis that meets the definition for principal diagnosis? Yes or No

20-1l. If yes, what is the other diagnosis? _____

20-1m. Is there any opportunity for physician query?

_____

_____

20-1n. What is the drug Zofran used to treat? _____

20-2. CASE STUDY

History and Physical

CC: ARF, anuria.

HPI: The patient is a very pleasant 68-year-old gentleman who was first diagnosed with IgG kappa multiple myeloma about 6 years ago. He has had treatments consisting of thalidomide and dexamethasone, which he last received 2 years ago. He has also received 6 cycles of melphalan plus prednisone. He then went on to receive 4 cycles of Velcade plus dexamethasone; his last cycle was received last year. More recently, the patient received 3 cycles of Cytoxan. His most recent therapy consisted of Revlimid, which had to be held because of cytopenias. He was admitted in this instance for acute renal failure and anuria ×2 days in the setting of taking norfloxacin and Bactrim recently as an outpatient. Additionally, on admission, the patient was noted to be febrile, with an absolute neutrophil count of 570.

251

Past medical history: Progressive multiple myeloma.

Hypertension

Past surgical history: None.

Social history: Married. Retired. Quit smoking 20 years ago. Social alcohol.

Allergies: NKDA.

REVIEW OF SYSTEMS:

The patient has fever and diarrhea. Review of systems is otherwise negative, including review of HEENT, cardiovascular, lungs, GU, skin, and neurologic.

PHYSICAL EXAMINATION:

Vitals: Febrile. Rest of vitals stable.

General: Patient appears weak. NAD.

HEENT: Atraumatic.

Eye: Clear.

Neck: Supple. No masses.

Oropharynx: Benign.

Chest: Clear to auscultation.

CV: RRR. No murmur, rub, or gallops.

Abdomen: Soft. No masses or hepatosplenomegaly.

Extremities: Within normal limits.

Neuro: Intact.

A/P: Patient with progressive multiple myeloma in acute renal failure. Patient will be pan-cultured because of neutropenic fever. Patient will be started on empiric antibiotics.

Discharge Summary

DIAGNOSES/PROBLEMS:

1. Acute-on-chronic renal failure.
2. Multiple myeloma.
3. Nosebleed.
4. Neutropenic fever.
5. Hypertension.

PROCEDURES:

1. CT scan of chest showing increased lung markings consistent with mild congestion, but with no evidence of pneumonia.
2. CT scan of the L-spine showing multilevel degenerative disc disease, most severe at L4 and L5, with no significant central canal stenosis and moderate to severe L4-L5 neural foraminal stenosis.
3. CT scan of the sinuses showing no evidence of sinus disease; however, moderate soft tissue density is seen along the inferior tip of the left inferior turbinate, narrowing the inferior turbinate, the significance of which is unclear.

4. Renal ultrasound shows echogenic kidneys bilaterally, compatible with medical renal disease and a small septated cortical cyst in the lateral left kidney.

HISTORY, MAJOR FINDINGS, AND HOSPITAL COURSE:

The patient is a very pleasant 68-year-old gentleman who was first given the diagnosis of IgG kappa multiple myeloma about 6 years ago. He has been given treatments that consisted of thalidomide and dexamethasone, which he last received 2 years ago. He has also received 6 cycles of melphalan plus prednisone. He then went on to receive 4 cycles of Velcade plus dexamethasone; his last cycle was received last year. More recently, he received 3 cycles of Cytoxan. His most recent therapy has consisted of Revlimid, which had to be held because of cytopenias. He was admitted in this instance for acute renal failure and anuria ×2 days in the setting of taking norfloxacin and Bactrim recently as an outpatient. Additionally, on admission, the patient was noted to be febrile, with an absolute neutrophil count of 570.

HOSPITAL COURSE BY SYSTEMS:

1. Oncologic: The patient has a longstanding history of multiple myeloma and has had multiple therapies. Unfortunately, his most recent therapy consisting of Revlimid was held because of cytopenias. While in the hospital, the patient's regular oncologist met with him and his family and also discussed his case with us. We all decided that his myeloma was significantly refractory, and that no other therapies were available for his myeloma. Given his grim prognosis and new renal failure, which is likely secondary to his myeloma, discussions were had regarding hospice care. Initially, the patient was wary of this and wanted to progress with more therapy; however, after additional discussions and after discussions involving his children and his wife, it was decided that home hospice care would be best for him because additional therapies would probably do more harm than good. In this light, we worked with a social worker to arrange for home hospice, and the patient was discharged to home with home hospice follow-up.

2. Renal: On admission, his creatinine was 2.8, up from a baseline of 1.4. It quickly then went up to 5.4 by the second day of admission, and he was anuric. A Foley catheter was placed, which did not result in any urine output. Electrolytes remained normal. However, the patient progressively became more and more azotemic while in the hospital and had a worsening creatinine. There were never any indications for dialysis. The renal team was consulted for their input, and a renal ultrasound was performed that showed no obstructive disease. Additionally, we considered that his renal failure may have been secondary to norfloxacin or Bactrim. However, this seemed less likely when his renal function failed to return to normal after these medications were held on admission. Additionally, urine eosinophils were collected and were negative. All in all, given the complete picture, it was thought that his renal failure was secondary to multiple myeloma.

3. Infectious disease: On admission, the patient was noted to have a fever in the setting of leukopenia. Blood cultures were collected on admission; no growth was revealed on any microorganisms. Upon admission, the patient was empirically treated with Zosyn 2.25 g every 4 hours. Once it was clear that his cultures were negative and his fever had resolved, the antibiotic was stopped. Additionally, a stool C. diff antigen was tested for, but findings were negative; C. diff as a cause for his fever was ruled out. Upon discharge, the patient had no active infectious disease issues and therefore was discharged with no antibiotics.

4. Nosebleed: While in the hospital, the patient had a mild nosebleed. CT of the sinus showed a soft tissue density at the left inferior turbinate. An ENT was consulted, and this lesion was cauterized. This significantly helped the patient's nosebleed, which was likely secondary to this soft tissue density, as well as to uremic platelets in the setting of his renal failure.

We had multiple discussions with the patient and his family, including his children and wife, and it was decided that the best care for him would be to involve home hospice because effective treatment for his myeloma was not possible. In this regard, the social worker was able to arrange for home hospice, and the patient was discharged to home in fair condition.

DISCHARGE MEDICATIONS:

Compazine 10 mg every 6 hours as needed for nausea.
Ambien 5 mg nightly as needed for sleep.
Afrin 2 sprays twice daily in the nose.
Allopurinol 100 mg daily.
Renagel 1600 mg 3 times daily.
Metoprolol 25 mg twice daily.
Imodium as needed for diarrhea.

FOLLOW-UP CARE:

Discharged to home hospice.

Progress Note

DAY 1

Patient with progressive multiple myeloma presents with ARF. Will need renal consult.

Cr increased from 1.4 to 2.8 to 5.4. Minimize nephrotoxins. No acute need yet to start dialysis. Patient has diarrhea. Watch potassium levels.

DAY 2

This is a patient with end-stage myeloma and renal failure. His diarrhea continues with blood-stained stool. He required several units of RBCs. The patient has also had a nosebleed (after ENT cauterized him). After extensive discussions with patient and family, we are not proceeding with dialysis at the present time. Ordered CT sinuses.

DAY 3

Patient was admitted with ARF. No evidence of sinus disease per CT. Add loperamide for diarrhea. Check C diff. Continue bicarb for nongap acidosis.

DAY 4

Diarrhea is improving. Patient continues to have nosebleeds. Neutropenic fever on Zosyn.

Cultures are negative.

DNR/DNI DISCUSSION

I had a discussion with the patient and his family regarding DNR and DNI status. After further discussion with their son, family members agree with DNR/DNI code status, and an order has been placed in the chart. I also discussed hemodialysis. At this time, we are not going to pursue. The patient's wife agrees with this because it is not likely to change his prognosis in light of refractory multiple myeloma.

Patient with refractory multiple myeloma admitted with ARF. Home hospice arrangements are under way. Patient has no complaints. Diarrhea is better. Nosebleeds have subsided. Afebrile.

CV: RRR.

Lungs: Diffuse crackles.

Abd: +BS.

Discharge when hospice arrangements are complete.

CASE STUDY QUESTIONS

20-2a.   Admit diagnosis: _____

20-2b.   Discharge disposition: _____

20-2c.   Principal diagnosis: _____

20-2d.   Secondary diagnoses (indicate POA status for secondary diagnoses):

_____

_____

_____

_____

_____

20-2e.   Principal procedure: _____

20-2f.   Secondary procedures: _____

_____

20-2g.   Assign MS-DRG: _____

20-2h.   Relative weight of MS-DRG: _____

20-2i.   Can this MS-DRG be optimized with the addition of a CC? Yes or No
         Can this MS-DRG be optimized with the addition of an MCC? Yes or No

20-2j.   Is there a main guideline pertinent to selection of the principal diagnosis in this case study?

_____

_____

20-2k.   Is there another diagnosis that meets the definition for principal diagnosis? Yes or No

20-2l.   If yes, what is the other diagnosis? _____

20-2m. Is there any opportunity for physician query?

_____

_____

20-2n. What is the drug Lisinopril 20/HCTZ 12.5 used to treat? _____

20-3. CASE STUDY

History and Physical

CC: Right flank pain.

HPI: The patient is an 80-year-old female who presented to the emergency department with severe, 8 out of 10, right flank pain that radiated to the right upper quadrant. The pain was associated with nausea and several episodes of vomiting. She had at least one of her typical seizures prior to admission. It was believed that the seizure occurred because she was unable to hold down her antiepileptic medication. CT scan of the abdomen and pelvis in the emergency department showed numerous diverticula in the cecum and descending colon with minimal surrounding fat stranding, possibly representing mild diverticulitis, although no evidence suggested diverticular abscess or perforation. No renal stones were seen. Ultrasound showed two cysts in the right kidney. Increased echogenicity of the kidneys was noted, consistent with medical renal disease. Again, no stones were seen. The gallbladder was normal. The patient's examination was remarkable for right flank pain and hypertension, and morphine was required to control her pain. No evidence of an acute cardiac event was seen. Evidence of diverticulitis was not found on physical examination.

Past medical history: Hypertension, hyperlipidemia, seizure disorder, osteoarthritis, trigeminal neuralgia, and GERD. History of lacunar infarcts.

Past surgical history: Cervical fusion.

Social history: Retired seamstress. Lives with son. No tobacco or alcohol.

REVIEW OF SYSTEMS:

Constitutional: No fever or chills. Appetite is good. Some weight gain over past year.

Neuro: Seizures. No headache, syncope, weakness, or tremor.

HEENT: No vision change or hearing loss. No sore throat.

CV: No chest pain, palpitations, orthopnea, PND, or edema.

Respiratory: SOB with exertion. No wheezing, cough, or hemoptysis.

GI: No dysphagia or hematemesis.

GU: No dysuria, frequency, or urgency.

Skin: No rashes or bruising.

PHYSICAL EXAMINATION:

Vitals: T 100.3, HR 76, BP 126/66, RR 20, SaO_2, 94% RA.

General: NAD.

HEENT: PERRL. EOMI. MMM. Oropharynx clear. Neck is supple. JVP not elevated.

Chest: Bibasilar rales.

Heart: RRR. No m/r/g.

Abd: Obese, slightly distended. Umbilical hernia.

Neuro: Intact. Alert and oriented ×3.

256

A/P: Patient is admitted with right flank pain and nausea. Treat with pain medications, IVs, antiemetics, and strain urine.

Discharge Summary

DIAGNOSES/PROBLEMS:

1. Right flank pain, probably secondary to nephrolithiasis.
2. Nausea and vomiting.
3. Urinary tract infection.
4. Complex partial seizures with secondary generalization.
5. Hypertensive heart disease with left ventricular hypertrophy.
6. Gastroesophageal reflux.
7. Hyperlipidemia.
8. Diverticulosis.
9. Trigeminal neuralgia.

PROCEDURES:

CT scan and ultrasound of the abdomen and pelvis.

HISTORY, MAJOR FINDINGS, AND HOSPITAL COURSE:

History: The patient is an 80-year-old female who presented to the emergency department with severe, 8 out of 10, right flank pain that radiated to the right upper quadrant. The pain was associated with nausea and several episodes of vomiting. She had at least one of her typical seizures prior to admission. It was believed that the seizure occurred because she was unable to hold down her antiepileptic medication. CT scan of the abdomen and pelvis in the emergency department showed numerous diverticula in the cecum and descending colon with minimal surrounding fat stranding, possibly representing mild diverticulitis, although no evidence of diverticular abscess or perforation was found. No renal stones were seen. Ultrasound showed two cysts in the right kidney. Increased echogenicity of the kidneys was noted, consistent with medical renal disease. Again, no stones were seen. The gallbladder was normal. The patient's examination was remarkable for right flank pain and hypertension, and morphine was required to control her pain. No evidence of an acute cardiac event was noted. Evidence of diverticulitis was not found on physical examination.

Lab studies were remarkable for a BUN of 25 and a creatinine of 1.4, along with a baseline creatinine of 1.2. Hematocrit 48.3. Urinalysis was initially unremarkable; however, repeat urinalysis showed significant pyuria. No hematuria was noted. The patient's white count remained normal throughout her hospitalization.

The patient was able to take her Keppra orally, and she had no additional seizures. She had been on hydrochlorothiazide prior to admission; this was held secondary to her vomiting and elevated renal function studies. Her blood pressure was elevated during the hospitalization, and she was restarted on HCTZ at discharge. She has a history of angioneurotic edema on ACE inhibitors and has not tolerated beta blockers in the past. She has been maintained on verapamil because of significant left ventricular hypertrophy and end-systole cavity obliteration, which was documented on prior echocardiograms. She was taken off Lipitor prior to this admission because of an elevated CK, which was believed to be due to statin therapy. CK elevation was associated with extremity discomfort, which has resolved since the patient came off of the Lipitor. She was initially kept NPO on IV fluids. Her diet was then advanced as tolerated. By day 2, she was eating well and holding down her medications. She was believed to be stable for discharge. Although no nephrolithiasis was documented on her radiologic studies, her clinical course was believed to be consistent with that of passing a renal stone. She was placed on Bactrim DS one 2 times a day for treatment of a urinary tract infection. Her potassium level was 3.3, and she was treated with oral potassium. Her BUN was 15 and baseline creatinine was 1.2 on the day of discharge. Her estimated GFR was 52 mL/min.

257

Reportable diseases: None.

Allergies: Penicillin and ACE inhibitors (prior history of angioneurotic edema on enalapril). Possible CK elevation due to Lipitor.

Condition on discharge was good.

DISCHARGE MEDICATIONS:

Bactrim DS 1 by mouth 2 times a day to complete treatment for her UTI.

Keppra 500 mg 2 times a day, alternating with 500 mg 3 times a day.

Verapamil SR 240 mg nightly.

Nexium 40 mg every day for GERD.

Nortriptyline 10 mg nightly for trigeminal neuralgia.

Lorazepam 0.5 mg nightly as needed.

ASA 81 mg every day.

Tylenol as needed for pain.

Lipitor 40 mg is on hold at the time of discharge.

She is restarted on hydrochlorothiazide 12.5 mg every day.

DISCHARGE INSTRUCTIONS:

Diet: No added salt, low cholesterol.

Activity: As tolerated.

Other: She is to notify her physician about any recurrent pain or seizures.

FOLLOW-UP CARE:

Follow up care with primary physician in 1 week.

Progress Notes

DAY 1

The patient states that she feels better this morning. She has some lingering pain in the right flank area but with no radiation. VSS except for mild elevation of BP.

Lungs: Clear.

CV: Regular S1 and S2.

Abd: Soft. Bowel sounds present.

Labs show significant pyuria despite normal UA yesterday. This points to a renal stone source, although no hematuria is evident. Advance diet as tolerated. Patient must be able to hold down her seizure meds before she can be discharged.

DAY 2

Patient is significantly better today. She is tolerating liquids. No additional seizures. Her abdominal examination is benign. No RUQ or flank pain is reported today. Morning labs are remarkable for a low potassium of 3.3. This will be replaced with oral supplements. The patient can be discharged home today if she tolerates her lunch. Follow up in 1 week.

CASE STUDY QUESTIONS

20-3a. Admit diagnosis: _____

20-3b. Discharge disposition: _____

20-3c. Principal diagnosis: _____

20-3d. Secondary diagnoses (indicate POA status for secondary diagnoses):

_____

_____

_____

_____

_____

_____

20-3e. Principal procedure: _____

20-3f. Secondary procedures: _____

_____

20-3g. Assign MS-DRG: _____

20-3h. Relative weight of MS-DRG: _____

20-3i.   Can this MS-DRG be optimized with the addition of a CC? Yes or No

Can this MS-DRG be optimized with the addition of an MCC? Yes or No

20-3j.   Is there a main guideline pertinent to selection of the principal diagnosis in this case study?

_____

_____

20-3k. Is there another diagnosis that meets the definition for principal diagnosis? Yes or No

20-3l.   If yes, what is the other diagnosis? _____

20-3m. Is there any opportunity for physician query?

_____

_____

20-3n. What is a "statin" drug used to treat? _____

21 Pregnancy, Childbirth, and the Puerperium (ICD-10-CM Chapter 15, Codes O00-O9a)

ABBREVIATIONS/ACRONYMS

Without the use of reference materials, define the following abbreviations or acronyms.

1. SVD _____
2. OB _____
3. EDC _____
4. AROM _____
5. VBAC _____
6. PTL _____
7. PP _____
8. PIH _____
9. IUD _____
10. FTP _____
11. IOL _____

GLOSSARY DEFINITIONS

Match the glossary term to the correct definition.

1. _____ Primigravida
2. _____ Preeclampsia
3. _____ Labor
4. _____ Gravid
5. _____ Antepartum

A. Process by which the products of conception are expelled from the uterus

B. Complication of pregnancy characterized by hypertension and edema

C. First pregnancy

D. Pregnant

E. Before delivery

CODING

Using the code book, code the following.

1. Ruptured ectopic with removal of right fallopian tubal pregnancy _____

2. Therapeutic abortion secondary to chromosomal defect in fetus; D&C was performed _____

3. Vaginal delivery at 43 weeks; baby was stillborn _____

4. Low forceps delivery at 39 weeks; baby was large for gestational age _____

5. Delivered 1 week PTA; presents with postpartum pyrexia _____

6. Incomplete abortion with D&C _____

7. Pregnancy at term; baby delivered by gas station attendant as patient was unable to make it to the hospital _____

8. Patient delivered by low transverse C section because of malpresentation of twins at 38 weeks; patient also has a fibroid uterus _____

9. Missed abortion _____

10. Toxemia of pregnancy at 28 weeks, seen in physician office. _____

11. Uterine rupture during labor at 39 weeks. Patient delivered by classical cesarean section _____

CASE SCENARIOS

Using the code book, code the following cases.

1. The patient is admitted to the hospital in preterm labor. She is 27 weeks pregnant. Terbutaline is administered, and the patient remained on bed rest. On the second week of bed rest, her water breaks and she is taken to the delivery room. She vaginally delivers a baby girl.

   _____

   _____

2. The patient is admitted in labor at term. She labors for 24 hours when it is noted that the baby is in fetal distress. The patient is taken to the OR for an emergency C-section (LTCS).

   _____

   _____

3. The patient is admitted in labor at term. After lab work is completed, it is noted that the patient has a UTI and appears to be preeclamptic. The patient goes on to vaginally deliver a healthy baby boy.

   _____

   _____

4. The patient is 9 weeks pregnant. She is admitted for an elective abortion. The physician performs a suction D&C to terminate the pregnancy.

   _____

   _____

5. The patient presents to the hospital with high fever and hypotension. Three days PTA, she had undergone an elective abortion. Upon completion of the lab work, it is determined that she has sepsis due to retained placental tissue A D&C is performed.

   _____

   _____

6. The patient presents to the hospital in labor at term. She labors for 5 hours with the help of an epidural and goes on to deliver a healthy baby girl.

_____

_____

7. A patient with known breech presentation presents to the hospital in labor at term. After an attempt at manual rotation is made, the patient is taken to the delivery room for a low transverse C-section. She delivers a healthy baby boy.

_____

_____

8. The patient is admitted to the hospital in week 12 of pregnancy. She is vomiting and dehydrated. She is administered IV fluids and is sent home with a diagnosis of hyperemesis gravidarum.

_____

_____

9. The patient is admitted to the hospital in labor at 33 weeks. She has a known twin pregnancy. She has premature rupture of her membranes and goes on to deliver twin boys. On the second day after delivery, she develops a pulmonary embolism.

_____

_____

10. A 42-year-old mother with a previous CS delivers vaginally at 39 weeks. Because of the large size of the baby (more than 4000 g), the physician uses low forceps to deliver. The physician performs an episiotomy, but because of the baby's size, a 4 degree laceration occurs. The tears and the episiotomy are repaired.

_____

_____

CASE STUDIES

Using the code book, code and answer questions about the following case studies.

21-1. CASE STUDY

History and Physical

CC: SROM

HPI: History: The patient is a 32-year-old para 0-0-1-0 who presented at 40-6/7 weeks as determined by dates examination and 7-week sonogram. She presented with spontaneous rupture of membranes in active labor. Antenatal course notable for the following laboratories: blood type A, Rh positive, antibodies negative. STS nonreactive. GC negative. _Chlamydia_ negative. Rubella immune. Hepatitis negative. AFP screen normal. Hemoglobin type AA, HIV negative, GBS negative, and glucose screen 120. Total weight gain, 36 pounds.

History of previous pregnancies: 9-week blighted ovum a couple of years ago.

Past medical history: Migraines, a history of positive PPD, treated with 6 months of isoniazid for prophylaxis and with a negative chest x-ray. Drainage of thyroid cyst.

Gynecologic history: D&C for blighted ovum. No history of sexually transmitted diseases.

Medications: Prenatal vitamins.

Allergies: No known drug allergies.

Blood transfusion history: None.

Family history: Maternal grandmother with thalassemia major.

Social history: The patient denies smoking cigarettes, drinking alcohol, and using illicit drugs during this pregnancy. Her urine tox has been negative.

Physical Examination:

Vitals: Ht: 66, Wt: 176, afebrile, P 85, RR 18, BP 125/75, FHR 130s.

General: Patient is in early labor.

HEENT: NCAT.

Chest: CTAB.

CV: RRR.

Abd: Gravid abdomen.

Ext: No edema. 2+ reflexes.

GU/Rectal: Deferred.

Neuro: Alert and oriented ×3.

Assessment/Plan: Patient with 40 6/7-week gestation with SROM in early labor. Admitted for management of her labor and anticipated vaginal delivery. Patient has requested epidural. Prenatal course has been unremarkable. GBS negative.

OB Delivery Summary

Delivery Hospital: Hospital A.

OB Attending of Record: John Smith, MD.

Name: OB Patient.

Medical Record Number: 1234567.

Date of Birth: 12/01/79.

Gestational Age, weeks: 40.

Gestational Age, days: 6.

Number of Fetuses: Singleton.

Mode of Delivery: Spontaneous vaginal delivery.

VBAC: N/A.

Delivery Date/Time: 12/16/11 @ 14:10.

1st Stage of Labor, hours: 11.

1st Stage of Labor, minutes: 17.

2nd Stage of Labor, hours: 1.

2nd Stage of Labor, minutes: 44.

3rd Stage of Labor, hours: 0.

3rd Stage of Labor, minutes: 10.

Stages of Labor Total, hours: 13.

Stages of Labor Total, minutes: 11.

Membranes Monitoring

ROM: Spontaneous.

Amniotic Fluid at ROM: Clear.

Total Time Ruptured, days: 0.

Total Time Ruptured, hours: 13.

Total Time Ruptured, minutes: 1.

Amniotic Fluid at Delivery: Clear.

FHR Monitoring: EFM continuous.

Uterine Activity Monitoring: External.

Delivery Information

Infant Medical Record Number: 012345.

Born Prior to Arrival to L&D: No.

Infant Sex: Male.

Infant Birthweight, g: 3654.

Infant Status: Liveborn.

Apgar Score 1 Minute: 7.

Apgar Score 5 Minutes: 8.

Baby Disposition: NICU.

Labor Analgesia: Epidural.

Delivery Analgesia/Anesthesia: Epidural.

Placenta Delivery: Spontaneous.

Placenta Intact: Yes.

Postpartum Uterotonics: Pitocin IV.

Episiotomy/Laceration Information

Episiotomy: None.

Laceration Type: Perineal-midline.

Perineal Laceration Degree: Second degree.

Laceration Repaired: Yes.

Inspections: Cervical.

Inspections: Vaginal.

EBL, cc: 300.

Suture Used: 3-0.

Suture Used: Chromic.

Repair Details: Patient with second-degree midline laceration repaired with 3-0 chromic suture in the normal fashion with good hemostasis noted.

Delivery Diagnosis

Fetal Presentation: Vertex.

Position at Birth: OA.

Temperature: Intrapartum fever.

GBS: Negative.

Laceration Type: Perineal-midline.

Laceration/Extension: Second degree.

VBAC: N/A.

Nuchal Cord: N/A.

Delivery Diagnosis: History of positive PD S/P INH treatment, migraines, and chorioamnionitis.

Delivery Procedures

Delivery Type: Spontaneous vaginal delivery.

Analgesia Labor: Epidural.

Analgesia/Anes at Delivery: Epidural.

Labor: Spontaneous labor.

Maneuvers at Delivery: Ritgen's.

Perineum: Laceration repair.

Repair Details: Patient with second-degree midline laceration repaired with 3-0 chromic in the normal fashion with good hemostasis noted.

Delivery Procedures: AMP/Gent, ob sono, EFM/TOCO.

Delivery Comments: The patient is 32 yo P0010 @ 40.6 weeks S/P FTSVD with second-degree laceration. Infant has some grunting, so Peds was called and child was transported to NICU for further evaluation.

Discharge Summary

1. Intrauterine pregnancy at 40-6/7 weeks, delivered.
2. Chorioamnionitis.
3. Migraines.
4. History of positive PPD.
5. History of isoniazid prophylaxis.
6. Second-degree midline laceration.

PROCEDURES:

1. Full-term spontaneous vaginal delivery.
2. External fetal monitoring.
3. Tocodynamometry.
4. Anesthesia consult/epidural anesthesia.
5. Sonogram.
6. Intravenous Pitocin.
7. Ampicillin and gentamicin.
8. Second-degree laceration repair.

History: The patient is a 32-year-old para 0-0-1-0 who presented at 40-6/7 weeks as determined by dates examination and 7-week sonogram. She presented with spontaneous rupture of membranes in active labor.

History of previous pregnancies: 9-week blighted ovum a couple of years ago.

Past medical history: Migraines, history of positive PPD treated with 6 months isoniazid for prophylaxis and with a negative chest x-ray.

Gynecologic history: D&C for blighted ovum. Drainage of thyroid cyst. No history of sexually transmitted diseases.

Medications: Prenatal vitamins.

Allergies: No known drug allergies.

Blood transfusion history: None.

Family history: Maternal grandmother with thalassemia major.

Social history: The patient denies smoking cigarettes, drinking alcohol, and using illicit drugs during this pregnancy. Her urine tox has been negative.

Antenatal course notable for the following laboratories: Blood type A, Rh positive, antibodies negative. STS nonreactive. GC negative. *Chlamydia* negative. Rubella immune. Hepatitis negative. AFP screen normal. Hemoglobin type AA, HIV negative, GBS negative, and glucose screen 120. Total weight gain, 36 pounds.

Examination on admission: Height 66 inches, weight 176 pounds, heart rate 85, respiratory rate 18, blood pressure 125/75, fetal heart rate 130s and reactive. HEENT examination was within normal limits. The lungs were clear to auscultation bilaterally, the heart was regular rate and rhythm, no edema was noted in bilateral extremities, and reflexes were 2 plus bilaterally and symmetric. Fundal height was 38 cm, estimated fetal weight 3200 g; fetus was in vertex presentation as determined by sonogram. Sterile vaginal examination identified pelvic dilatation of 5 cm, 90% effacement, and negative 2 station, with rupture of membranes with positive ferning and nitrazine.

The patient was started on Pitocin as needed for augmentation of labor and received an epidural for her anesthesia when she became uncomfortable. Of note, the patient became febrile intrapartum with a T$_{max}$ of 38.2 degrees and was started on ampicillin and gentamicin for chorioamnionitis. She progressed to become fully dilated and delivered a male infant, with birth weight of 3654 g and Apgar scores of 7 at 1 minute and 8 at 5 minutes. The patient sustained a perineal midline second-degree laceration, which was repaired with 3-0 chromic suture with good hemostasis. Please see Delivery Summary for full delivery details.

Her postpartum course was unremarkable. The patient was ambulating, voiding, and tolerating regular diet at the time of discharge. She had minimal lochia. Her fundus was firm and nontender. Her pain was well controlled with Motrin. She chose to breastfeed her infant and to defer selection of birth control method until she visits her OB physician at 4 to 6 weeks post partum. The patient was discharged home on postpartum day 2 with no active issues.

Condition on discharge: Stable.

Discharge medications: Colace 100 mg 1 tablet by mouth 2 times a day, Motrin 600 mg 1 tablet by mouth every 6 hours as needed for pain, prenatal vitamins 1 tablet by mouth.

DISCHARGE INSTRUCTIONS:

Diet: Regular

Activity: Pelvic rest, meaning no intercourse, tampons, or douching for 4 to 6 weeks. No driving for 2 weeks or until the patient can safely press the brake pedal.

FOLLOW-UP CARE:

The patient is to follow up with her primary OB-GYN in 4 to 6 weeks after discharge from the hospital.

Progress Notes

Last examination, 6 to 7 cm dilated. Vertex presentation. Continue to monitor. Expectant management. FHR stable. Pitocin was started to augment labor. The patient is febrile with a temp of 38.2. Ampicillin and gent will be given for chorioamnionitis.

DAY 1

Patient is S/P FTSVD with second-degree laceration repair. She is doing well this AM. Tolerating po, ambulating, voiding. Denies shortness of breath or chest pain. No calf tenderness, no n/v, + flatus. Breastfeeding, lactation consult ordered.

DAY 2

S/P FTSVD complicated by intrapartum fever. Afebrile. Patient has some perineal pain that is relieved with Motrin. No BM, + flatus. Tolerating diet, ambulating. Lochia is decreasing. Discharge to home today.

CASE STUDY QUESTIONS

21-1a. Admit diagnosis: _____

21-1b. Discharge disposition: _____

21-1c. Principal diagnosis: _____

21-1d. Secondary diagnoses (indicate POA status for secondary diagnoses):

_____

_____

_____

_____

_____

_____

21-1e. Principal procedure: _____

21-1f. Secondary procedures: _____

_____

21-1g.   Assign MS-DRG: _____

21-1h.   Relative weight of MS-DRG: _____

21-1i.   Can this MS-DRG be optimized with the addition of a CC? Yes or No
         Can this MS-DRG be optimized with the addition of an MCC? Yes or No

21-1j.   Is there a main guideline pertinent to selection of the principal diagnosis in this case study?

_____

_____

21-1k.   Is there another diagnosis that meets the definition for principal diagnosis? Yes or No

21-1l.   If yes, what is the other diagnosis? _____

21-1m. Is there any opportunity for physician query?

_____

_____

21-1n.   What is the drug ampicillin used to treat? _____

21-2. CASE STUDY

History and Physical

CC: Fetal hydrops with nonreassuring FHT

HPI: This is a 26-year-old, para 0-1-1-1, presenting at 32 and 5/7th weeks by dates, examination, and a 29-week sono with a history of antibody positive for anti-C, anti-O, and anti-Kell, whose prenatal course is significant for severe Rh and Kell sensitization, noncompliance with obstetrical care visits, substance abuse, and the following labs: blood type A negative, antibody screen positive, Pap low-grade SIL, STS nonreactive, gonorrhea and *Chlamydia* negative, GBS negative, PPD negative, RhoGAM was given at 20 weeks, urine culture negative, rubella immune, hepatitis negative, AFP within normal limits, HIV negative, hepatitis C less than 35, anti-O antibody titer 35, anti-C at 8, anti-Kell 1:128, anti-c 1:16, 1-hour Glucola 95, hematocrit 30% to 31%, blood pressures 80-125/90-66, and total weight gain of 16 pounds. Her last sono showed an MCA Doppler of 3. History of previous pregnancies 4 years ago, preterm SVO at 36 weeks, 5 pounds; then, one 10 years ago, a 7-week termination.

Family history: Father of the baby was heterozygous for C, O, and E, homozygous for Kell; RhO-antigen carrier.

Transfusions: None.

Allergies: No known drug allergies.

Current medications: Methadone 85 mg and prenatal vitamin.

Medical history: Red cell alloimmunization noted above, hepatitis C, and anemia.

Past surgical history: D&C 9 years ago.

Past GYN history: No history of STDs except the above-mentioned hepatitis and low-grade SIL Pap.

PHYSICAL EXAMINATION:

_____

Vitals: Stable. General: NAD. HEENT: PERRLA. EOMI. Trachea is midline. Neck is supple without masses.

Chest: CTA.

CV: RRR.

Abd: Gravid; FHT 140s.

Ext: WNL.

GU/Rectal: Deferred.

Skin/Musculoskeletal: Normal.

Neuro: Alert and oriented.

Assessment/Plan: Fetal hydrops and nonreassuring fetal heart tones. The plan is to proceed with an intrauterine transfusion for possible severe fetal anemia in the setting of some fetal scalp edema and ascites.

OB/Delivery Summary

Delivery Hospital: Hospital A.

OB Attending of Record: John Smith, MD.

Name: OB Patient.

Medical Record Number: 2345671.

Date of Birth: 11/29/85.

Gestational Age, weeks: 32.

Gestational Age, days: 4.

Mode of Delivery: Low segment transverse cesarean.

Cesarean Type: Primary.

VBAC: N/A.

Delivery Date/Time: 09/03/11 @ 18:00.

3rd Stage of Labor, hours: 0.

3rd Stage of Labor, minutes: 1.

Membranes/Monitoring

ROM: Artificial ROM.

Amniotic fluid at ROM: Bloody.

Total Time Ruptured, days: 0.

Total Time Ruptured, hours: 0.

Total Time Ruptured, minutes: 0.

Amniotic Fluid at Delivery: Clear.

FHR Monitoring: EFM continuous.

Uterine Activity Monitoring: External.

Delivery Information

Infant Medical Record Number: 3456712.

Born Prior to Arrival to L&D: No.

Infant Sex: Female.

Infant Birthweight, g: 1790.

Infant Status: Liveborn.

270

Apgar Score 1 Minute: 5.

Apgar Score 5 Minutes: 7.

Baby Disposition: NICU.

Labor Analgesia: None.

Delivery Analgesia/Anesthesia: Spinal.

Placenta Delivery: Manual.

Placenta Intact: Yes.

Postpartum Uterotonics: Pitocin IV.

EBL, cc: 1000.

Delivery/Diagnosis

Fetal Presentation: Vertex.

GBS Status: Unknown.

VBAC: N/A.

Primary Indication for C-Section: Placenta abruption, suspected.

Secondary Indication for C-Sec: Fetal testing/tracing, nonreassuring.

Nuchal Cord: N/A.

Delivery Diagnosis: Rh isoimmunization, Kell isoimmunization, Fetal hydrops.

Delivery Procedures

Delivery Type: Low segment transverse cesarean.

C-Section Incidence: Primary.

Analgesia Labor: None.

Analgesia/Anes at Delivery: Spinal.

Placenta: Manual removal of placenta.

Delivery Comments: Uncomplicated primary LSTCS for NRFHTs and placental abruption.

Discharge Summary

DIAGNOSES/PROBLEMS:

1. A 32 and 5/7th weeks intrauterine pregnancy, delivered.
2. Nonreassuring fetal heart tracing.
3. Placental abruption.
4. Red cell alloimmunization, anti-O, anti-C, and anti-Kell.
5. Anemia.
6. Polysubstance abuse.
7. Limited prenatal care.
8. Hepatitis C.
9. Low-grade squamous intraepithelial lesion Pap.
10. Hydrops fetalis.

PROCEDURES:

1. Primary low-segment transverse C section.
2. Fetal blood transfusion.
3. EFM/toco.
4. Foley.
5. Epidural.
6. Spinal.

271

7. Methadone.
8. Social Work consult.

HISTORY, MAJOR FINDINGS, AND HOSPITAL COURSE:

This is a 26-year-old, para 0-1-1-1, presenting at 32 and 5/7th weeks by dates, examination, and a 29-week sono with a history of antibody positive for anti-C, anti-O, and anti-Kell, whose prenatal course is significant for severe Rh and Kell sensitization, noncompliance with obstetric care visits, substance abuse, and the following labs: blood type A negative, antibody screen positive, Pap low-grade SIL, STS nonreactive, gonorrhea and *Chlamydia* negative, GBS negative, PPD negative, RhoGAM was given at 20 weeks, urine culture negative, rubella immune, hepatitis negative, AFP within normal limits, HIV negative, hepatitis C less than 35, anti-O antibody titer 35, anti-C at 8, anti-Kell 1:128, anti-C 1:16, 1-hour Glucola 95, hematocrit 30% to 31%, blood pressures 80-125/90-66, and total weight gain of 16 pounds. Her last sono showed an MCA Doppler of 3. History of previous pregnancies 4 years ago, preterm SVD at 36 weeks, 5 pounds; then, one 10 years ago, a 7-week termination.

Family history: Father of the baby heterozygous for C, O, and E, homozygous for Kell; RhO-antigen carrier.

Transfusions: None.

Allergies: No known drug allergies.

Current medications: Methadone 85 mg and prenatal vitamin.

Medical history: Red cell alloimmunization noted above, hepatitis C, and anemia.

Past surgical history: D&C 9 years ago.

Past GYN history: No history of STDs except the above-mentioned hepatitis and low-grade SIL Pap.

On presentation, her vital signs were stable, heart tones in the 140s. EFW 1781. She was 1, 50, and minus 3. On pelvic sono, evidence of ascites with scalp edema. The fetus was vertex with an AFI of 4.2. The patient was admitted with a hydropic fetus and hydropic placenta by sono with history of red cell alloimmunization. Repeat antibody titers were drawn. After counseling as to risks and benefits, the plan was to proceed with intrauterine transfusion on hospital day number 2 secondary to probable severe fetal anemia in the setting of some fetus scalp edema and ascites. Betamethasone number 1 was given at 4 PM. Gonorrhea and *Chlamydia* cultures were pending, and the NICU was made aware. Regarding her polysubstance abuse, she was continued on methadone, and nicotine patch was placed. Regarding hepatitis C, a CMP was drawn for viral load. On the day of admission, she underwent an intrauterine fetal blood transfusion of a total of 80 cubic centimeters of blood via cordocentesis to bring fetal Hct to 35%; higher volumes not given because of hydrops present and load on the fetal cardiovascular system. Initial fetal hemoglobin and hematocrit were 2.6 and 6.5%, respectively (confirmed initial results on separate samples as 2.6 [Hgb] and 6.4% [Hct]), with an MCV of 180 and platelets 70,000. Fetal heart rate was in the 130s after the procedure and stable. Prior to the procedure, minimal fetal tricuspid regurgitation was visualized in the ductus arteriosus, but no reverse flow was visualized. She was placed on Ancef. No streaming was noted. At about 1700, the patient began complaining of vaginal bleeding with moderate blood. Speculum examination showed about 20 to 30 cubic centimeters of clot in the os, uterus was firm, and fetal heart tone in the 120s with good variability, but there was a concern for possible abruption, especially given the hydropic placenta. Therefore, a decision was made to proceed with C section for nonreassuring fetal heart tracing in the presence of possible placental abruption. She underwent a primary low-segment transverse C section with an EBL of 1000 cubic centimeters. Findings include a female infant, 1.97 kg, Apgars 5 and 7; clot was documented between the placenta and the membranes. She had an uncomplicated postoperative course. Her hematocrit remained stable postoperatively at 32%. She was without complaints,

272

was tolerating oral, ambulating, and passing flatus. By postoperative day number 4, blood pressures remained stable, slightly elevated at 130 to 150/83 to 88. Otherwise, her fundus was firm, 2 cm below the umbilicus, and her incision was clean, dry, and intact. She was discharged home and was told to follow up in the clinic in 1 week for blood pressure check; however, her urine protein had been negative throughout this admission.

Discharge medications: Tylox 1 to 2 tablets by mouth every 4 to 6 hours as needed for pain, Motrin 600 mg by mouth every 6 hours as needed for pain, Colace 100 mg by mouth 2 times a day, prenatal vitamin 1 tablet by mouth every day.

DISCHARGE INSTRUCTIONS:

Activity: Pelvic rest times 4 to 6 weeks, no driving while on narcotics, and no heavy lifting greater than 10 pounds.

FOLLOW-UP CARE:

She was told to follow up in the clinic in the next day or two for repeat blood pressure check and for her methadone.

Operative Report

Primary low-segment transverse cesarean section.

Indications for Surgery: The patient is a 26-year-old para 0-1-1-1 at 32-5/7 weeks, by dates, examination, and 29-week sonogram who had had cramping and vaginal bleeding, which prompted concern about placental abruption in conjunction with nonreassuring tel tones.

Preoperative diagnosis: A 32-5/7th-week intrauterine pregnancy. Placental abruption. Nonreassuring fetal heart tone.

Postoperative diagnosis: A 32-5/7th-week intrauterine pregnancy, delivered. Placental abruption. Nonreassuring fetal heart tone.

Specimen (bacteriologic, pathologic, or other): Placenta.

Surgeon's Narrative

EBL: 1000 cubic centimeters.

Fluids: 2000 cubic centimeters.

Urine output: 400 cubic centimeters.

Findings: A female infant weighing 1.97 kg, Apgar scores of 5 and 7, cord gas pH 7.15, pO_2 9.0, pCO_2 76, bicarbonate 26, base excess of minus 3. Other findings included a clot that was revealed upon incision of the uterus and a clot between the placenta and membranes.

Narrative: The patient was taken back to the Operating Room and was prepped and draped in the usual sterile fashion. Spinal anesthesia was found to be adequate. A low Pfannenstiel skin incision was made and was taken down to the fascia with a scalpel. The fascia was dissected and separated with Mayo scissors. The anterior aspect of the fascia was resected off the rectus muscle with the use of Kocher and Mayo scissors, and a similar procedure was used on the posterior edge of the fascia. The rectus muscles were separated bluntly at the midline. The peritoneum was entered bluntly. The bladder blade was inserted to reveal the vesicouterine reflection. Using pickups and Metzenbaum scissors, the bladder flap was created at this junction. The bladder blade was then replaced, showing the lower uterine segment. At this point, a transverse incision on the lower uterine segment was made and carried superiorly with bandage scissors. The infant's head was brought to the incision and suctioned. Shoulders and body were then delivered. The cord was clamped and cut, and the infant was handed off to waiting pediatricians. Attention was then turned to prenatal cord gas, and the placenta was removed with massage and gentle traction. It was revealed that between the placenta and membranes, blood clot was found. The uterus was exteriorized and was cleared of all clot and debris. The uterine incision was closed in two layers with 0 Vicryl suture. It was found to be hemostatic. The uterus was returned to the abdominal cavity. The gutter was cleared of all clots. The uterine incision was observed again and again and was found to be hemostatic. The fascia was closed with 1-0 Vicryl suture in a running fashion, and the skin was closed with staples. The patient tolerated the procedure well and was sent to the recovery room in stable condition.

Complications: None.

Operative Report

Title of operation: Intrahepatic vein blood sampling. Cordocentesis. Fetal blood transfusion via cordocentesis (loop).

Indications for surgery: Severe Rh isoimmunization, positive anti-Kell (K1) and anti-C antibodies; fetal hydrops.

Preoperative diagnosis: 32-5/7 weeks intrauterine pregnancy, undelivered. Rh isoimmunization. Anti-K1 and C antibodies. Fetal hydrops.

Postoperative diagnosis: Same. Fetal anemia: Hematocrit 6.5%, elevated MCA Doppler 113.4 cm/s, status post fetal blood sampling and intrauterine transfusion via cordocentesis.

Anesthesia: Local 1% lidocaine (10 cc), IV Fentanyl and Versed.

Specimen (bacteriologic, pathologic, or other): To laboratory, fetal blood for CBC, ABO type, HCV IgG/IgM.

Surgeon's Narrative

The patient is a 26-year-old 83 P0111 at 32-5/7 weeks' gestation. Pregnancy significant for positive anti-D, K1, and C antibodies. The patient is an IV drug user and admits to sharing needles with the father of the baby. His red blood cell antigen status is homozygous for K1, heterozygous for C, and positive for O (Rh). On initial presentation, the patient's anti-D titer was 1:32, anti-K1 titer was 1:128, and anti-C titer was 1:8. The patient was noncompliant with prenatal care. Repeat titer a few months ago was unchanged for K1; however, anti-D titer increased to 1:512. The patient underwent ultrasonography at that time without evidence of fetal hydrops. The patient did not show for ultrasound appointments. However, the patient saw a physician, and ultrasound showed no evidence of fetal hydrops at that time. On the day of admission, the patient underwent fetal testing with findings of decreased variability and occasional decelerations. She was sent to Labor and Delivery for prolonged monitoring and underwent ultrasound that showed oligohydramnios and fetal ascites. The patient was transferred to our facility for fetal blood transfusion. This is her first fetal blood transfusion.

Findings: On ultrasonography, fetal ascites and skin edema were appreciated. Minimal tricuspid regurgitation was seen and reverse flow in the ductus arteriosus was not visualized. Estimated fetal weight 1957 g, MCA Doppler 113.4 cm/s (66.6 cm/s is 1.5 MOM for 32-week fetus), oligohydramnios, fetal heart rate during and after procedure was stable. No streaming was visualized.

Total volume drawn via intrahepatic vein blood sampling: 0.4 cc.

Total volume drawn via cordocentesis: 4 cc.

Fetal blood sample #1: Hgb 2.6, hct 6.5%, MCV 158.5 fL, Plts 71 K; fetal sample #2: Hgb 2.6 mg/dL, hct 6.4%, MCV 150 fL, Plts 70 K.

Calculated final fetal hematocrit: 35%.

Antibiotics: Patient was on Ancef prior to the procedure and will be continued on Ancef after the procedure.

Estimated blood loss: Minimal.

After informed consent was obtained, the patient was taken to the operating room, and ultrasonography revealed that the fetus was in a satisfactory position. The patient was prepped and draped in the usual sterile fashion. Under ultrasound guidance, a 20-gauge needle was inserted and guided directly into the fetal intrahepatic vein. Initially, a total of 0.4 cc of fetal blood was obtained. However, additional fetal blood could not be obtained because of uterine contractions that moved the needle tip. A second 20-gauge needle was inserted and was guided directly into the intrahepatic vein; however, fetal blood could not be accessed because of uterine contractions. The first two needles did not traverse the placenta. The patient had uterine contractions throughout the procedure, which changed the location of the targeted fetal intrahepatic vein. This, along with the position of the fetal arm and fetus, necessitated insertion of a third 20-gauge needle; from this insertion site, a portion of the placenta was traversed before it was guided into the fetal intrahepatic vein. However, an adequate fetal blood sample could not be obtained; the intrahepatic vein seemed to be collapsed. Therefore, a fourth 20-gauge needle was inserted, which traversed a portion of the anterior placenta; the needle was guided into the umbilical vein within a loop of cord. A total of 4 cc of fetal blood was obtained and was sent to the laboratory for a stat CBC and for ABO type and HCV IgM and IgG. A total of 80 cc of O negative, CMV negative, irradiated blood was transfused to correct to approximate fetal final hematocrit of 35% (transfusion purposely limited to 35% secondary to fetal hydropic status).

After each of the needle insertions, the needle was removed under direct visualization, and no evidence of streaming was found. The fetus tolerated the procedure well with no evidence of bradycardia or tachycardia. The total time of the procedure was 90 minutes.

After the procedure, the patient was continued on Ancef for prophylaxis. The patient was transferred back to Labor and Delivery for prolonged fetal heart rate and uterine activity monitoring.

Complications: None.

Condition: Mother and fetus stable.

Progress Notes

DAY 1

Explained risks to the patient and her fetus due to fetal transfusion procedure. Also discussed the risk of transmission of Hep C. The patient understands the risks and agrees to proceed. NICU and anesthesia are aware.

DAY 2

Feels mild cramping, denies contractions. FHT 120s. Continue to monitor. Patient is having some vaginal bleeding. Vaginal examination showed a 20 cc to 30 cc clot in the os. US was done. Clinically consistent with abruption. Will proceed to OR for C section. Now is having decelerations with contractions and decreased uterine tone by palpation.

DAY 3

The patient is S/P primary LSTCS for placental abruption. Minimal lochia. No complaints. Has elevated BP but no proteinuria. Will continue to monitor. If remains elevated, will consider labetalol. Routine postop CBC. Social Work consult.

Day 4

Routine postop. No complaints. Regular diet. Pain is controlled with Tylox/Motrin. BP is still elevated.

Day 5

Surgical wound is c/d/i. Minimal lochia. On daily dose of methadone 85 mg. Doing well.

Day 6

The patient is doing well. No headache, SOB, or CP. Follow-up regarding elevated BP in clinic. Ready for discharge home.

CASE STUDY QUESTIONS

21-2a.   Admit diagnosis: _____

21-2b.   Discharge disposition: _____

21-2c.   Principal diagnosis: _____

21-2d.   Secondary diagnoses (indicate POA status for secondary diagnoses):

_____

_____

_____

_____

_____

_____

_____

21-2e.   Principal procedure: _____

21-2f.   Secondary procedures: _____

21-2g.   Assign MS-DRG: _____

21-2h.   Relative weight of MS-DRG: _____

21-2i.   Can this MS-DRG be optimized with the addition of a CC? Yes or No
         Can this MS-DRG be optimized with the addition of an MCC? Yes or No

21-2j.   Is there a main guideline pertinent to selection of the principal diagnosis in this case study?

_____

_____

21-2k.   Is there another diagnosis that meets the definition for principal diagnosis? Yes or No

21-2l.   If yes, what is the other diagnosis? _____

21-2m. Is there any opportunity for physician query?

_____

_____

21-2n.   What is the drug Colace used to treat? _____

21-3. CASE STUDY

History and Physical

CC: Leaking fluid.

HPI: The patient is a 23-year-old, para 0-0-1-0, who presented at 26-2/7 weeks. The patient presented to the hospital with complaints of PPROM at 2:30 AM on the day of admission. She was 26-2/7 weeks by dates examination and 8 week sono. Her prenatal laboratory results are as follows: Blood type A positive, antibody negative, STS nonreactive, GC negative, *Chlamydia* negative, HIV negative, hepatitis C negative, hepatitis B negative, rubella immune. The patient has pregestational diabetes, and her hemoglobin A1C was 6.3. Sono at 20 weeks demonstrated an AFI of 11.43, no fetal anomalies, and a cervical length of 4.28 cm. Repeat sono last week revealed an AFI of 9.67 and a cervix of 2.8 cm in length with funneling. She had a fetal echo that was within normal limits. She was started on bed rest a few weeks ago for decreased fluid.

As a type 2 diabetic patient, she was on metformin and Actos for control of her diabetes. In pregnancy, she is on NPH of 30 units in the morning and 58 units in the evening, and 18 units of regular insulin in the morning and 34 units in the evening. She is on prenatal vitamins and is also on nifedipine for the funneling. The patient has a history of migraines and asthma. The patient states that her fasting Dextrostix have been between 90 and 104 over the past 10 days.

History of previous pregnancy: First-trimester miscarriage.

Past GYN history: The patient denies any abnormal Pap smears or STDs.

Past medical history: Type II diabetes, asthma, migraines. The patient denies blood transfusions.

Family history: No mental retardation, birth defects, or cerebral palsy.

Social history: During this pregnancy, the patient denies alcohol and illegal drug use. She states that she does smoke half a pack a day of cigarettes.

Allergies: She has no known drug allergies.

Physical examination: Vitals: Afebrile. BP 135/85, HFR 150. Fasting blood sugar 163 General: NAD. Denies contractions.

HEENT: NCAT. PERRL. EOMI. TMs clear. Oropharynx clear.

Chest: CTA bilaterally.

CV: RRR.

Abd: Gravid. Soft, nontender.

Ext: No edema.

GU/Rectal: Deferred.

Neuro: A&O.

Assessment/Plan: The patient is 26-2/7 weeks pregnant with preterm PROM, type II diabetes currently on insulin. She is admitted for a course of betamethasone, ampicillin, and erythromycin ×7 days. Continue to monitor fingersticks, and adjust insulin accordingly. Asthma is stable.

Discharge Summary

DIAGNOSES/PROBLEMS:

1. Principal diagnosis: Intrauterine pregnancy at 26-6/7 weeks.

2. Other diagnoses: Preterm, premature rupture of membranes, pregestational diabetes, hyperglycemia, asthma, migraine headaches, cervical funneling, demoralization, high-risk pregnancy.

PROCEDURES:

Strict bed rest, T-berg; OB sono; Doppler tones; NICU consult; external fetal monitoring/tocodynamometry; PT consult; Psych consult; Nutrition consult; fingerstick sugar paneling; betamethasone; latency antibiotics; Social Work consult; and insulin administration.

HISTORY, MAJOR FINDINGS, AND HOSPITAL COURSE:

The patient is a 23-year-old, para 0-0-1-0, who presented at 26-2/7 weeks. The patient presented to the hospital with complaints of PPROM at 2:30 AM on the day of admission. She was 26-2/7 weeks by dates examination and 8 week sono. Her prenatal laboratory results are as follows: Blood type A positive, antibody negative, STS nonreactive, GC negative, *Chlamydia* negative, HIV negative, hepatitis C negative, hepatitis B negative, rubella immune. The patient has pregestational diabetes, and her hemoglobin A1C was 6.3. During this pregnancy, she denies alcohol and illegal drug use. She states that she does smoke half a pack a day of cigarettes. Sono at 20 weeks demonstrated an AFI of 11.43 and no fetal anomalies, and her cervical length was 4.28 cm. Repeat sono last week revealed an AFI of 9.67 and a cervix of 2.8 cm in length with funneling. She had a fetal echo that was within normal limits. The patient was started on bed rest a few weeks ago for decreased fluid.

History of previous pregnancy: First-trimester miscarriage.

Family history: No mental retardation, birth defects, or cerebral palsy. The patient denies blood transfusions. She has no known drug allergies. As a type 2 diabetic she was on metformin and Actos for control of her diabetes. In pregnancy, she is on NPH of 30 units in the morning and 58 units in the evening, 18 units of regular insulin in the morning and 34 units in the evening. She is on prenatal vitamins and is also on nifedipine for the funneling. The patient has a history of migraines and asthma. The patient states that her fasting Dextrostix have been between 90 and 104 over the past 10 days.

Past GYN history: The patient denies any abnormal Pap smears or STDs. On examination, the patient was afebrile with stable vital signs. Fetal heart tones were in the 150s with moderate variability. Fundal height measured 23 cm. Estimated fetal weight was 767 grams, presentation was vertex by sono. The patient had positive fern, positive nitrazine, with negative pooling, and on sterile speculum examination, her cervix was visually closed. The patient was admitted and was given her first dose of betamethasone to complete a full course of steroids and latency antibiotics. The patient was found not to be contracting on admission and was sent to the floor. She was on strict bed rest in T-berg position and had no complaints other than a continuous leakage of fluid. She was afebrile with stable vital signs. She was on ampicillin and erythromycin for latency antibiotics and had received her first dose of betamethasone. She was continued on the paneling and was written for sliding scale to cover, given the fact that her sugars were less controlled secondary to steroid administration. The patient remained stable throughout most of her hospital stay and on bed rest. She was seen by Nutrition, who recommended a carb-controlled

278

diet. Her sugars remained very well controlled on her NPH and regular regimen as described earlier. The patient completed her course of latency antibiotics. Gonorrhea and *Chlamydia* cultures were obtained and were negative. Fetal assessment sono demonstrated oligohydramnios and estimated fetal weight of 935 g. During part of her hospital stay, her postprandial sugar increased, and upon further investigation, it was found that the patient was not abiding by her carb-controlled diet. The patient had a long discussion with Nutrition and the OB team; she understood the importance of trying to stay within the boundaries of a carb-controlled diet. After that, her sugars were very well controlled. During her stay, the patient was seen by Social Work because, at times, she became very tearful when her husband was not around during the week. She was bored and tired, and she was unhappy. The baby always had good fetal heart tones, and reassuring if not reactive NSTs that were done on a daily basis. The patient remained afebrile; she had no fundal tenderness and no complaints of contractions or vaginal bleeding. Her only complaint was of continued leakage of fluid. The patient will remain on strict bed rest at home with weekly clinic appointments to monitor her condition.

Discharge medications: NPH and regular insulin as taken above, prenatal vitamins, Motrin, Colace.

DISCHARGE INSTRUCTIONS:

Diet: Continue with her diabetic diet.

Activity: She is to have strict bed rest until the delivery of her baby.

FOLLOW-UP CARE:

She is to follow up with her primary OB-GYN.

Ultrasound Examination

EXAMINATION INDICATIONS:

1. Fetal anatomy screen.
2. PPROM.
3. Evaluate amniotic fluid volume.

GENERAL RESULTS:

Fetus #1 of 1

Cephalic presentation.

Placenta location = Anterior.

No placenta previa.

Placenta grade = I.

Largest vertical pocket = 1.3 cm.

Amniotic fluid = Oligohydramnios.

Regarding fetal measurements:

*Indicates measurement included in average gestational age.

Abdom circ	21.2 cm c/w	25 weeks 4 day(s)* (18%)
Femur	5.0 cm c/w	27 weeks 0 day(s)* (40%)
Humerus	4.3 cm c/w	25 weeks 5 day(s) (21%)
FL/AC	24.0 (22 ± 2)	
EFW	935 g (AC & FL)	(27%)

Average gestational age is 26 weeks 2 day(s) ± 14 days.

FETAL DOPPLER STUDIES:

	S/D	PI	RI	PSV cm/s	AEDV
	RF				
Umbilical artery:	3.38	1.17	0.70		

Anatomy details: Visualized, appearing sonographically normal:

STOMACH, RIGHT KIDNEY, LEFT KIDNEY, BLADDER, SPINE (thoracic spine, lumbar spine, sacrum); EXTREMITIES (lt femur, rt femur, lt humerus); PLACENTA, UMBILICAL CORD.

Visualized:

EXTREMITIES (lt lower leg, lt forearm)

Not adequately visualized:

HEAD (calvarium, BPD level, lateral ventricles, choroid plexus, cerebellum, cisterna magna); FACE AND NECK (profile, orbits, nose/lips, palate, face); THORACIC CAVITY (diaphragm); HEART (4-chamber view, LVOT, RVOT, cardiac axis, cardiac position); ABDOMINAL WALL, SPINE (cervical spine); EXTREMITIES (rt lower leg, lt foot, rt foot, rt humerus, rt forearm, lt hand, rt hand); GENITALIA, PLACENTAL CORD INSERTION.

Impression: Singleton IUP. Cephalic presentation. Regular FHR of 146 bpm. Anterior placenta. 27 weeks 1 day(s) by dates. 26 weeks 2 day(s) by this ultrasound. Estimated fetal weight = 935 g. Estimated fetal weight = 2 lb 1 oz. Oligohydramnios.

Comments: This study was technically difficult because of oligohydramnios, maternal habitus, and fetal position. Fetal head measurements cannot be obtained because of fetal position. Fetal abdominal circumference and lengths of femur and humerus are consistent with menstrual dating. Unable to complete anomaly screen at this time because of oligohydramnios and fetal position.

Social Work Progress Note

Patient was seen today to evaluate progress at the request of the OB resident staff in assisting with symptoms of homesickness and frustration with hospitalization requirements.

The patient is a 23-year-old married female who is currently experiencing difficulties surrounding required hospitalization. She was admitted at 26 weeks for PROM and was required to remain on bed rest until the completion of 34 weeks. She stated during initial assessment that this experience was difficult because of the lack of consistent family support. Her family currently resides at 2 hours' driving distance and cannot travel for visits until the weekend arrives.

Exploration with the patient regarding possible progress with hospital stay revealed persistent feelings of loneliness but an effort to adapt to hospital stay. Patient recognized health risk factors involved in early discharge and still presents a desire to cooperate with medical staff recommendations. She expressed relief in maintaining a single room and an interest in the patient/staff library for possible entertainment. This worker discussed possible bedside activities to aid with relaxation and to provide comfort with stay.

Patient presents a good understanding of the consequences for early discharge and anticipates the arrival of her husband tomorrow. He will continue his stay for the duration of the weekend. This will provide support for the patient and will assist in her transition. She remained easily engaged and receptive to Social Work intervention. This worker will follow up with the patient periodically to assist with any needs.

Progress Notes

DAY 1

Patient is lying comfortably. Reports minimal fluid loss and no bleeding. Denies contractions. FHR 150 to 160. Physical examination is negative. Continue antibiotics and strict bed rest. Sliding scale insulin for DM.

280

Day 2

No regular contractions. No vaginal bleeding. Continue bed rest.

Day 3

No signs or symptoms of chorio. Continue antibiotics. All dexis were elevated likely because of steroids. Insulin adjusted accordingly. GBS unknown. Continue close observation because of increased risk of preterm labor and delivery.

Day 4

Afebrile. No tachycardia. No fundal tenderness. Reminded of the importance of strict bed rest. Social Work consult ordered.

Day 5

Afebrile. Antibiotics continued for PPROM. DM and asthma stable. Bed rest.

Day 6

No complaints. Afebrile. No signs and symptoms of chorio. No contractions or vaginal bleeding. Continue DM monitoring and bed rest.

Day 7

Status much the same. No specific complaints. Continue bed rest.

Day 8

Will discharge to home with strict bed rest until at least 34 weeks.

CASE STUDY QUESTIONS

21-3a. Admit diagnosis: _____

21-3b. Discharge disposition: _____

21-3c. Principal diagnosis: _____

21-3d. Secondary diagnoses (indicate POA status for secondary diagnoses):

_____

_____

_____

_____

_____

_____

21-3e. Principal procedure: _____

21-3f.   Secondary procedures: _____

_____

21-3g.   Assign MS-DRG: _____

21-3h.   Relative weight of MS-DRG: _____

21-3i.   Can this MS-DRG be optimized with the addition of a CC? Yes or No
         Can this MS-DRG be optimized with the addition of an MCC? Yes or No

21-3j.   Is there a main guideline pertinent to selection of the principal diagnosis in this case study?

_____

_____

21-3k.   Is there another diagnosis that meets the definition for principal diagnosis? Yes or No

21-3l.   If yes, what is the other diagnosis? _____

21-3m.   Is there any opportunity for physician query?

_____

_____

21-3n.   What is the drug betamethasone used to treat? _____

22 Certain Conditions Originating in the Perinatal Period and Congenital Malformations, Deformations, and Chromosomal Abnormalities (ICD-10-CM Chapter 16, Codes P00-P96, and Chapter 17, Codes Q00-Q99)

ABBREVIATIONS/ACRONYMS

Without the use of reference materials, define the following abbreviations or acronyms.

1. TOF _____
2. LGA _____
3. BPD _____
4. NICU _____
5. PDA _____
6. RDS _____
7. IUGR _____
8. CHD _____
9. TTN _____
10. VSD _____

GLOSSARY DEFINITIONS

Match the glossary term to the correct definition.

1. _____ Apgar
2. _____ Tachycardia
3. _____ Perinatal
4. _____ Congenital
5. _____ Trisomy
6. _____ Hypertrophy
7. _____ Tachypnea
8. _____ Bradycardia
9. _____ Meconium
10. _____ Hypoxia

A. Test to measure the condition of a newborn at birth
B. Insufficient oxygen in the blood
C. Fast breathing
D. Material in the intestine of a fetus
E. Condition present at birth
F. Extra chromosome
G. Slow heart rate
H. Fast heart rate
I. Excessive growth
J. Around birth

CODING

Using the code book, code the following.

1. Baby born via vaginal delivery _____
2. Twins born via C section _____

3. Baby stillborn _____

4. Small for gestational age; delivered via C section at 38 weeks. Birth weight was 5 lbs _____

5. Fetal alcohol syndrome _____

6. Premature infant born at 30 weeks weighing 1800 g; vaginal birth _____

7. Newborn with meconium below the vocal cords; vaginal birth _____

8. Trisomy 21 _____

9. Cryptorchidism _____

10. Supernumerary toe _____

11. Indeterminate sex _____

12. Cleft lip _____

13. Pyloric stenosis, congenital _____

14. Exstrophy of the bladder _____

15. Jaundice due to ABO incompatibility _____

CASE SCENARIOS

Using the code book, code the following cases.

1. Baby born by C section. Mother was 40 weeks pregnant at time of birth. Baby was born with Down syndrome. During the hospital stay, the baby was diagnosed with thrush and anemia.

_____

_____

2. Baby was born vaginally. Mother tested positive for group B strep and was given antibiotics during labor. The day after birth, the newborn developed a fever and was lethargic. Treatment was begun for presumed pneumonia due to group B strep.

_____

_____

3. Baby was born vaginally to Mother on methadone. Shortly after birth, the baby became jittery and inconsolable. The physician documents withdrawal from methadone.

_____

_____

4. A 3-month-old infant who was born with unilateral cheiloschisis is admitted for repair.

_____

_____

5. A 55-year-old man is taken to the OR for removal of a port wine stain on the face by laser.

_____

_____

6. Baby is born in Hospital A and is transferred to the University Hospital with a diagnosis of Tetralogy of Fallot. A repair of the VSD as well as ventricular stenosis.

_____

_____

7. Patient is a 4 1b, 8 oz male born by spontaneous vaginal delivery at 32 weeks. The pregnancy was complicated by premature rupture of the membranes for over 24 hours prior to delivery. The baby is treated with antibiotics for possible sepsis. The infant's blood work is negative, and antibiotics are discontinued.

_____

_____

8. This 40-year-old woman with Marfan's syndrome and mitral valve prolapse is admitted to the hospital for a mitral valve replacement. A mechanical valve is used.

_____

_____

9. A child born with a right club foot is admitted to the hospital for repair. A release of the tendons is performed.

_____

_____

10. Patient is a 1250-g premature female born by SVD at 28 weeks. Immediately after birth, the baby was given a synthetic surfactant for presumed RDS.

_____

_____

CASE STUDIES

Using the code book, code and answer questions about the following case studies.

22-1. CASE STUDY

History and Physical Examination

CC: Scalp AVM

History of present illness: The patient is a 40-year-old male who had a long history of a mass on the vertex of his scalp. This mass was pulsatile, and the patient was referred to me after an MRI scan revealed an AVM or an AV fistula. The patient underwent 4-vessel cerebral angiogram, which confirmed this as an AV fistula consisting primarily of one large varix supplied by both occipital arteries. The patient ultimately opted for embolization of the lesion.

285

Past medical history: The patient's past medical history is remarkable for hypertension and hepatitis B.

Family history: Noncontributory.

Social history: The patient does not smoke and does not drink.

Review of systems: A complete review of systems is remarkable only for mild discomfort.

Medications: Medications at home include Avalide, Norvasc, vitamin K, and Hepsera.

Allergies: The patient has no known drug allergies.

Physical examination: The patient has stable vitals with a heart rate in the 80s and systolic blood pressures in the 120 to 130 range. He is alert and oriented with intact language and cognition. Cranial nerves are grossly unremarkable, and he has normal strength in all 4 extremities. His groin site is normal without hematoma, and both his lower extremities are neurovascularly intact. Scalp lesion is now sessile, and no pulsation is palpated.

Imaging studies: I reviewed the patient's 4-vessel cerebral angiogram from today, which reveals little if any flow through the lesion any longer. I was unable to appreciate early venous drainage on any of the images, and even the previously enlarged occipital arteries are somewhat now regressed in size.

Assessment/Plan: Admit for embolization of scalp AVM.

Discharge Summary

1. Scalp arteriovenous malformation, spontaneously obliterated.
2. Hypertension.
3. Hepatitis B.

PROCEDURES:

Cerebral angiogram under general anesthesia.

HISTORY, MAJOR FINDINGS, AND HOSPITAL COURSE:

The patient is a 40-year-old male with long-standing history of scalp AVM, who was admitted because he was scheduled to undergo embolization of his AVM under general anesthesia. However, diagnostic angiogram performed prior to embolization revealed that the lesion had spontaneously thrombosed and was for the most part obliterated. The patient remained hemodynamically stable overnight with no complications to his groin site and resumed diet and activity as tolerated; he was discharged to home on the following day.

Discharge medications: The patient is to resume his regular medications.

Discharge instructions: He should also resume diet and activity as tolerated with the exception of observing standard post-angio limitations for the next several days.

Follow-up care: The patient should contact my office to arrange follow-up in 3 to 4 weeks.

Angio Carotid Cerebral Bilat

Cerebral angiogram of 40-year-old with a scalp AVM for embolization. The technical aspects of the procedure, as well as its potential risks and benefits, were reviewed with the patient, who understood and agreed to proceed.

The patient was placed in the supine position on the angiography table, and the skin of the groin was prepped in the usual sterile fashion. The procedure was performed with the patient under general anesthesia. A 6-French sheath was introduced into the right common femoral artery.

Heparin: None.

Contrast agent: Omnipaque 300, 30 mL.

Catheters and wire: 5-French MPC guide catheter and 0.035 Glidewire.

Vessels catheterized: Right femoral artery; right common carotid artery; left common carotid artery.

Vessels studied: Right femoral artery RAO; right common carotid artery AP and lateral; left common carotid artery AP and lateral.

Findings:

Right common femoral artery: Unremarkable.

Right common carotid: The large scalp varix noted on the previous angiogram has now thrombosed. Slow flow is noted in the right occipital artery, but no evidence of significant shunt or early draining veins is found.

Left common carotid: Thrombosed varix since previous angiogram. The left occipital artery no longer supplies the malformation.

Disposition: After completion of the study, the femoral sheath was removed. No evidence of bleeding or hematoma was noted. The procedure was well tolerated, and no early complications were reported. The patient was transferred to PACU.

Impression: Spontaneous thrombosis of the large scalp varix since the previous study. No significant shunt or early draining veins are visualized.

Progress Note

The patient has done very well. Vitals are stable. He is alert and oriented. Cranial nerves are grossly unremarkable, and the patient has normal strength in all 4 extremities. His groin site is normal without hematoma, and both lower extremities are neurovascularly intact. The scalp lesion is now sessile, and no pulsation is palpated. I discussed with the patient that his lesion is now gone, and he will require further follow-up in the future and may require a plastic surgery procedure to remove the mass itself. The risk of bleeding or catastrophic complication of the lesion is now minimal or none. The patient can be discharged to home with instructions for follow-up.

CASE STUDY QUESTIONS

22-1a. Admit diagnosis: _____

22-1b. Discharge disposition: _____

22-1c. Principal diagnosis: _____

22-1d. Secondary diagnoses (indicate POA status for secondary diagnoses):

_____

_____

_____

_____

_____

22-1e. Principal procedure: _____

22-1f. Secondary procedures: _____

_____

22-1g. Assign MS-DRG: _____

22-1h. Relative weight of MS-DRG: _____

22-1i. Can this MS-DRG be optimized with the addition of a CC? Yes or No
Can this MS-DRG be optimized with the addition of an MCC? Yes or No

22-1j. Is there a main guideline pertinent to selection of the principal diagnosis in this case study?

_____

_____

22-1k. Is there another diagnosis that meets the definition for principal diagnosis? Yes or No

22-1l. If yes, what is the other diagnosis? _____

22-1m. Is there any opportunity for physician query?

_____

_____

22-1n. What is the drug Hepsera used to treat? _____

22-2. CASE STUDY

Admission Examination

General: Active and alert.

Skin: No jaundice.

Head/Neck: Neck supple + molding/caput.

EENT: Nares patent. Palate intact.

Chest/Lungs: Breath sounds clear.

Heart: Normal heart sounds.

Abdomen: Soft + bowel sounds. No HSM.

Genital/Anus: Normal male genitalia; testes are descended; anus patent.

Skeletal: No spinal deformity; no hip clicks.

Neurologic: Normal tone + reflexes.

Impression: 41-week gestation. Monitored in NICU for 2 hours for delayed transition.

Plan: Amp and Gent × 48 hours. Blood culture pending.

General: Vigorous male infant.

Skin: Jaundice with erythema toxicum.

Head/Neck: Neck supple.

EENT: PERRL, palate intact, sclera white.

Chest/Lungs: Clear.

Heart: No murmur. Femoral pulses strong.

Abdomen: Soft + bowel sounds.

Genital/Anus: Normal male.

Skeletal: No hip click. Clavicle without crepitus.

Neurologic: WNL.

Impression: Stable AGA male infant with mild feeding problems.

Plan: Discharge to home with parents.

Circumcision Note

After informed consent was obtained from the mother, newborn circumcision was performed with sterile technique and a 1.3 Gomco clamp. Tolerated well with minimal EBL.

Discharge Summary

DIAGNOSES/PROBLEMS:

1. Full-term male.
2. Delayed transition.
3. Maternal chorioamnionitis.
4. Sepsis, ruled out.

PROCEDURES:

1. Circumcision.
2. Distortion product otoacoustic emissions hearing screen.

HISTORY, MAJOR FINDINGS, AND HOSPITAL COURSE:

The patient is a 3654-g male, born by spontaneous vaginal delivery at 40 weeks' gestation to a 32-year-old P0-0-1-0 A-positive mother. The pregnancy was uncomplicated. Maternal toxicology screen was negative.

The delivery was complicated by maternal chorioamnionitis. Ampicillin and gentamicin were administered prior to the birth. Pediatrics was called to the delivery because of grunting. The baby received bulb suction, blow-by oxygen, and was taken to the Newborn Intensive Care Unit, where he was observed for 2 hours. Apgar scores were 7 and 8.

The nursery course was complicated. CBC and blood cultures were obtained. CBC was within normal limits. Ampicillin and gentamicin were given for 48 hours, and blood cultures were negative. The baby remained stable, despite some initial breastfeeding problems related to sleepiness during maternal attempts to breastfeed every hour. Lactation support is being provided. Total bilirubin level at 38 hours of life was 8.7. The baby's discharge examination is remarkable for jaundice and erythema toxicum.

Hearing screen: The baby passed the DPOAE hearing screen bilaterally.

Medications: Recombivax 0.5 cc given.

Discharge medications: None.

DISCHARGE INSTRUCTIONS: _____

Extensive review of routine newborn care was discussed with the parents.

FOLLOW-UP CARE: _____

Follow-up care in 2 weeks with pediatrician

CASE STUDY QUESTIONS

22-2a. Admit diagnosis: _____

22-2b. Discharge disposition: _____

22-2c. Principal diagnosis: _____

22-2d. Secondary diagnoses (indicate POA status for secondary diagnoses):

_____

_____

_____

_____

_____

_____

22-2e. Principal procedure: _____

22-2f. Secondary procedures: _____

_____

22-2g. Assign MS-DRG: _____

22-2h. Relative weight of MS-DRG: _____

22-2i. Can this MS-DRG be optimized with the addition of a CC? Yes or No
Can this MS-DRG be optimized with the addition of an MCC? Yes or No

22-2j. Is there a main guideline pertinent to selection of the principal diagnosis in this case study?

_____

_____

22-2k. Is there another diagnosis that meets the definition for principal diagnosis? Yes or No

22-2l. If yes, what is the other diagnosis? _____

22-2m. Is there any opportunity for physician query?

_____

_____

22-2n. What is the drug gentamicin used to treat? _____

22-3. CASE STUDY

Admission Examination

General: Alert and vigorous.

Skin: Pink, no lesions, no jaundice.

Head/Neck: Neck supple.

EENT: Nares patent. Palate intact.

Chest/Lungs: Breath sounds clear and equal bilaterally.

Heart: Normal heart sounds, no murmurs. Femoral pulses ± bilaterally.

Abdomen: Soft + bowel sounds. No HSM. No palpable masses.

Genital/Anus: Normal female genitalia. Anus patent.

Skeletal: No spinal deformity. No hip clicks. No crepitus.

Neurologic: Normal tone + reflexes.

Impression: 37-week well female.

Plan: Routine newborn care.

Discharge Examination

General: Vigorous female infant.

Skin: Pink; no jaundice.

Head/Neck: Neck supple.

EENT: PERRL, palate intact.

Chest/Lungs: Clear.

Heart: No murmur. Fem pulses strong.

Abdomen: Soft + bowel sounds.

Genital/Anus: Normal female. Anus patent.

Skeletal: No hip click. Clavicle without crepitus.

Neurologic: Tone symmetric + Moro.

Impression: 37-week female infant.

Plan: Discharge to home with parents. Failed hearing test on the right. Follow-up hearing test in 1 month.

Discharge Summary

DIAGNOSES/PROBLEMS:

1. 37-week newborn female delivered via C section.
2. Size appropriate for gestational age.
3. Failed right ear hearing screen.

PROCEDURES:

Distortion product otoacoustic emissions hearing screen.

HISTORY, MAJOR FINDINGS, AND HOSPITAL COURSE:

The infant is a 2794-g newborn female delivered by cesarean section at 37 weeks' gestation to a 33-year-old, para 0, A-positive mother. Maternal history is remarkable for vasodepressor syncope. Maternal serologies included a nonreactive RPR, negative HBsAg, and negative HIV. Cultures for GC, *Chlamydia*, and group B strep were negative. The maternal toxicology screen was not obtained prior to delivery. The pregnancy was unremarkable except for breech presentation. The delivery was uncomplicated. The infant was delivered 1½ hours after rupture of membranes and required no resuscitation. Apgars were 9 and 9.

Nursery course: The nursery course was unremarkable. A bilirubin obtained on DOL #2 was 8.0 mg/dL.

Medications: Recombivax declined.

Hearing screen: The DPOAE was administered and failed on the right. A 1-month hearing follow-up is recommended.

Metabolic screen: Pending.

Condition at discharge: Stable. The baby's discharge weight is 2609 g; head circumference is 33 cm at the time of discharge. She is breastfeeding on demand. Vital signs are stable, and good urinary and stool output have been established.

Discharge medications: None.

DISCHARGE INSTRUCTIONS:

Diet: Breastfeed on demand every 1 to 3 hours.

Activity: Routine newborn care.

Other: Mother was advised regarding routine newborn care, safety, signs and symptoms of illness, jaundice, and expected intake and output.

FOLLOW-UP CARE:

Follow-up care will be arranged by the mother with the pediatrician.

CASE STUDY QUESTIONS

22-3a. Admit diagnosis: _____

22-3b. Discharge disposition: _____

22-3c. Principal diagnosis: _____

22-3d. Secondary diagnoses (indicate POA status for secondary diagnoses):

_____

_____

_____

22-3e. Principal procedure: _____

22-3f. Secondary procedures: _____

_____

22-3g. Assign MS-DRG: _____

22-3h. Relative weight of MS-DRG: _____

22-3i. Can this MS-DRG be optimized with the addition of a CC? Yes or No
       Can this MS-DRG be optimized with the addition of an MCC? Yes or No

22-3j. Is there a main guideline pertinent to selection of the principal diagnosis in this case study?

_____

_____

22-3k. Is there another diagnosis that meets the definition for principal diagnosis? Yes or No

22-3l. If yes, what is the other diagnosis? _____

22-3m. Is there any opportunity for physician query?

_____

_____

22-3n. What is the drug Recombivax used to treat? _____

Injury and Certain Other Consequences of External Causes and External Causes of Morbidity (ICD-10-CM Chapters 19 and 20, Codes S00-Y99)

23

ABBREVIATIONS/ACRONYMS

Without the use of reference materials, define the following abbreviations or acronyms.

1. TBI _____

2. FB _____

3. CT _____

4. ATV _____

5. LOC _____

6. MVA _____

7. SLAP _____

8. ORIF _____

9. CHI _____

10. SCI _____

GLOSSARY DEFINITIONS

Match the glossary term to the correct definition.

1. _____ Air embolism

2. _____ Closed reduction

3. _____ Sprain

4. _____ Concussion

5. _____ Open reduction

6. _____ Loss of consciousness

7. _____ Subluxation

8. _____ Dislocation

9. _____ Closed fracture

10. _____ Suture

11. _____ Open fracture

12. _____ Contusion

13. _____ External skeletal fixation

14. _____ Traumatic brain injury

15. _____ Colles' fracture

16. _____ Strain

A. The bone is broken, but the skin remains intact

B. Common fracture in adults in which the lower end of the radius is fractured and the wrist and hand are displaced backward

C. Any mechanical injury resulting in hemorrhage beneath unbroken skin

D. Form of fracture treatment that involves insertion of percutaneous pins proximal and distal to the fracture and application of a frame that connects the pins externally

E. Injury to the brain that results from a significant blow to the head

F. Patient is unable to respond to people or other stimuli

G. Bone exits and is visible through the skin, or a deep wound exposes the bone through the skin

H. The surgeon makes an incision at the fracture site to reduce or manipulate the fracture into anatomic position

I. When air or gas bubbles get into the bloodstream and obstruct the circulation

Continued

295

J. Stretch and/or tear of a ligament

K. Displacement of the bones that form a joint. It is the separation of the end of a bone from the joint that it meets.

L. Injury to a muscle or a tendon

M. Method for closing cutaneous wounds

N. Injury to the brain that may result in interference with the brain's normal functions

O. Partial or incomplete dislocation

P. The surgeon manipulates or reduces fractured bones into anatomic alignment without making an incision through the skin and subcutaneous tissue

CODING

Using the code book, code the following.

1. Sprained right wrist due to fall from bicycle while riding on street   _____

2. Broken left scapula due to snowboarding injury at ski resort   _____

3. Cut left big toe on glass. Big piece of glass removed from laceration; patient was walking on the beach; removal of glass from subcutaneous tissue   _____

4. Anterior dislocation of right elbow due to ski injury; patient fell from ski lift   _____

5. Open fracture of left shaft femur; patient was pedestrian struck by car while trying to cross the street; fracture was repaired with ORIF   _____

6. Crush injury to fingers with laceration of right index finger; patient's hand was slammed in door of house   _____

7. Anterior dislocation of the left radial head and fracture of the ulna due to fall while running; closed reduction of the Monteggia fracture/ dislocation   _____

8. Abrasion and laceration of left eyebrow; hit head on cabinet door in kitchen; suture repair of laceration   _____

9. Infected mosquito bite on left calf   _____

10. Observation following MVA; patient complained of some neck pain   _____

11. Healing traumatic fracture of left femur   _____

12. Head injury with LOC for 70 minutes; fall from slide on school playground   _____

13. History of left BKA   _____

14. Piece of metal in right cornea; patient works at an industrial warehouse; removed by physician with use of a magnet   _____

15. Blunt trauma due to multivehicle accident on interstate; patient has hematuria that was due to contusion of right kidney   _____

CASE SCENARIOS

Using the code book, code the following cases.

1. The patient is a 2-year-old child who was admitted after falling down four steps and hitting his head on concrete. The accident occurred at the patient's home. There was about 5 minutes' LOC with continued lethargy per paramedics. CT of the head and neck revealed no abnormality. The patient is on oral antibiotics for pneumonia and AOM, and these were continued during the hospital stay. He will follow up with pediatrician.
   Final Diagnosis: Closed head injury due to fall.

   _____

   _____

2. The patient is a 12-year-old female who was involved in an MVC. She was a restrained back seat passenger in a car that was rear ended. Initial examination in the ER indicated that she was hemodynamically stable but was complaining of left arm and right leg pain. X-rays revealed a nondisplaced tibial diaphyseal fracture and a nondisplaced proximal humerus fracture. Orthopedic consult was obtained, and a sling was applied to the arm and a cast to the leg. The patient was discharged and will receive physical therapy as an outpatient.
   Final Diagnoses: Nondisplaced humerus fracture, left.
   Fracture of tibial diaphysis, right.

   _____

   _____

3. The patient fell down four steps at his house and sustained a compression fracture of T12. On chest x-ray, the patient also had acute fracture of two ribs. Other medical conditions include Alzheimer's dementia, CAD with history of three-vessel CABG, and osteoporosis. The injuries were treated conservatively. Arrangements were made for the patient to be discharged to a nursing home.
   Final Diagnoses: Compression fracture, T12.
   Fracture of two ribs on the left side.
   Alzheimer's.
   Coronary artery disease.
   Osteoporosis.

   _____

   _____

4. The patient was admitted for observation after an accident at work. The patient fell into a trench but was quickly rescued by coworkers. CT scan and x-rays were taken to evaluate for internal injury. No respiratory issues were noted. On the following morning, the patient had no complaints and was discharged to home.
   Discharge Diagnosis: Contusion on forehead.

   _____

   _____

5. The patient was assaulted by an unknown assailant and had stab wounds to the chest and neck. Shortly after arrival in the ER, the patient's condition deteriorated with the development of acute respiratory distress. CT scan showed a left hemothorax, and a chest tube was inserted. Wounds to the neck were superficial and were closed with sutures. The patient has a history of IV drug abuse and is HIV positive.

   _____

   _____

6. The 6-year-old patient was seen by orthopedics for right supracondylar elbow fracture with posterior displacement of the fracture fragment. The patient fell off monkey bars at the park. The patient was taken to surgery for an open reduction and internal fixation of the fracture. A posterior long-arm splint was applied. Intravenous antibiotics were continued for 24 hours postoperatively. The patient was comfortable with oral pain medications and was discharged.

_____

_____

7. The patient had an amputation of the right middle finger from a grain auger while working on the farm. The patient was able to find the missing finger, and it was put on ice. After consultation with a hand specialist, the decision was made to not reattach the finger. The bone was amputated farther in order to have a favorable closure of the skin around the finger stump. The patient received a tetanus shot and a prescription for pain medications and antibiotics.
Discharge Diagnosis: Traumatic amputation of right middle finger.
Procedure: Reamputation with primary closure, mid level.

_____

_____

8. The patient was shot in the back during a robbery attempt at a convenience store. After admission, it was evident that there was significant injury to the spinal cord in the T7 region. The patient will receive physical and occupational therapy for his paraplegia. The patient was discharged to a rehab center for continued therapy.
Final Diagnosis: Paraplegia due to spinal cord injury.

_____

_____

9. The patient was the driver in an ATV rollover. The patient was intoxicated at the time of the accident and was not wearing a helmet. CT of the head revealed a contusion of the brain with small hemorrhage. The patient was observed closely for any change in mental status, and neurology was consulted. There was no need for operative intervention at this time. The patient was stable and was given instructions for follow-up.

_____

_____

10. The patient was on military patrol and received injuries from a roadside bomb. The patient had severe multiple fractures of the tibia and fibula with no hope of saving the leg. The patient was taken to surgery for a right above-knee amputation. The patient's amputation site looked good, and the patient was discharged on oral pain meds and antibiotics.
Discharge Diagnosis: Severe trauma to right lower leg.
Procedure: Right above-knee amputation (low level).

_____

_____

11. The patient is a 75-year-old man who fell while going down the stairs at his house. The patient heard a pop and immediately felt pain and was unable to straighten his left knee. After x-rays confirmed that the quadriceps tendon had ruptured, the patient was taken to the OR for quadricepsplasty. The patient's past medical history includes a remote history of smoking (quit 2 years ago). COPD, and restless leg syndrome.

_____

_____

Using the code book, code and answer questions about the following case studies.

23-1. CASE STUDY

History and Physical

CC: Fall down the stairs at home.

HPI: The patient is an active 2 y/o who was walking with the dog down a flight of stairs and fell and hit her face. No LOC per Mom.

Past medical history: None. Full-term infant. Up to date on vaccinations and has achieved normal developmental milestones. No exposure to tobacco.

Allergies: NKDA.

Physical examination: T 96.3, HR 120, RR 24, BP 133/93, GCS 15, O_2 Sats 99% on RA, Wgt 30 pounds. Patient's airway, breathing, and circulation are all intact.

HEENT: PERRL, TMs are clear. EOMI. Loss of upper and lower teeth (#9 and #15). No other injury to mouth. C-spine has no tenderness or deformity.

Chest: CTA.

Heart: RR.

Abd: Soft, nontender.

Extremities: Good pulses in all extremities.

Neuro: GCS 15.

A/P: Status post fall with loss of 2 teeth. Obtain CT exams, and admit for observation for cervical spine and head injury.

Discharge Summary

DIAGNOSES/PROBLEMS:

Status post fall down stairs.

PROCEDURES:

CT face/head/C-spine.

HISTORY, MAJOR FINDINGS, AND HOSPITAL COURSE:

The patient is an active 2 y/o female with no significant PMH who presented as a trauma to the ED. She was walking her dog down the stairs, and the dog pulled her down the steps. She hit her face on the wooden steps, losing some of her teeth. There was no LOC. On presentation, the child was alert and oriented with a GCS of 15 with normal vital signs. Her primary and secondary surveys were intact with the exception of loss of a single maxillary and a single mandibular incisor. She was appropriately upset but otherwise normal. Her workup included a head and face CT, of which the final reads were negative for intracranial abnormality, fracture of the face, and fracture or subluxation of the C-spine.

The patient was admitted for overnight observation with a C-collar intact until the final reads returned. She was alert and oriented the morning after and was deemed stable for discharge home. The patient was instructed, however, to follow up with her family dentist for cosmetic dental care. There was no concern regarding the mechanism, and Social Services was not contacted.

Discharge medications: Tylenol: Use as directed on bottle for aches/pains.

DISCHARGE INSTRUCTIONS:

Call if fever >101, any change in mental status including disorientation, change in eyesight/hearing, any weakness, problems eating, or other concerns.

FOLLOW-UP CARE:

Please follow up in clinic in 2 weeks.

Brain Without IV Contrast CT

Indication: S/P fall.

Technique: Unenhanced axial CT scan images were performed from the foramen magnum to the vertex.

Contrast: None.

Comparisons: None.

Findings: The ventricles are normal in size, evidence for mass, mass effect, or midline shift. There is no evidence of acute intracranial hemorrhage. No abnormal extra-axial fluid collections are noted. Bone windows reveal no obvious or depressed skull fracture. Visualized portions of the paranasal sinuses and mastoid air cells are well aerated.

Impression: Unremarkable unenhanced CT of the head.

CT of the Maxillofacial Bones with Contrast

Indication: S/P fall.

Technique: Axial CT images were obtained through the maxillofacial bones without IV contrast. Sagittal and coronal 2D reformations were obtained from this data set.

Comparisons: None.

Findings: There is no evidence of fracture. The left central upper incisor and the second left lower incisor are absent. There is high attenuation soft tissue swelling in the midline maxillary region. The paranasal sinuses and mastoid air cells are well aerated and anatomic. No mass lesions are identified. The osteomeatal complex is patent bilaterally. Note is made of secretions within the left choanal region. The orbits are unremarkable. Contents are unremarkable. Visualized portions of the intracranial contents are unremarkable.

Impression: Absence of the upper left central and lower second left incisors, likely posttraumatic. There is soft tissue contusion overlying these regions.

CT Cervical Spine Without Contrast

Indication: S/P fall.

Technique: Contiguous axial images of the cervical spine were obtained from the skull base through T1. Data were reconstructed into thinner slices, and 2D multiplanar reformations were obtained.

Contrast: None.

300

Comparisons: None.

Findings: The craniocervical junction has an unremarkable appearance. The cervical vertebrae are normal in height and alignment. There is no evidence of fracture or subluxation. There is slight rotation of C1 on C2, which is positional. The intervertebral disc spaces are well preserved. No significant degenerative change is present. The central canal and neural foramina are patent. The facet joint alignment is anatomic bilaterally.

Impression: Unremarkable CT of the cervical spine with no acute fracture or subluxation.

Progress Note

The patient was observed overnight. The final reads to CT exams are negative. The C-collar was removed. The patient is alert and oriented. She is stable for discharge.

CASE STUDY QUESTIONS

23-1a. Admit diagnosis: _____

23-1b. Discharge disposition: _____

23-1c. Principal diagnosis: _____

23-1d. Secondary diagnoses (indicate POA status for secondary diagnoses):

_____

_____

_____

_____

_____

23-1e. Principal procedure: _____

23-1f. Secondary procedures: _____

23-1g. Assign MS-DRG: _____

23-1h. Relative weight of MS-DRG: _____

23-1i. Can this MS-DRG be optimized with the addition of a CC? Yes or No
Can this MS-DRG be optimized with the addition of an MCC? Yes or No

23-1j. Is there a main guideline pertinent to selection of the principal diagnosis in this case study?

_____

_____

23-1k. Is there another diagnosis that meets the definition for principal diagnosis? Yes or No

23-1l. If yes, what is the other diagnosis? _____

23-1m. Is there any opportunity for physician query?

_____

_____

23-1n. What is the drug Tylenol used to treat? _____

23.2. CASE STUDY

History and Physical

CC: Pain in right leg.

HPI: This 33-year-old female twisted her right leg when she fell into a hole while walking her dog. She immediately felt pain and was unable to bear weight on her leg. There were no other injuries.

Past medical history: Obesity.

Past surgical history: None.

Family history: Noncontributory.

Social history: Smokes 10 cigarettes per day. Occasional alcohol use. Married.

Allergies: NKDA.

ROS: All systems are negative except for HPI.

Physical examination: VS are stable.

General: Appears to be some distress due to right leg pain.

HEENT: Unremarkable. Neck without JVD, lymphadenopathy, thyromegaly, or bruit.

Lungs: CTA.

Heart: RRR.

Abd: Soft. Obese. No organomegaly.

Extremities: There is some swelling in the right leg.

Neuro: Intact.

X-ray shows a spiral fracture of tibial midshaft.

A/P: The patient will need to be taken to the OR for reduction of her tibial fracture. Surgery will be scheduled for the AM.

Operative Report

Title of operation: Intramedullary rod fixation of right tibial shaft fracture.

Indications for surgery: The patient is a 33-year-old female who sustained a twisting injury to her right leg. She complained of immediate pain and was unable to bear weight. The patient presented to the Emergency Department, where physical examination and radiographic workup revealed a diagnosis of closed right tibial shaft fracture. She is recommended to undergo surgical treatment. Informed consent was obtained after the risks, benefits, alternatives, and potential complications including, but not limited to, pain, bleeding, infection, scarring, damage to blood vessels, nerves, muscles, or tendons, nonunion, malunion, delayed union, painful hardware,

hardware failure, compartment syndrome, failure of surgery, need for further surgery, risk of anesthesia, thromboembolic complications, and anterior knee pain were explained at length to the patient. She agreed to proceed. She was admitted to the orthopedic service after a long-leg bulky Jones splint was applied. Compartment checks were performed serially throughout hospital day 1. She was ultimately taken to the Operating Room for fixation.

Preoperative diagnosis: Closed right tibial shaft fracture.

Postoperative diagnosis: Closed right tibial shaft fracture.

Anesthesia: General endotracheal.

Specimen (bacteriologic, pathologic, or other): None.

Prosthetic device/implant: Striker T2 tibial nail measuring 10 × 315 mm with 5-mm locking screws measuring 32.5, 42.5, and 47.5, respectively.

Surgeon's Narrative

Intravenous fluid: 1600 mL of crystalloid.

Estimated blood loss: 100 mL.

Urine output: 200 mL.

Drains: None.

Complications: None.

Disposition: Stable to PACU.

Procedure note: The patient was identified in the preoperative holding area, and the right lower extremity was identified and marked. The patient was then taken back to the Operating Room and was placed supine on the operating table, where a general endotracheal anesthetic was administered. She received preoperative prophylactic antibiotics. The right lower extremity splint was then removed. The right lower extremity was prepped and draped in the usual sterile fashion after a Foley catheter was inserted. An approximately 5-cm longitudinal incision was made over the patellar tendon from the level of the inferior pole of the patella to the tibial tubercle. The incision was made with a 15-blade scalpel. Bovie electrocautery was used to dissect the subcutaneous tissues down to the level of the paratenon. The paratenon was incised with a 15-blade scalpel. Metzenbaum scissors were used to dissect medially and laterally around the patellar tendon. A 15-blade scalpel was then used to make a longitudinal incision through the patellar tendon. The starting guidewire was taken by hand and was placed on the medial border of the lateral tibial spine, on the proximal shaft of the tibial plateau. AP and lateral fluoroscopic images confirmed the appropriate starting point of the guidewire. The guidewire was advanced approximately 5 cm into the tibial metaphysis, and the T-handle reamer was used to open up the proximal tibia. The T-handled reamer was then used to create a track down the tibial intramedullary canal to the level of the fracture site. AP and fluoroscopic images confirmed appropriate passage of the T-handled reamer. A long bottle-tip guidewire was then advanced down to the level of the fracture site. AP and lateral fluoroscopic images were used to confirm that the bottle-tip guidewire had passed across the fracture site to the level of the ankle. Care was taken to ensure that the bottle-tip guidewire was in the center position on the AP and lateral views of the distal tibia. The guidewire was then measured just under 330 mm; therefore, we chose a 315-mm nail. Reaming began sequentially with a size 8-mm reamer up to an 11.5-mm reamer. This was noted to give excellent cortical chatter.

During the reaming process, care was taken to image the fracture site, and the reamer was pushed manually across the fracture site. After an 11.5 reamer was passed down the canal, we inserted the real 10 × 315–mm Stryker T2 tibial nail. AP and lateral fluoroscopic images of the knee, fracture site, and ankle were obtained to confirm appropriate fracture reduction and nail placement both proximally and distally. Once

303

the nail was sunk proximally to an appropriate level, attention was turned to applying proximal locking screws. The proximal locking assembly was used, and two medial-to-lateral static proximally locked screws were placed under fluoroscopic guidance. Attention was taken to ensure that both screws were bicortical and of appropriate length. AP and lateral fluoroscopic images confirmed that this was true. The fracture site was then visualized and was noted to be near anatomic reduction. Clinically, the rotation looked appropriate. Attention was taken to inserting the two distal locking screws. Perfect circle technique was used to insert two medial-to-lateral distal tibial locking screws in the usual fashion. AP and lateral fluoroscopic images confirmed appropriate screw length and positioning. Final AP and lateral images of the knee, fracture site, and ankle were obtained to confirm appropriate positioning of all hardware and reduction of the fracture. Attention was turned to closure. All wounds were copiously irrigated with sterile saline. Stab incisions for the proximal and distal locking screws were closed with 2-0 Vicryl interrupted simple sutures followed by skin staples. The incision for insertion of the nail was closed with number 1-0 Vicryl running through the tendon, a 2-0 running Vicryl through the paratenon, and interrupted simple 2-0 subcutaneous Vicryl sutures. The skin was then closed with staples. The wounds were filled with Xeroform 4 × 4 gauze, and a sterile soft on an ACE wrap was applied. The patient was then extubated and was taken to the recovery room in stable condition with no apparent complications. At the completion of the case, all sponge, needle, and instrument counts were correct.

The plan will be for the patient to return to the orthopedic service, where she will conduct toe touch weight bearing. She should be monitored for compartment syndrome. The patient should receive 24 hours of routine prophylactic antibiotics and should be placed on Lovenox for DVT prophylaxis.

Discharge Summary

DIAGNOSES/PROBLEMS:

Right tibia shaft fracture.

PROCEDURES:

1. Intramedullary nailing, right tibia.
2. Physical Therapy consultation.
3. CAM walking boot placement.

HISTORY, MAJOR FINDINGS, AND HOSPITAL COURSE:

This is a very pleasant 33-year-old female who fell into a hole while walking her dog. She immediately complained of right leg pain. She denied any other injury. She denied any past medical history and is not allergic to any medications. The patient is an active smoker. She was seen and evaluated in the Emergency Room and was found to have a right tibia fracture. She was initially placed in a long leg splint for immobilization and consented to surgery.

The patient was brought to the Operating Room on the day after admission for an intramedullary nail of her right tibia. She tolerated this procedure without complications. She remained neurovascularly intact and afebrile. The patient was seen by Physical Therapy on postoperative day 1 and was able to ambulate with toe touch weight bearing to the right lower extremity. A CAM walking boot was placed on her right lower extremity; she may remove this as needed. She is allowed only toe touch weight bearing to the right lower extremity. She was trained with crutches and has been deemed safe for discharge to home.

Her pain has been fairly well controlled on OxyContin and oxycodone. The patient will wean off OxyContin over a 7-day course and will follow up in the Orthopedic Clinic in 1 week. The discharge plan has been discussed with the patient, and all questions have been answered.

Discharge medications: Colace 100 mg by mouth twice daily, Oxycodone 5 mg 1 to 3 tablets by mouth every 4 hours as needed for pain, OxyContin 10 mg by mouth every 12 hours × 7 days, then 1 tablet by mouth at bedtime × 7 days, Lovenox 40 mg subcutaneous injections daily × 14 days.

DISCHARGE INSTRUCTIONS:

Diet: Regular.

Activity: She is toe touch weight bearing to the right lower extremity with boot.

Other: She needs dry dressing changes once a day with 4 × 4 and Ace wrap. She will wear the boot as tolerated.

FOLLOW-UP CARE:

The patient has an orthopedic appointment for follow-up in the Outpatient Center. If she has any questions or problems with this appointment, she may call.

Pelvis and Hip, Right

Indication: Pain

Impression: Limited examination, the right femoral neck is not visualized. Few pelvic phleboliths. No fracture visualized.

Tibia and Fibula, Right

Indication: Pain, trauma.

Impression: Spiral fracture of tibial midshaft with minimal posterolateral displacement of distal fragment.

Progress Notes

DAY 1

Patient with fx of right tibia.

No paresthesia. Pain controlled with IV morphine.

VS: 36.5, 75, 114/65, 20.

Pulses are symmetric. No pallor. Full motor strength. Sensation is intact.

No evidence of compartment syndrome. Continue to monitor. To OR tomorrow morning.

DAY 2

Preop and postop diagnosis: R tibia fx.

Proc: IM rod R tibia.

EBL: 100.

IVF: 1600.

UO: 200.

Complications: None.

Drain: None.

DAY 3

Patient is recovering from surgery. Pain is 3/10. On PCA.

No paresthesia.

VS: 36.8, 93, 125/62, 18.

Dressing: C/D/I.

No evidence of compartment syndrome.

DAY 4

Doing well. Pain under control.

PT/OT. Compartments soft.

Continue elevation, ice.

Ready for discharge.

CASE STUDY QUESTIONS

23-2a. Admit diagnosis: _____

23-2b. Discharge disposition: _____

23-2c. Principal diagnosis: _____

23-2d. Secondary diagnoses (indicate POA status for secondary diagnoses):

_____

_____

_____

_____

_____

23-2e. Principal procedure: _____

23-2f. Secondary procedures: _____

_____

23-2g. Assign MS-DRG: _____

23-2h. Relative weight of MS-DRG: _____

23-2i.   Can this MS-DRG be optimized with the addition of a CC? Yes or No
         Can this MS-DRG be optimized with the addition of an MCC? Yes or No

23-2j.   Is there a main guideline pertinent to selection of the principal diagnosis in this case study?

_____

_____

23-2k.   Is there another diagnosis that meets the definition for principal diagnosis? Yes or No

23-2l.   If yes, what is the other diagnosis? _____

23-2m. Is there any opportunity for physician query?

_____

_____

23-2n.   What is the drug Lovenox used to treat? _____

23-3. CASE STUDY

History and Physical

CC: Fall from bed; LOC.

HPI: This active 20-month-old male child was jumping on the bed and fell off, hitting his head on the floor at his home. There was a brief loss of consciousness according to the mother, maybe for about 5 minutes. The ambulance was called, and the child was brought to the Emergency Room. The child was crying and was difficult to examine.

Past medical history: None. 38-week gestation. Vaccinations up-to-date. No exposure to secondhand smoke. No illness or surgeries.

Allergies: NKDA.

Physical Examination:

Vital signs are stable. The patient's airway, breathing, and circulation are intact.

HEENT: PERRLA. EOMI. TMs show evidence of otitis media, right greater than left. Contusion forehead. C-spine is normal.

Chest: CTA.

Heart: RRR.

Abd: Soft. No guarding or rigidity.

Extremities: Moves all extremities. No obvious injury.

Neuro: GCS 15.

A/P: Closed head injury with loss of consciousness. Admit for serial neuro examinations.

Discharge Summary

DIAGNOSES/PROBLEMS:

1.   Closed head injury, fall with loss of consciousness.

2. Acute ethmoid and maxillary sinusitis.
3. Otitis media.

PROCEDURES:

CTs

HISTORY, MAJOR FINDINGS, AND HOSPITAL COURSE:

This is a 20-month-old child who was jumping on the bed and fell off, hitting his head. According to the mother, the child was unconscious for about 5 minutes. The patient was admitted and underwent CT to determine whether he had an intracranial abnormality. CT showed that there was nothing wrong. He did have some acute sinus inflammation. CT of the neck also showed that there was no problem. He did well after the C-spine was cleared and there was no evidence of acute spinal fracture. He was cleared clinically. He was given fluids, then oral drinks, and he did quite well.

Reportable disease: None.

Adverse drug reactions: None.

Condition on discharge: Stable.

Discharge medications: None.

Discharge instructions: Closed head injury sheet given.

Other: Return to clinic.

Follow-up care: Follow up with primary care provider.

Progress Note

Patient is eating breakfast. No headache or drowsiness. Neuro status is stable. CT results are negative for any acute injury. CT did indicate acute ethmoid and maxillary sinusitis. Will treat with oral antibiotics. Patient can be discharged with parents. Give head injury instruction sheet.

CASE STUDY QUESTIONS

23-3a. Admit diagnosis _____

23-3b. Discharge disposition: _____

23-3c. Principal diagnosis: _____

23-3d. Secondary diagnoses (indicate POA status for secondary diagnoses):

_____

_____

_____

_____

_____

_____

23-3e.   Principal procedure: ———————————————————————————————————————

23-3f.   Secondary procedures: ——————————————————————————————————————

———

23-3g.   Assign MS-DRG: ———————————

23-3h.   Relative weight of MS-DRG: ———————————

23-3i.   Can this MS-DRG be optimized with the addition of a CC? Yes or No
         Can this MS-DRG be optimized with the addition of an MCC? Yes or No

23-3j.   Is there a main guideline pertinent to selection of the principal diagnosis in this case study?

———

———

23-3k.   Is there another diagnosis that meets the definition for principal diagnosis? Yes or No

23-3l.   If yes, what is the other diagnosis? ——————————————————————————————

23-3m.   Is there any opportunity for physician query?

———

———

Burns, Adverse Effects, and Poisonings (ICD-10-CM Chapters 19 and 20, Codes S00-Y99)

24

Without the use of reference materials, define the following abbreviations or acronyms.

1. AKA _____

2. UTI _____

3. CC _____

4. OR _____

5. MVA _____

GLOSSARY DEFINITIONS

Match the glossary term to the correct definition.

1. _____ Epidermis

2. _____ Residual effect

3. _____ Erythema

4. _____ Adverse effect

5. _____ Necrosis

6. _____ Dermis

7. _____ Corrosion

A. The death of cells

B. Outermost layer of skin

C. Redness of the skin

D. Pathologic manifestation due to ingestion or exposure to drugs or other chemical substances

E. The acute phase of an illness or injury has passed, but a residual condition or health problem remains

F. Layer of skin below the epidermis

G. Burn due to chemical

CODING

Using the code book, code the following.

1. Patient has a history of Redman's syndrome due to vancomycin _____

2. Anaphylactic shock due to accidental ingestion of shellfish _____

3. Inhalation of chlorine gas at warehouse; patient admitted with pulmonary edema due to accidental chlorine exposure on the job _____

4. Carbon monoxide poisoning due to malfunction of home furnace; patient had headache, nausea, and dizziness _____

5. Frostbitten fingers on the left hand due to cold weather exposure; patient is homeless; amputation of gangrenous fingertip little finger _____

6. Nonunion of right tibia fracture _____

7. Observation following rape, adult patient _____

8. Thrombocytopenia due to Bactrim taken for prophylaxis in patient with AIDS _____

9. Burns to face and eyes due to car battery explosion; patient had blistering corrosive burns to entire face and eyelids; from caustic acid; the eyes appear undamaged; the accident happened at a garage where the patient works _____

10. Polyneuropathy due to chemotherapy drugs; patient is on chemotherapy for cancer of the left kidney that has metastasized to the left adrenal gland _____

11. Child with cigarette burns on buttocks (bilateral) and multiple contusions on body; on skeletal survey, there are numerous old healed fractures; child was injured by mother _____

12. Patient was admitted in a coma; it was determined that the patient accidentally overdosed on heroin; he recovered following administration of Narcan _____

13. Patient is on Coumadin for a previous PE; patient accidentally took twice the prescribed dosage; there is no evidence of abnormal bleeding; the patient's coagulation profile is abnormal, and adjustments to medication were made _____

14. Patient was admitted with intentional overdose of Dilantin, taken for seizure disorder, and diazepam, taken for anxiety disorder _____

15. Hypothyroidism due to amiodarone, taken for atrial fibrillation _____

CASE SCENARIOS

Using the code book, code the following cases.

1. A child was brought to the ER after sustaining burns after pulling a kettle of hot soup from the stove. The patient had second- and third-degree burns to the chest and abdomen. The patient was sedated, and the burn area was debrided. The burns were covered with an antibiotic cream, then sterile bandages. These bandages are changed frequently, and the burned area is carefully monitored for signs of infection. About 11% of the patient's body was burned, 4% with third-degree burns. A Social Work consult was obtained to evaluate the safety of the patient's home situation.
   Final Diagnosis: Second- and third-degree burns of chest and abdomen due to accidental injury.
   Procedure: Excisional debridement.

   _____

   _____

2. The patient was admitted from the ER after being mugged while walking on the sidewalk downtown. The patient was thrown to the ground and kicked. The patient had a number of contusions of the head, abdomen, and thighs. X-rays were taken, vitals were monitored, and no hematuria was noted. The patient was observed overnight with no complications and was discharged to home.
   Final Diagnosis: Observation following an assault.

   _____

   _____

3. The patient was admitted for treatment of his sacral pressure ulcer, Stage IV. The patient has been in a nursing home for the past 3 years because of paraplegia due to spinal cord injury at T9, incomplete, from an MVA. The patient has a neurogenic bladder and suffers from depression. The patient's ulcer was debrided by the physician until viable pink tissue was visible. The wound care nurse saw this patient for daily dressing changes.
   Final Diagnoses: Ulcer of sacrum.
   Paraplegia with neurogenic bladder.
   Procedure: Excisional debridement.

   _____

   _____

4. The patient in case scenario 1 has now returned to the hospital with an infected third-degree burn of the chest area. The patient's burns on the abdomen are healing well. A wound care consult was ordered, and the wound care nurse did a nonexcisional debridement. The chest burns started to look much better, and the patient was discharged.
   Final Diagnosis: Infected burns of chest area.
   Procedure: Nonexcisional debridement.

   _____

   _____

5. The patient was admitted with hematemesis. The patient has been taking NSAIDs as directed by the physician for arthritis pain. EGD showed that the patient had an acute erosive gastritis most likely due to NSAIDs that is the likely cause of the bleeding. The patient has IBS and bipolar disorder.

Final Diagnoses: Erosive gastritis with hemorrhage due to NSAIDs.

Irritable bowel syndrome.

Bipolar disorder.

Procedure: EGD with gastric biopsy.

_____

_____

6. The patient reported to the ER with nausea/vomiting and weakness. The patient is on OxyContin for chronic pain due to unresectable pancreatic cancer. The patient was in extreme pain and decided to double the OxyContin dosage. When this did not relieve the pain, the patient decided to drink a couple of shots of whiskey. The patient got very weak and called 911. The patient was volume depleted and was treated with IVs; his pain medications were adjusted.

Final Diagnoses: Accidental overdose of OxyContin.

Pain due to pancreatic cancer.

_____

_____

7. The patient was brought to the ER by her mother. The patient admits to being beaten by her husband and has bruises on her abdomen, back, buttocks, and upper arms. X-rays showed three fractured ribs on the right and a spiral fracture of the right humerus. The humeral fracture was manipulated and was found to be in alignment on follow-up x-rays. The patient was given pain medications and was discharged to the care of her mother.

Final Diagnosis: Fracture of 3 ribs and shaft of humerus due to spousal abuse.

Procedure: Closed reduction of fracture of right humerus.

_____

_____

8. The patient was admitted with acute renal failure. The patient had been treated by Home Health with IV gentamicin for *Pseudomonas* pneumonia. The patient was experiencing some edema and decreased urine output. Labs were drawn, and the physician admitted the patient for IV fluids and investigation of the patient's renal status. Gentamicin was stopped, and chest x-ray revealed adequate clearing of the patient's pneumonia. The patient's renal function returned to normal. Conditions that are treated with medications include chronic gastritis, hiatal hernia, and seizure disorder.

Final Diagnoses: Acute renal failure due to gentamicin.

History of pneumonia.

Chronic gastritis.

Hiatal hernia.

Seizure disorder.

_____

_____

9. The patient is a college student who was partying with friends and passed out. The patient's friends noticed that she was vomiting and was having seizure-like activity and called 911. In the Emergency Room, the patient was hypothermic; breathing was slow and shallow, and the patient had a seizure. The patient was intubated for acute respiratory failure and was taken to the ICU. The patient was stabilized and was treated for aspiration pneumonia. The patient recovered and was counseled on the dangers of alcohol.

Final Diagnoses: Acute respiratory failure due to accidental alcohol poisoning.

Aspiration pneumonia.

Procedure: Mechanical ventilation for 2 days.

_____

_____

10. A 2-year-old child was admitted with an accidental electrical burn to the upper lip. The child was at home and had bitten on an electrical cord. The mother immediately sought medical attention. The burn was a full-thickness burn. Local wound care was performed. The patient was not having any breathing problems. Further intervention will depend on how the burn heals.

Final Diagnosis: Full-thickness burn to upper lip due to electrical current.

Procedure: Local wound care.

_____

_____

CASE STUDIES

Using the ICD-9-CM code book, code and answer questions about the following case studies.

24-1. CASE STUDY

History and Physical

CC: Electrocution.

HPI: The patient was working in the garage at his house. He was up on a ladder, was shocked from a 220-volt A/C line, and fell 4 to 6 feet from the ladder. His wife found him lying on the garage floor and called 911. He is complaining of pain in his right side and numbness in his right hand. No LOC is reported.

Past medical history: None.

Medications: None.

Allergies: NKDA.

Social history: Married. Quit tobacco 10 years ago. No drugs or alcohol.

ROS: General: No fever or chills. Resp: No cough or dyspnea. CV: No chest pain, DOE, or edema. GI: No abd pain, N/V/D. Musculoskeletal: Pain neck, back, and right arm.

Physical examination:

Vital signs: BP 180/110, HR 63, O_2 sat 98% on RA.

General: NAD.

HEENT: Atraumatic. PERRL. Trachea midline. MM moist.

Chest: CTA.

CV: RRR.

GI: Bowel sounds present. Abdomen is soft and nontender.

Back: Tenderness of neck and thoracic spine.

Extremities: Cannot make a fist with R hand. Left hand normal. No obvious soft tissue injury to the right hand.

A/P: Electrical injury to right hand with no obvious external injury. Fall from ladder. Obtain hand and spine x-rays.

Discharge Summary

DIAGNOSES/PROBLEMS:

Electric shock with fall.

PROCEDURES:

None.

HISTORY, MAJOR FINDINGS, AND HOSPITAL COURSE:

The patient is a 55-year-old man who presented to the Emergency Room after he was shocked with a 220-volt A/C line and fell 4 to 6 feet off a ladder. He was found lying supine on the ground with complaints of dizziness, back pain, and a burning sensation in his right hand. He did not lose consciousness. EKG was normal. CT scan of chest, abdomen, pelvis, and brain were all unremarkable. The patient was transferred to the floor for overnight observation. Orthopedics was consulted and splinted his right hand. After an uneventful night, the patient was discharged in stable condition with instructions to follow up with orthopedics.

Discharge medications: Oxycodone 5 to 10 mg PO q 4h prn pain. Continue all home medications as previously.

Discharge instructions: Diet is regular. Activity as tolerated. Please contact physician for any increase in chest pain, dizziness, nausea/vomiting, increased numbness or tingling in right hand, shortness of breath, or difficulty breathing. Wear right arm splint for comfort.

Follow-up care: Please follow up in clinic in 1 week.

Progress Note

Patient comfortable. Pain resolved. Burning resolved. Mild wrist soreness. No swelling. No erythema. No obvious soft tissue injury. Splint hand for rest. Ready for discharge.

CASE STUDY QUESTIONS

24-1a. Admit diagnosis: _____

24-1b. Discharge disposition: _____

24-1c. Principal diagnosis: _____

24-1d. Secondary diagnoses (indicate POA status for secondary diagnoses):

_____

_____

_____

24-1e. Principal procedure: _____

24-1f. Secondary procedures: _____

24-1g. Assign MS-DRG: _____

24-1h. Relative weight of MS-DRG: _____

24-1i. Can this MS-DRG be optimized with the addition of a CC? Yes or No
Can this MS-DRG be optimized with the addition of an MCC? Yes or No

24-1j. Is there a main guideline pertinent to selection of the principal diagnosis in this case study?

_____

_____

24-1k. Is there another diagnosis that meets the definition for principal diagnosis? Yes or No

24-1l. If yes, what is the other diagnosis? _____

24-1m. Is there any opportunity for physician query?

_____

_____

24-2. CASE STUDY

Clinic Note/History and Physical

Reason for visit: Follow-up evaluation of low back pain and left ankle pain.

History of present illness: This is a 46-year-old female with a history significant for pain in the paraspinous area of her mid back with radiation around the right middle rib cage. Prior to history taken for her follow-up, the patient informed us upon triage that she was experiencing a "racing heart." At that time, an EKG reviewed by our office concluded that the patient's heart rate was 145 beats per minute with a regular rhythm. No signs of major axis deviation were noted. The QRS was not widened; however, some questionable Q waves were noted in the inferior leads with no discernible P waves. The patient states that she has been experiencing intermittent episodes of these palpitations over the past week. The patient presently denies chest pain; however, she admits to some shortness of breath. She denies any jaw pain but states that she is presently experiencing some episodes of dizziness and light-headedness. The patient states that she just increased her nortriptyline approximately 5 days prior to the onset of these palpitations from 25 mg to 50 mg.

Past medical history: The patient denies any past medical history of cardiac problems. She states that several years ago, she was experiencing these episodes; however, workup was negative. She states that at no time was she ever present at a physician's office when she experienced these palpitations. The patient has a long history of systemic lupus erythematosus, which was previously treated with prednisone; now, she is on Plaquenil. Prednisone was discontinued due to osteoporosis. The patient has GERD and spastic bowel.

Past surgical history: Cholecystectomy.

ROS: See HPI. Mild weight loss. Chronic diarrhea.

Physical examination:

Vital signs: T 100, HR 145, BP 160/78, and RR 22.

General: NAD. Slightly anxious.

HEENT: PERRL, EOMI, sclera anicteric, MMM. Neck is supple without masses or LAD. Slight R carotid bruit.

Chest: CTA.

Heart: Tachy.

Abd: Positive bowel sounds. Soft, not distended.

Ext: Good cap refill. No edema.

GU/Rectal: Deferred.

Neuro: Walks with a walker.

A/P: Palpitations.

The patient was brought to our postprocedure recovery area and was placed on a monitor. The Emergency Room was called, and the attending physician was informed that we would be transferring the patient to the Emergency Room. At that time, we instructed the patient to follow up in our office as needed. A copy of the EKG was provided to the patient to be transported with her to the Emergency Room.

Discharge Summary

DIAGNOSES/PROBLEMS:

1. Drug-induced sinus tachycardia.
2. Systemic lupus erythematosus diagnosed in 1989; patient previously on prednisone but discontinued secondary to osteoporosis; now on Plaquenil (flares consistent with rash, fatigue, and myalgias).
3. Gastroesophageal reflux disease.
4. Spastic bowel.
5. Status post open cholecystectomy.

PROCEDURES:

1. PE protocol CT. Preliminary reading showed no pulmonary embolism. No mediastinal, hilar, or axillary lymphadenopathy. No focal consolidation or pulmonary nodule; upper abdomen made of well-circumscribed fluid density structure. The medial edge of the spleen may represent a posttraumatic cyst.
2. Chest x-ray; no infiltrate, no effusions.
3. Continuous telemetry.

HISTORY, MAJOR FINDINGS, AND HOSPITAL COURSE:

The patient is a 46-year-old female with a history of chronic pain and lupus, who presented to the Emergency Department after feeling palpitations and was found to have a heart rate of 145 in the clinic. The patient reports a history of palpitations in the distant past but has not had palpitations during the year prior to this onset. She describes increasing episodes of palpitations over the 4 days prior to her admission. The patient describes these palpitations as sensations of heart racing, feeling flushed, and shortness of breath, similar to when she yawns, with only mild light-headedness. The patient denies any syncope or chest pain associated with the palpitations. She denies any vision changes or headaches. She is unable to provide any possible provoking events or agents. However, she does report that she just increased her nortriptyline approximately 5 days prior to the onset of these palpitations from 25 to 50 mg.

In the Emergency Department, the patient's vital signs were as follows: temperature 100°, heart rate 145, blood pressure 160/78, respirations 22, and saturating 100% on room air. The patient received 1 mg of Ativan without benefit, a liter of normal saline without improvement, and 650 mg of Tylenol; she was admitted for further workup.

Past medical history: As noted above.

Medications on admission: Atenolol 150 mg by mouth every day, clonidine 0.1 mg patch, Ativan 1 mg every day, baclofen 20 mg by mouth 3 times a day, Plaquenil 200 mg by mouth 2 times a day, Nexium, Neurontin 300 mg by mouth every 6 hours, Actonel 35 mg every week, and nortriptyline 50 mg recently increased just 5 days prior to onset of palpitations.

Social history: No tobacco, no alcohol, no illicits. She works as a retail manager.

Family history: Notable for mother who passed away about a year ago and died secondary to MRSA status post CABG. Father underwent CABG in late 60s and had hypertension. Of three brothers, one had hypertension, and one underwent CABG at age 48.

Clinical examination was significant for a flat JVP and a tachy heart rate with 1/6 left lower sternal border murmurs. No rubs or gallops. Examinations were essentially unremarkable. Creatinine of 0.6, bicarbonate 26. Cardiac enzymes were negative times 4 over 6 hours. EKG consistent with sinus tach with a rate of approximately 119 beats per minute. Possible different T-wave morphology. PR less than 0.2, QRS less than 0.12. Non-path Q waves and aVF in V4 and V6, but no ST elevation or depression. No T-wave inversion appreciated on EKG.

Hospital Course by System:

1. Urine. Toxicology was negative; the patient denied any herbal therapies or caffeine. TSH was checked and was found to be 1.3; in addition, positive metanephrines were sent off to rule out pheochromocytoma.

2. Cardiovascular. The patient was admitted on continuous telemetry. EKGs showed no evidence of any arrhythmias. EKGs were notable for sinus tachycardia without the presence of any arrhythmias. The patient's atenolol was increased, given ample blood pressure and tachycardic pulse with excellent resolution of tachycardia to pulses approximately 80s to 90s. Tachycardia was felt not to be associated with fever, given the fact that the patient was afebrile. Dehydration was unlikely because the patient's heart rate did not respond to intravenous boluses. In addition, this was felt less likely to be triggered with clonidine withdrawal, given the fact the patient was compliant with all medicines, as noted by the clonidine patch.

3. Hypertension. The patient was mildly hypertensive in-house, 150s/80s. Therefore, lisinopril 10 mg by mouth every day was initiated. Given her increased risk of coronary artery disease, both in light of her family history and her diagnosis of lupus, the patient was initiated on lisinopril 10 mg and was started on aspirin 81 mg by mouth every day. While in-house, her medicines were titrated up, and the patient will be discharged on increased levels of atenolol 150 mg by mouth every day.

Allergies: Colchicine, Prevacid (causes hives), Zocor, and Darvocet.

Discharge medications: Atenolol 150 mg by mouth every day, lisinopril 10 mg by mouth every day, aspirin 81 mg by mouth every day, baclofen 20 mg by mouth 3 times a day, Plaquenil 200 mg by mouth 2 times a day, Nexium 20 mg by mouth every day, Ativan 1 mg by mouth 2 times a day, Neurontin 300 mg by mouth every 4 to 6 hours,

Actonel 35 mg by mouth every week, clonidine 0.1 mcg patch weekly; recommended titrating clonidine patch off as lisinopril was increased.

Chest PA and Lateral

Indication: Chest pain.

Impression: Normal except for cholecystectomy clips.

Progress Note

The patient is feeling better this morning. No specific arrhythmias on telemetry or EKG. It is thought that the patient's tachycardia is due to her increase in nortriptyline. Will discontinue the medication and monitor her symptoms. Patient can be discharged home this evening.

CASE STUDY QUESTIONS

24-2a. Admit diagnosis: _____

24-2b. Discharge disposition: _____

24-2c. Principal diagnosis: _____

24-2d. Secondary diagnoses (indicate POA status for secondary diagnoses):

_____

_____

_____

_____

_____

_____

24-2e. Principal procedure: _____

24-2f. Secondary procedures: _____

_____

24-2g. Assign MS-DRG: _____

24-2h. Relative weight of MS-DRG: _____

24-2i.   Can this MS-DRG be optimized with the addition of a CC? Yes or No
         Can this MS-DRG be optimized with the addition of an MCC? Yes or No

24-2j.   Is there a main guideline pertinent to selection of the principal diagnosis in this case study?

_____

_____

24-2k. Is there another diagnosis that meets the definition for principal diagnosis? Yes or No

24-2l. If yes, what is the other diagnosis? _____

24-2m. Is there any opportunity for physician query?

_____

_____

24-2n. What is the drug nortriptyline used to treat? _____

24-3. CASE STUDY

History and Physical

CC: Chest pain; SOB.

HPI: The patient is a 40-year-old gentleman who presents with chest pain and shortness of breath since the previous day. The pain came all of a sudden; it was 7 out of 10 and constant and had not abated since yesterday afternoon. The patient does admit to a cough with productive green sputum over the past week. At the time of the chest pain, the patient was watching TV and sitting; the pain was nonpositional and nonpleuritic in nature. His toxicology was positive for cocaine and barbiturates upon arrival at the Emergency Department.

Past medical history: Atrial fibrillation with RVR, chronic hepatitis C, chronic renal insufficiency, hypertension, and anemia.

Past surgical history: Repair of left inguinal hernia.

Allergies: NKDA.

Medications: Lisinopril 10 mg by mouth every day; aspirin 325 mg by mouth every day; diltiazem TR 240 mg by mouth every day. The patient states that he was compliant with his medications until 2 days ago.

Social history: The patient has a 20-pack-year history of smoking and is currently smoking. Uses intranasal heroin and cocaine and currently uses on a regular basis.

Family history: Mom passed away at an unknown age from cardiac causes. The father passed away at 75 from cardiac causes as well. His sister also has coronary artery disease; age unknown.

Review of systems: ROS was positive for chills. The patient denies fevers. No nausea, vomiting, abdominal pain. Some shortness of breath in association with chest pain for the past several days; the patient again reports productive cough. The patient denies any dysuria or hematuria. No constipation or diarrhea.

Physical examination:

Vitals: Blood pressure was 145/95, temperature 99.1°, 98% on room air, respiratory rate 12, heart rate 65.

General: The patient was in no apparent distress but was frequently requesting morphine.

HEENT: Had some mildly injected sclerae, but no icteric sclerae. Jugular venous pulsation was mildly elevated.

Chest: Lungs were clear to auscultation bilaterally with good air movement.

CV: Heart examination was significant for regular rate and rhythm; positive S1, S2; no S3, S4, or murmur.

Abd: Slight tenderness to palpation throughout his abdomen but normoactive bowel sounds.

321

Extremities: No lower extremity edema.

Neurologic: Examination was nonfocal.

A/P: Cocaine-induced chest pain. Because of the patient's positive family history and other risk factors such as male gender and smoking, will investigate cardiac cause for the chest pain.

Discharge Summary

DIAGNOSES/PROBLEMS:

1. Multiple admissions for cocaine chest pain with narcotic-seeking behavior.
2. Atrial fibrillation with rapid ventricular response in the setting of cocaine use.
3. Hepatitis C, chronic.
4. Hypertension.
5. Left inguinal hernia, status post repair.
6. Chronic renal insufficiency with a baseline creatinine of 1.2 to 1.5.
7. Anemia.

PROCEDURES:

Chest x-ray. Punctate radiodensities superimposed on the left upper and lower lungs, most likely artifact.

HISTORY, MAJOR FINDINGS, AND HOSPITAL COURSE:

The patient is a 40-year-old gentleman with the previously mentioned past medical history who presents with chest pain and shortness of breath since the previous day. The pain came all of a sudden; it was 7 out of 10 and constant, and it had not abated since yesterday afternoon. The patient does admit to a cough with productive green sputum for the past week. At the time of the chest pain, the patient was watching TV and sitting; the pain was nonpositional and nonpleuritic in nature.

Review of systems was positive for chills. The patient denies fevers. No nausea, vomiting, abdominal pain. Some shortness of breath in association with chest pain for the past several days, and the patient again reports productive cough. The patient denies any dysuria or hematuria. No constipation or diarrhea.

Past medical history: As previously described.

Allergies: NKDA.

Medications: Lisinopril 10 mg by mouth every day; aspirin 325 mg by mouth every day; diltiazem TR 240 mg by mouth every day. The patient states that he was compliant with his medications until 2 days ago.

Social history: The patient has a 20-pack-year history of smoking and is currently smoking. Uses intranasal heroin and cocaine and currently uses on a regular basis. His toxicology was positive for cocaine and barbiturates upon arrival at the Emergency Department.

Family history: Mom passed away at an unknown age from cardiac causes. The father passed away at 75 from cardiac causes as well. His sister also has coronary artery disease, age unknown.

Physical examination: The patient's blood pressure was 145/95, temperature 99.1°, 98% on room air, respiratory rate 12, and heart rate 65. The patient was in no apparent distress but was frequently requesting morphine. The patient had some mildly injected sclerae, but no icteric sclerae. His jugular venous pulsation was mildly elevated. His lungs were clear to auscultation bilaterally with good air movement. Heart examination was significant for regular rate and rhythm; positive S1, S2; no S3, S4, or murmur. The patient had slight tenderness to palpation throughout his abdomen but had normoactive bowel sounds; he had no lower extremity edema. Neurologic examination was nonfocal.

322

Laboratory evaluation: Significant for a creatinine of 1.4, which is consistent with baseline creatinine clearance. Mild elevation in AST and ALT to 69 and 64, hematocrit of 38 with an MCV of 77. UA was negative but did include 9 RBCs. Urine toxicology positive for cocaine and barbiturates. The patient had troponin separated by 12 hours, all of which were less than 0.06.

EKG, which showed sinus bradycardia at a rate of 57, normal axis, normal intervals. The patient did have some peaked T waves in V2 to V3, but upon repeat EKG, the patient no longer had those PT waves in V2 to V3. The patient also had LVH by voltage criteria in V2 and V5. PT waves may be associated with the LVH.

HOSPITAL COURSE BY SYSTEM:

Cardiovascular: The patient's chest pain remained stable throughout the patient's hospitalization. It was believed that the chest pain was noncardiac in nature and was associated with cocaine use. No evidence of ischemic damage was found. The patient was subsequently put back on his medications, but the patient was not to be put on beta blockers because he actively used cocaine. During his stay, the patient's blood pressure remained elevated in the 150s to 180s for systolic blood pressure, at which point, his lisinopril was titrated up with improvement of his blood pressure to systolics in the 140s to 150s at the time of discharge on lisinopril 20 mg by mouth every day.

Pulmonary: The patient had a productive cough, and initial thoughts centered on pneumonia. The patient was initially given antibiotics in the Emergency Department, even though there was no chest infiltrate. The patient's blood cultures showed no growth to date. The antibiotic was discontinued.

Endocrine: The patient had a lipid profile that was quite good with HDL of 60 and LDL of 97.

Ophthalmology: The patient was thought to have a bacterial conjunctivitis that caused his erythematous sclera. Therefore, he was put on gentamicin drops for 5 to 7 days, 1 drop every 4 hours.

Reportable diseases: None.

Adverse drug reactions: None.

Allergies: None.

Complications to procedures: None.

Condition on discharge: Stable.

Discharge medications: Lisinopril 20 mg by mouth every day, aspirin 325 mg by mouth every day, Atorvastatin 20 mg by mouth every day, diltiazem TR 240 mg by mouth every day, gentamicin ophthalmic solution 1 drop both eyes every 4 hours.

DISCHARGE INSTRUCTIONS:

Diet: The patient is to eat a diet that is low in fat and low in salt.

Other: The patient is to abstain from intranasal cocaine and heroin.

FOLLOW-UP CARE:

The patient is to follow up at the clinic.

Progress Notes

DAY 1

The patient was admitted with CP. ACS rule-out followed. EKG and cardiac enzymes are normal. Chest x-ray is normal without infiltrate. Advance diet. Watch for signs of withdrawal. It appears that the patient had a bacterial conjunctivitis; gentamicin drops were started.

323

Chest pain has resolved. The patient is encouraged to abstain from drug use and is given a list of local NA meetings. Blood pressure has been somewhat elevated. Increase lisinopril from 10 to 20 mg. The patient is ready for discharge home.

CASE STUDY QUESTIONS

24-3a. Admit diagnosis: _____

24-3b. Discharge disposition: _____

24-3c. Principal diagnosis: _____

24-3d. Secondary diagnoses (indicate POA status for secondary diagnoses):

_____

_____

_____

_____

_____

_____

24-3e. Principal procedure: _____

24-3f. Secondary procedures: _____

_____

24-3g. Assign MS-DRG: _____

24-3h. Relative weight of MS-DRG: _____

24-3i. Can this MS-DRG be optimized with the addition of a CC? Yes or No
        Can this MS-DRG be optimized with the addition of an MCC? Yes or No

24-3j. Is there a main guideline pertinent to selection of the principal diagnosis in this case study?

_____

_____

24-3k. Is there another diagnosis that meets the definition for principal diagnosis? Yes or No

24-3l. If yes, what is the other diagnosis? _____

24-3m. Is there any opportunity for physician query?

_____

_____

24-3n. What is the drug diltiazem TR used to treat? _____

324

25 Complications of Surgical and Medical Care

ABBREVIATIONS/ACRONYMS

Without the use of reference materials, define the following abbreviations or acronyms.

1. TPN _____

2. DVT _____

3. THR _____

4. ECT _____

5. TURP _____

6. PO _____

GLOSSARY DEFINITIONS

Match the glossary term to the correct definition.

1. _____ Iatrogenic

2. _____ Aspiration

3. _____ Stent

4. _____ Oliguric

5. _____ Dehiscence

6. _____ Neuroma

7. _____ Intractable

A. Small amount of urine

B. Tumor of the nerve cells

C. Breathing in a foreign object

D. Not manageable

E. Caused by medical treatment

F. Opening of a surgical wound

G. Device inserted into areas of the body such as arteries to assist in keeping them open

CODING

Using the code book, code the following.

1. Acute renal failure due to obstructed Foley catheter _____

2. Cardiac biopsy of the right atrium via percutaneous approach shows mild rejection of heart transplant _____

3. Ventilation pneumonia caused by pseudomonas _____

4. Fracture of right hip prosthesis _____

5. Fever likely due to postoperative atelectasis _____

6. Severe nausea and vomiting postop _____

7. Acute respiratory insufficiency due to surgery _____

8. Neuroma of amputation stump; patient has left AKA _____

9. Infected stitches post appendectomy _____

10. Restenosis of cardiac stent _____

CASE SCENARIOS

Using the code book, code the following cases.

1. Patient with decreased visual acuity due to right corneal graft rejection. Admitted for cadaver keratoplasty.

   _____

   _____

2. Patient admitted with an infected seroma of abdominal surgical wound. Cultures were positive for *Streptococcus*. The seroma was incised and drained.

   _____

   _____

3. Patient was admitted for TAH due to symptomatic fibroids. The bladder was accidentally lacerated during the procedure and was repaired with suture.

   _____

   _____

4. Patient had an outpatient procedure this morning and was discharged in stable condition. Patient returns because of inability to void. A Foley catheter was inserted.
   Diagnosis: Postoperative urinary retention.

   _____

   _____

5. Patient had bariatric surgery 2 years ago and has lost 150 pounds. She was admitted for panniculectomy and repair of incisional hernia. Surgery was performed without complications. On postop day 2, the patient became short of breath with chest pain. Emergency CT showed numerous PEs. The patient's condition deteriorated, and she expired. Autopsy was ordered.

   _____

   _____

6. Patient was seen for outpatient colonoscopy because of Crohn's disease. In the days following, the patient had increasing abdominal pain. Patient was admitted because CT showed perforation of the colon.

   _____

   _____

7. Patient was admitted to donate a right kidney to his son. Surgery was performed without complications. Recovery was slowed by postoperative ileus.

   _____

   _____

8. Patient had an outpatient ERCP for extraction of a bile duct stone. At home the patient developed acute abdominal pain and was admitted to rule out post ERCP pancreatitis.
   Impression: Post ERCP pancreatitis.

   _____

   _____

9. Patient previously had a laparoscopic partial right nephrectomy for RCC. The patient recovered and was discharged in stable condition. The patient returns now with fever and flank pain. CT showed a perinephric abscess. The patient had percutaneous drainage performed.
   Impression: Postoperative abscess.

   _____

   _____

10. Patient was admitted with a right lung nodule for an outpatient transbronchial lung biopsy. After the procedure, the patient developed a pneumothorax and was admitted. A chest tube was inserted and serial chest x-rays performed. The pathology of the nodule was squamous cell carcinoma.

    _____

    _____

CASE STUDIES

Using the code book, code and answer questions about the following case studies.

25-1. CASE STUDY

History and Physical

CC: Fevers

History of present illness: This is a 62-year-old white female with a history of a 5 × 6 splenic artery aneurysm. Other medical history includes portal hypertension, history of gastrointestinal bleeding, and biliary cirrhosis. The patient underwent splenic artery aneurysm coil embolization a few months ago; a total of 35 coils were deployed. Postoperatively, the patient developed pneumonia. Currently, the patient states that she had pain postoperatively for approximately 2 weeks in her abdomen. It gradually went away. It did return recently. She states that she had a low-grade fever ranging from 99 to 100.

Past medical history: Asthma, portal hypertension, history of gastrointestinal bleeding, and primary biliary cirrhosis. She has osteoporosis. Has a history of pneumonia following splenic artery embolization a few months ago. The patient is on the transplant list at two different facilities for a liver transplantation.

Social history: No tobacco or alcohol.

Family history: History of diabetes.

Allergies: Percocet causes hives.

REVIEW OF SYSTEMS:

Constitutional: Fever and chills. No change in weight. No night sweats.

Neuro: Headache, but no dizziness or syncope.

HEENT: Negative. No change in vision.

CV: Negative. No chest pain.

Respiratory: SOB with cough related to her asthma.

GI: Negative. No dysphagia, reflux, or heartburn.

GU: No dysuria, frequency, urgency, or hematuria.

Skin/Skeletal: No rashes or myalgias.

PHYSICAL EXAMINATION:

Vital signs: Blood pressure on right arm 166/90, pulse 98, oxygen saturation 98% on room air.

General: Patient is alert and oriented in no acute distress. Well nourished.

HEENT: Normocephalic, atraumatic. PERRLA. EOMI. Trachea is central, and tongue is midline. No lymphadenopathy.

Chest: CTA, bilaterally.

CV: RRR.

Abd: Positive bowel sounds. Soft and slightly tender to palpation in the suprapubic region, left lower quadrant and left flank. No rebound tenderness noted.

Extremities: No cyanosis, clubbing, or edema. Good capillary refill.

Neuro: Alert and oriented ×3. Cranial nerves intact.

Assessment/Plan: The patient is admitted for fever workup. Cultures of blood, urine, and sputum will be taken. Chest x-ray will be done. MRI of abdomen to rule out abscess of spleen. Restart routine home meds.

Discharge Summary

DIAGNOSES/PROBLEMS:

Cellulitis abdomen most likely due to Lovenox injections.

PROCEDURES:

IV antibiotics.

HISTORY, MAJOR FINDINGS, AND HOSPITAL COURSE:

The patient is a 62-year-old female who presents with fever, S/P splenic embolization approximately 2 months ago. CT scan shows the known necrotic area in the spleen, encompassing about 40% of the spleen with no evidence of abscess. Given fevers and concern for abscess, she was started on cefepime, and an MRI was ordered. She was shortly thereafter noted to have an abdominal cellulitis, for which she was started on vancomycin. While awaiting MRI, the cellulitis improved markedly and the patient defervesced without additional fevers. Given her improvement, it was decided to hold on the MRI, treat cellulitis with oral Keflex, and follow up in clinic in 1 week. This was all discussed with the patient, who reported feeling much better and was ready to return home. She was also instructed to administer Lovenox in other subcutaneous areas beside her abdomen until her cellulitis resolves.

Discharge medications: Resume all home medications as previously prescribed. Keflex 500 mg PO BID × 7days.

Discharge instructions: Call MD for fever >101, worsening redness, swelling, or pain along abdomen.

Diet: Per routine.

328

Activity: As tolerated.

Follow-up care: Follow up in clinic.

Progress Notes

DAY 1

Patient is feeling better. Abdominal pain has subsided. Afebrile. Abdominal cellulitis is slightly improved. Still awaiting MRI. Continue IV antibiotics.

DAY 2

Patient is much improved with decreased cellulitis. Will cancel MRI. Patient is tolerating a regular diet. Start oral Keflex 500 mg BID. Instructed patient to administer Lovenox injections to other sites until her cellulitis has completely resolved.

CASE STUDY QUESTIONS

25-1a. Admit diagnosis: _____

25-1b. Discharge disposition: _____

25-1c. Principal diagnosis: _____

25-1d. Secondary diagnoses (indicate POA status for secondary diagnoses):

_____

_____

_____

_____

_____

_____

25-1e. Principal procedure: _____

25-1f. Secondary procedures: _____

_____

25-1g. Assign MS-DRG: _____

25-1h. Relative weight of MS-DRG: _____

25-1i. Can this MS-DRG be optimized with the addition of a CC? Yes or No
        Can this MS-DRG be optimized with the addition of an MCC? Yes or No

25-1j.   Is there a main guideline pertinent to selection of the principal diagnosis in this case study?

_____

_____

25-1k.   Is there another diagnosis that meets the definition for principal diagnosis? Yes or No

25-1l.   If yes, what is the other diagnosis? _____

25-1m. Is there any opportunity for physician query?

_____

_____

25-1n.   What is the drug Keflex used to treat? _____

25-2. CASE STUDY

History and Physical

CC: N/V, anorexia.

HPI: The patient is a 75-year-old male who is known to Surgical Service because a central pancreatectomy/mucosa pancreaticogastrotomy reconstruction was performed a couple of weeks ago for a serous cyst adenoma. About 1 week ago, the patient's JP was pulled at home accidentally, during which time the output was roughly 100 to 200 cc/day. CT did not show any abscess formation. However, the patient began to decline with symptoms of nausea, vomiting, and anorexia, and CT scan on the day of admission showed an intra-abdominal fluid collection.

Past medical history: Hypercholesterolemia, hypothyroidism, CAD with MI, COPD, history of gallstone pancreatitis, BPH, seizure disorder, and subdural hematoma.

Past surgical history: Central pancreatectomy for serous cyst adenoma a few weeks ago. CABG×3, TURP, and craniotomy for subdural hematoma.

Social history: Stopped tobacco 30 years ago. No alcohol. Retired.

Allergies: NKDA.

Review of systems:

Constitutional: Weight loss of 13 pounds since operation. No fever or chills.

Neuro: No headache or syncope. Patient has seizure disorder.

HEENT: No hearing loss or visual disturbance. No glaucoma.

CV: No CP or palpitations.

Respiratory: No SOB or cough. No sputum production.

GI: Belching and heartburn. No dysphagia.

GU: Nocturia ×2.

Skin/Skeletal: No rashes.

Physical examination:

Vitals: T 97.1, HR 92, BP 118/81.

General: Well-developed and well-nourished man in no acute distress.

HEENT: Normocephalic, atraumatic. PERRL, EOMI, sclera anicteric, and MMM.

Chest: CTA.

CV: RRR; no murmurs, gallops, or rub. Normal S1 and S2.

Abd: Normal bowel sounds, soft, nontender, nondistended. No masses. Surgical wound is healing and looks good.

Ext: No cyanosis, clubbing, or edema.

GU/Rectal: Normal rectal tone.

Neuro: Alerted and oriented ×3.

Assessment/Plan: Patient is admitted for drainage of peripancreatic fluid collection and antibiotics.

Discharge Summary

DIAGNOSES/PROBLEMS:

1. S/P central pancreatectomy/mucosa pancreaticogastrotomy (serous adenoma).
2. History of seizure disorder.
3. History of myocardial infarction.
4. Stable angina.
5. Negative stress test 1 month ago.
6. Chronic obstructive pulmonary disease.
7. Benign prostatic hypertrophy; status post transurethral resection of prostate.
8. History of gallstone pancreatitis.
9. Hypothyroidism.
10. Hyperlipidemia.
11. Status post traumatic brain injury with a craniotomy.
12. Severe obstructive sleep apnea on continuous positive airway pressure at home.
13. Possible urethral strictures.

PROCEDURES:

Placement of 8-French locking all-purpose drainage catheter in mid abdomen.

HISTORY, MAJOR FINDINGS, AND HOSPITAL COURSE:

The patient is a 75-year-old male who is known to Surgical Service because of a central pancreatectomy/mucosa pancreaticogastrotomy reconstruction performed a couple of weeks ago for a serous cyst adenoma. About 1 week ago, the patient's JP was pulled at home accidentally, during which time the output was roughly 100 to 200 cc/day. CT that day showed no abscess formation. However, the patient began to decline with symptoms of nausea, vomiting, and anorexia, and CT scan on the day of admission showed an intra-abdominal fluid collection. The patient was admitted for drainage, IV antibiotics (Zosyn, Flagyl), and NG decompression. The drain was placed uneventfully, and purulent, thick fluid was expressed. The fluid was cultured and grew anaerobic bacteria that were sensitive to a number of antibiotics, including TMP/SMX. During hospital stay, insertion of a Foley was attempted because of low urine output by a resident then by a urologist; this was unsuccessful. After fluid boluses to improve apparent dehydration, urine output improved and placement of a Foley was unnecessary. Hospital stay proceeded well. On the date of discharge, the patient was feeling well, was ambulating and voiding without difficulty, and was excited about discharge. The patient was discharged with a JP drain, and home care referral was made.

Allergies: NKDA.

Discharge medications:

1. Metoclopramide 10 mg q 6 hours.
2. Bactrim OS 1 tablet q 12 hours for 14 days.

At-home meds included Synthroid 150 mcg daily, ASA 325 mg PO daily, atenolol 25 mg daily, Zetia 10 mg daily, Amiodarone 200 mg daily, Dilantin Caps 100 mg q 12 hours. Also, Nasacort Nasal Spray 2 puffs each nostril daily, Advair diskus 250/50 BID, Spiriva daily, Zocor 60 mg daily, Hytrin 5 mg daily, Dilantin 50 mg daily, Protonix 40 mg BID, Citracal, Centrum vitamin, vitamin C, and folic acid.

DISCHARGE INSTRUCTIONS:

1. Limited activity: No pushing, pulling, lifting greater than 20 pounds.
2. Continue Bactrim for full 2-week course.
3. No bathing, swimming; showering OK.
4. Resume at-home meds following discharge.
5. Notify physician's office if fever greater than 101°F, unremitting pain, nausea/vomiting, or diarrhea develops. Also, contact for any concerns/questions.
6. Regular diet.

FOLLOW-UP CARE:

Call physician's office for follow-up appointment within 2 weeks.

Abscess Drain Cath. Placement

History: The patient is a 75-year-old male S/P central pancreatectomy for serous cystadenoma who presents with a peripancreatic fluid collection.

Procedures:

1. Limited sonogram of mid abdomen.
2. Placement of 8-French locking all-purpose drainage catheter.
3. Tube sinogram.

Contrast: 30 cc Hypaque.

Complications: None.

Medications: 4 mg of Versed and 200 mcg of fentanyl, local lidocaine.

Description: After the patient was informed of the risks, benefits, and alternatives of the procedure, and informed consent was obtained and documented, the patient was brought to the interventional radiology suite and was prepped and draped in the usual sterile manner. After a mid-abdominal approach was selected with the use of fluoroscopic landmarks, the skin and subcutaneous tissues were anesthetized with lidocaine. With fluoroscopic landmarks, a 21-gauge trocar needle from a Jeffries set was used to access the collection. A 0.018-inch Microvena wire was placed into the collection, and location was confirmed with frank aspiration of pus and injection of contrast. The Jeffries set was placed into the collection under fluoroscopic guidance. The metal stiffener was removed, and a parallel 0.035 Rosen wire was placed alongside the Microvena wire. The set was removed, and an 8-French APDL catheter was placed under fluoroscopic guidance into the collection. Contrast was injected and images obtained to confirm placement. The drain was sewn into place with 2-0 Monosorb. The patient tolerated the procedure well.

Findings: Fluid collection located in mid abdomen with complex fluid. Aspiration of thick, purulent fluid from collection. Successful placement of 8-French locking all-purpose drainage catheter into collection.

Impression: Successful drainage of mid-abdominal collection with an 8-French locking all-purpose drainage catheter.

Plan: The tube should be left to external gravity drainage via drainage bag. The tube should be flushed twice daily with 15 cc normal saline. Patient was monitored and then was transferred to the floor in stable condition.

Clinical history: Abdominal pain, vomiting, status post partial pancreatectomy for serous cystadenoma.

Comparison: CT abdomen and pelvis from November and September.

Technique: Axial CT scan of the abdomen and pelvis was obtained following the administration of intravenous contrast without adverse reaction and the administration of oral contrast.

CT abdomen: Calcified and noncalcified pleurae are seen in the lung bases unchanged from prior studies. Slightly worsening dependent atelectasis noted in both lung bases. Several small subcentimeter low-attenuation lesions in the dome of the liver and the inferior aspect of the right lobe of the liver are too small to characterize but likely represent small cysts or hemangiomas. Hypodense lesions are unchanged compared with prior studies. The remainder of the liver appears unremarkable.

Areas of inflammation around the pancreatic resection site have worsened; an ill-defined collection of scattered small air bubbles within, now noted in the region of the pancreatic resection site collection, measures roughly 5.3 × 4.8 cm. The distal pancreas appears unremarkable.

The spleen, kidneys, and adrenals are normal. The stomach and small and large bowels are normal. No evidence of obstruction is seen. Mild tortuosity and mild other strut calcification of the abdominal aorta are noted. Infrarenal abdominal aorta reveals ectasia measuring up to 2.9 cm in diameter, with a small amount of mural thrombus along the right lateral aspect of the distal aorta.

CT pelvis: The urinary bladder appears unremarkable. Prosthetic calcifications are noted. Extensive atherosclerotic desiccation is noted of both common iliac arteries and internal iliac arteries. Sigmoid diverticulosis. The bony abdomen and pelvis are normal.

Impression: Ill-defined collection noted in the pancreatic resection bed worrisome for developing abscess. No evidence of obstruction is seen.

Progress Notes

DAY 1

Vitals stable. No events overnight. No nausea and vomiting. Abdomen is soft/NT/ND. Patient to have abscess drainage today. Continue IV antibiotics.

DAY 2

Admitted for nausea, vomiting, and anorexia S/P central pancreatectomy for benign pancreatic tumor. No leukocytosis or fever, but CT showed an evolving abscess. Drain was successfully placed to evacuate purulent material. Fluid was sent for culture.

DAY 3

Patient has had some oliguria, so Foley placement was attempted. Urology was called to place the Foley and staff were unable to place. IV fluids were increased and urine output improved. The patient will need to follow up as an outpatient with Urology for workup of possible urethral strictures. Repeat CT scan to assess fluid collection.

DAY 4

AF. HR 60s to 70s, BP 110/70, sats 95% on RA.
Ambulating. No complaints. Doing well. Abscess drain flushes easily.
Patient is ready for discharge.

333

CASE STUDY QUESTIONS

25-2a.   Admit diagnosis: _____

25-2b.   Discharge disposition: _____

25-2c.   Principal diagnosis: _____

25-2d.   Secondary diagnoses (indicate POA status for secondary diagnoses):

_____

_____

_____

_____

_____

25-2e.   Principal procedure: _____

25-2f.   Secondary procedures: _____

_____

25-2g.   Assign MS-DRG: _____

25-2h.   Relative weight of MS-DRG: _____

25-2i.   Can this MS-DRG be optimized with the addition of a CC? Yes or No
         Can this MS-DRG be optimized with the addition of an MCC? Yes or No

25-2j.   Is there a main guideline pertinent to selection of the principal diagnosis in this case study?

_____

_____

25-2k.   Is there another diagnosis that meets the definition for principal diagnosis? Yes or No

25-2l.   If yes, what is the other diagnosis? _____

25-2m. Is there any opportunity for physician query?

_____

_____

25-2n.   What is the drug Hytrin used to treat? _____

CC: DVT, weight loss, and coagulopathy.

HPI: The patient is an 18-year-old with ASCA-positive Crohn's diagnosed 1½ years ago. He presented to the clinic after he was hospitalized 2 times recently for pancreatitis, which resolved when he was made NPO. During a previous hospitalization, a femoral line was placed; the patient developed a left leg DVT and was started on Lovenox and Coumadin. He was discharged on NG feeds but has discontinued them. His weight continued to drop, and he appeared pale and malnourished in clinic. Additionally, he was discharged on Coumadin 5 mg every day, but because of an apparent miscommunication, he has been taking Coumadin 5 mg 2 times a day. He has been symptomatic from the DVT with pain and leg swelling. Because of his symptomatic clot, weight loss, and unclear coagulation status, the patient was admitted directly from clinic.

Past medical history: Significant for Crohn's disease diagnosed 1½ years ago, which has been treated with Pentasa and Remicade every 6 weeks. Further, the patient has a history of two prior hospitalizations—one for pancreatitis and one for thrombus.

Past surgical history: He has never had surgery before.

Medications: His current medications include Remicade every 6 weeks, Pentasa, iron, Lovenox, and Coumadin.

Social history: The patient is a senior in high school. He plans to go to a technical school.

Family history: Significant for a maternal aunt who has severe diabetes and subsequently developed renal failure secondary to her diabetes. She has a history of multiple lower extremity clots.

Allergies: NKDA.

Review of systems:

Constitutional: No fever or chills. Positive for weight loss.

Neuro: No headache or syncope.

HEENT: Benign.

CV: No chest pain or palpitation.

Respiratory: No shortness of breath.

GI: +heme stools.

GU: Negative.

Skin/Skeletal: Swelling, erythema, and edema of left leg.

Physical examination:

Vitals: Afebrile. HR 60, BP 100/60, RR 14, O_2 sats 97% on RA.

General: NAD. Appears comfortable.

HEENT: NCAT, MMM, oropharynx clear.

Chest: CTA bilaterally, normal respiratory effort.

CV: RRR, normal S1 and S2. No murmur.

Abd: BS+, S/NT/ND.

GU/Rectal: Guaiac positive.

Ext: Swelling of left thigh and lower extremity to the ankle. Good pulses. No evidence of skin breakdown.

Neuro: Alert and oriented.

335

Assessment/Plan: Patient is admitted for treatment of his DVT and assessment of coagulation and nutritional status.

Discharge Summary

DIAGNOSES/PROBLEMS:

1. Crohn's disease.
2. Left leg deep venous thrombosis now resolved.
3. Malnutrition.
4. Anemia.

PROCEDURES:

1. Packed red blood cells transfusion times 2.
2. Ultrasonography of left extremity.
3. Right upper quadrant ultrasonography.
4. Left popliteal, left iliac, and inferior vena cava venograms.
5. Trellis thrombolysis.
6. tPA thrombolysis.

HISTORY, MAJOR FINDINGS, AND HOSPITAL COURSE:

The patient is an 18-year-old with ASCA-positive Crohn's diagnosed 1½ years ago. He presented to the clinic after he had been hospitalized 2 times recently for pancreatitis, which resolved when he was made NPO. During previous hospitalizations, the patient had a femoral line placed, developed a left leg DVT, and was started on Lovenox and Coumadin. He was discharged on NG feeds but has discontinued them. His weight continued to drop, and he appeared pale and malnourished in clinic. Additionally, he was discharged on Coumadin 5 mg every day, but because of an apparent miscommunication, he has been taking Coumadin 5 mg 2 times a day. He has been symptomatic from the DVT with pain and leg swelling. Because of his symptomatic clot, weight loss, and unclear coagulation status, the patient was admitted directly from clinic. On admission, labs revealed hypoalbuminemia (2.0), anemia (hemoglobin of 6.1), malnutrition (a prealbumin of 6), inflammations (elevated erythrocyte sedimentation rate at 68 and CRP at 7.6), and a critically elevated INR of 11.3. He received multiple doses of vitamin K and a unit of FFP in an effort to return his INR to a more therapeutic range; by 11/01/06, it was 2.7, and by 11/04/06, it was 1.4. He received 2 units of packed red blood cells. Ultrasonography of his leg revealed a thrombus, which completely occluded the left common iliac, the common femoral, and the popliteal, as well as the nonocclusive thrombus of the left saphenous. He was brought to the Interventional Radiology suite, where he underwent a venogram, attempted mechanical lysis of the clot, and insertion of a catheter for intravenous tPA. After spending a night in the Pediatric Intensive Care Unit receiving tPA through the catheter, he returned to the Interventional Radiology suite, where a venogram revealed that the clot had completely resolved. Additionally, symptoms of pain and left leg swelling resolved. The patient was started on NG feeds as well and received his Remicade dose on 11/06/06. In terms of his pancreatitis, he had a normal amylase and only mildly elevated lipase. No symptoms of abdominal pain were reported, and no radiologic evidence of pancreatitis was seen on ultrasonography.

Allergies: Morphine (hives).

Condition on discharge fair.

Discharge medications: Iron 88 mg, Alimentum 2 times a day per NG tube, Lovenox 60 mg subcutaneous 2 times a day, Prednisone 60 mg per NG tube every day, Tylenol as needed for pain, and Neutra-Phos 250 mg per NG 2 times a day for 1 week.

DISCHARGE INSTRUCTIONS:

Diet: By mouth, ad lib with NG tube feeds of Nutren 1.5 at 175 cubic centimeters an hour for 10 hours daily.

Activity: Elevate left leg if it gets swollen. Wear compression stocking if the leg becomes swollen and when not walking. Do not take aspirin or aspirin-containing medicines.

FOLLOW-UP CARE:

Appointments have been made with Hematology and Gastroenterology.

Pediatric Inpatient Hematology Consultation

Chief complaint: Line-associated thrombus and excess anticoagulation secondary to Coumadin.

History of present illness: The patient is an 18-year-old male with Crohn's disease initially diagnosed 1½ years ago, who was admitted yesterday secondary to a 6-kg weight loss over the past 3½ months. The patient was recently in the hospital after experiencing abdominal pain, fevers, and vomiting. He was diagnosed with pancreatitis, which was treated with pain medications and NPO status with nutritional support times of approximately 1 week. It was difficult to gain access to the patient; therefore, the only line that could be obtained was a left femoral line, which remained in place throughout his hospitalization. His pancreatitis resolved, and the patient was discharged after line removal. While at home, he began experiencing significant left leg swelling, pain, and erythema. The patient subsequently was seen at an outside hospital, where he was readmitted; ultrasonography confirmed a left femoral thrombus. The patient was started on Lovenox and Coumadin at doses of Lovenox 70 mg subcutaneous 2 times a day and Coumadin 5 mg by mouth daily. He was discharged on the following day. The patient was seen by his pediatrician, and it was found that he had been taking only his Lovenox and not his Coumadin. Therefore, the pediatrician decided to start him on a loading dose of Coumadin at 5 mg 2 times a day ×2 days, then back to 5 mg daily. The patient misunderstood these instructions and had been taking Coumadin 5 mg by mouth 2 times a day. When the patient was seen in the clinic on the day of admission, again there was concern for his ongoing weight loss. Laboratory studies were sent off, and the patient was maintained on his home medications, including Coumadin. An INR that was sent off prior to his nighttime dose of Coumadin came back as 11.3. Repeat INR after his nighttime dose of Coumadin showed an INR of greater than 14.9. On his initial labs, his hemoglobin was 6.1. Upon repeat testing after his nighttime Coumadin dose, it was stable at 6.5. The patient was noted to be guaiac positive but was not having any evidence of bleeding elsewhere. He was given packed red blood cells early this morning. In addition, when his INR returned to greater than 14.9, Hematology was consulted, and the patient was given an oral dose of 5 mg of vitamin K. Repeat INR 4 hours after the dose of by mouth vitamin K showed that the INR was still greater than 14.9. Therefore, the primary team was instructed to give the patient an additional 2-mg intravenous dose of vitamin K; this is still pending at the present time.

The patient's past medical history is significant for Crohn's disease diagnosed 1½ years ago, which had been treated with Pentasa and Remicade every 6 weeks. The last dose was given in September.

Further, the patient has a history of two prior hospitalizations—one for pancreatitis and one for thrombus. He has never had surgery before.

Current medications include Remicade every 6 weeks (the last dose was in September) Pentasa, iron, Lovenox, and Coumadin.

Social history: The patient is a senior in high school. He plans to go to a technical school.

Family history: Significant for a maternal aunt who has severe diabetes and subsequently developed renal failure secondary to her diabetes. She has a history of multiple lower extremity clots.

On physical examination, the patient is afebrile with stable vital signs. He is awake, alert, and in no acute distress. He has a somewhat flat affect.

HEENT: Pupils are equal, round, and reactive to light. Sclerae and conjunctivae are clear. Mucous membranes are moist, and no oral lesions and no bleeding of the gums or epistaxis is noted. Lungs are clear to auscultation bilaterally.

Cardiovascular: The patient has a regular rate and rhythm with a normal S1, normal S2, and no murmurs, rubs, or gallops. Abdomen is soft, nontender, and nondistended, and the patient has normal bowel sounds and no hepatosplenomegaly. Extremity examination reveals significant swelling of the left lower leg. The left thigh measures 42 cm in circumference compared with 39 cm on the right. Significant edema, most notably around the right lower calf extending to and beyond the ankle, has been noted. There is no redness, warmth, or tenderness. The patient has full range of motion.

Laboratory studies from 10/31/06: The patient had a white blood cell count of 7760 with a hemoglobin of 6.1 and a platelet count of 866. PT was 93.7, with an INR of 11.3. PTT was 62 with a PTT ratio of 2.2. Repeat laboratory studies performed early in the morning on 11/01 showed a white blood cell count of 6070 with a hemoglobin of 6.5 and a platelet count of 871. INR was greater than 14.9. PTT was 69.2 with a PTT ratio of 2.4. The patient was subsequently given a one-time dose by mouth of vitamin K, along with a transfusion of packed red blood cells. Repeat labs done after these interventions showed a white blood cell count of 4890 with a hemoglobin of 9.1 and platelets of 829,000. His INR was still greater than 14.9 with a PTT of 61.7 and a PTT ratio of 2.1. The patient has had stool guaiac ×3, all of which were positive.

Ultrasonography with Doppler of the left lower extremity revealed a complete thrombus of the left common iliac and common femoral, femoral, and popliteal veins. Further, a nonocclusive thrombus of the left greater saphenous vein was noted.

Assessment: The patient is an 18-year-old male with Crohn's disease and now a line-associated thrombus and excessive anticoagulation secondary to Coumadin.

Recommendations:

1. We will continue to give vitamin K and to titrate the dose to his INR. The patient will get a repeat dose of 2 mg intravenously this evening, and we will follow up his INR status post that intervention. The INR will likely begin to significantly decrease within the next 24 hours. Once the INR approaches 3, we should restart his Coumadin at a dose of 5 mg by mouth daily for continued anticoagulation for line-associated thrombus.
2. We would recommend consulting interventional radiology for possible thrombolysis, given the size and extent of this clot and his risk for postclot valvular insufficiency with subsequent repeated episodes of edema and skin breakdown. Certainly, we would ask that he be in a more normal state of coagulation, given the risk of hemorrhage with this procedure, especially in the case of someone with continued GI bleeding.
3. For his coagulopathy workup, we can now send an anticardiolipin antibody panel, DRVVT, homocystine, MTHFR, PT 20210, and factor VIII. All other assays would be affected by Coumadin and would not be worth sending at this point.

The patient underwent catheter-directed thrombolysis with tPA at 0.7 mg per hour for about 24 hours. This resulted in near-total clot resolution; the patient was then transitioned to Lovenox 60 mg BID. The anti-Xa level 4 hours after a dose was therapeutic at 0.8. The patient was discharged on this dose.

Further workup for thrombophilia revealed a low protein S at 27%. However, this activity may have been affected by Coumadin. Antithrombin, protein C, and homocysteine were normal. DRVVT and anticardiolipin antibodies did not show the presence of an antiphospholipid antibody. The prothrombin mutation was negative.

Factor VIII was elevated. An activated protein C was not attained and will need to be done on an outpatient basis.

Given the difficulty of managing Coumadin previously, we have recommended management with Lovenox, initially at 60 mg BID. Once he is stable on this dose, we will consider transitioning the patient to a daily dose of 1.5 mg/kg with a target peak of 1.0 to 1.5. His thrombophilic evaluation identified the femoral line as a major reversible risk. Other factors identified include Crohn's disease, elevated FVIII, and possibly low protein S. Because FVIII and protein S may be affected by inflammation, and because protein S may be affected by Coumadin, these will need to be repeated. In addition, we will want to obtain an activated protein C, which is a screen for FV Leiden. We would plan to treat the patient for a minimum of 3 months, possibly longer depending on repeat assessment of the thrombus and thrombophilic risks.

Duplex Scan, Ven It Low Ext

Indication: History of femoral line clot at outside hospital 1 week ago. Now, with persistent pain, swelling, and warmth in the left lower extremity.

Technique: Gray scale, Color, and Duplex Doppler imaging of the left lower extremity veins was performed.

Findings: There is complete thrombosis of the left common iliac, common femoral, femoral, and popliteal veins. No blood flow is evident within these veins, and they are noncompressible. Echogenic thrombus is visualized within the left greater saphenous vein, which is noncompressible; however, there does appear to be flow within this vein. Flow is seen in the left profunda femoris vein. The right common iliac vein is patent. The visualized portion of the inferior vena cava is patent with normal venous waveform.

Impression: Complete thrombosis of the left common iliac, common femoral, femoral, and popliteal veins. Nonocclusive thrombus of the left greater saphenous vein.

Ultrasound, Single Quad

Indication: History of Crohn's disease with recent pancreatitis. Baseline study to assess the pancreas before high-dose steroids are begun.

Technique: Real-time ultrasound imaging of the right upper quadrant was performed.

Findings: The liver is normal in echotexture and size, measuring 16.9 cm in length. No evidence of intrahepatic biliary ductal dilatation is seen. The common bile duct is normal in caliber, measuring 3 mm. The gallbladder is decompressed and therefore is difficult to evaluate. The patient was not focally tender over the gallbladder. The well-visualized pancreas is normal in size and echogenicity. The main portal vein is patent and exhibits normal direction of flow. No ascites is noted within the right upper quadrant. The right kidney measures 10.1 cm in length and is normal in echotexture.

Impression: Normal right upper quadrant on ultrasonography. The gallbladder is decompressed and therefore is difficult to evaluate.

Mechanical Thrombolysis

History: Symptomatic left leg venous thrombosis.

List of procedures:

1. Ultrasound-guided access left popliteal vein.
2. Left popliteal, left iliac, and inferior vena cava venogram.
3. Trellis thrombolysis.
4. Placement of 40-cm infusion catheter.
5. Initiation of tPA infusion.

Medications: Versed, fentanyl, lidocaine, 4 mg TPA with Trellis.

Contrast: 80 cc Omnipaque.

Complications: None.

Procedure note: A "timeout" was provided in the room.

The procedure was explained in detail to the patient. With fully informed written consent, the patient was transferred to the procedure room and was prepared and draped in standard fashion. Sterile technique was used throughout.

With ultrasonography, guidance access into the left popliteal vein was accomplished with the ultimate placement of an 8-French vascular sheath. With a combination of glide wire and angled tapered catheter, access into the inferior vena cava was gained and a venogram was performed. Next, a pull-back venogram was performed to show the extent of thrombosis. An 8-French 30-cm Trellis thrombolysis system was advanced into the popliteal with the tip in the external iliac vein. Thrombolysis was performed for 10 minutes with injection of 6 mg tPA. A post-thrombolysis venogram was obtained. A 40-cm infusion catheter was advanced through the sheath with the tip of the catheter in the external iliac vein. Through the catheter, 0.75 mg tPA/hr was infused; in addition, through the sheath, 30 cc/hr of nonheparinized saline was infused overnight. The catheter and sheaths were sewn in, and the patient was transported to the PICU for monitoring.

Findings:

1. Diffuse clot involving the left popliteal to the origin of the inferior vena cava (acute from popliteal to CVF and chronic from CVF to common iliac vein).
2. Patent IVC.
3. Minimal effect of Trellis thrombolysis.
4. Successful placement of the infusion catheter with the tip in the external iliac vein.

Fluoroscopy time: 12 minutes.

Cumulative absorbed dose: 37,640 mGy/cm^2.

Impression: Diffuse clot involving the left popliteal to the origin of the inferior vena cava. Successful placement infusion tPA catheter overnight.

Disposition of patient: To monitored bed. Observe overnight. Check baseline and overnight fibrinogen. Follow-up CVD.

Angio: Infusion/embolized

History: Crohn's disease.

Status post lysis of left lower extremity clot.

List of procedures:

1. Left lower extremity venogram.
2. Pelvic venogram.
3. Completion lysis LLE.

Medications: Versed/fentanyl/lidocaine. See nursing notes.

Contrast: 10 cc Omnipaque.

Complications: None.

Procedure note: A "timeout" was provided in the room.

The procedure was explained in detail to the patient. With fully informed written consent, the patient was transferred to the procedure room and was prepared and draped in standard fashion. A sterile technique was used throughout. Contrast is injected into the left lower extremity venous sheath.

Venogram showed minimal clot at the insertion site in the region of the popliteal vein. However, no evidence of clot from the popliteal vein to the left common femoral vein was found. The sheath was therefore pulled, and manual pressure was applied.

Findings:

1. No evidence of significant thrombus from the left popliteal vein to the left common femoral vein with restoration of antegrade flow from popliteal vein into IVC.
2. Removal of left lower venous sheath.

Impression: Resolution of left lower extremity thrombus.

Disposition: To recovery and then to floor. Patient to wear compression stocking. Patient must keep left lower extremity elevated while sitting and lying down. Patient should be on anticoagulation for the next 6 months.

Progress Notes

DAY 1

Patient was admitted for DVT, Crohn's, malnutrition, and heme + stool and anemia. He was evaluated by Interventional Radiology, who recommended catheter-directed thrombolysis. Patient will require PICU stay because of postprocedure tPA continuous infusion. Monitor INRs. Give 2 U of PRBCs for anemia.

No evidence of recurrent pancreatitis. Afebrile. No antibiotics. Monitor for signs of respiratory distress.

DAY 2

Patient under venogram, Trellis thrombolysis, and tPA thrombolysis. Will be monitored in PICU overnight. Compression stockings, elevation of leg, and continued anticoagulation. NG tube feedings started. Dietary consult ordered. Vit K and 2 U of FFP were given prior to the procedure.

DAY 3

Patient is S/P lysis of left CFV clot. He tolerated the procedure well. Patient denies any pain or discomfort.

Vitals: HR 60, BP 100/60, RR 14.

Gen: In bed, appears comfortable.

HEENT: NCAT. MMM. Neck supple.

Chest: CTA.

CVS: RRR.

Abd: Soft. No tenderness.

Ext: Left LE wrapped from upper thigh to ankle in ACE. Right LE normal. No paresthesias. Mild edema left foot. Venogram shows restoration of flow from popliteal to IVC.

DAY 4

Patient is recovering nicely from thrombolysis. Will follow up with Gastroenterology and Hematology as an outpatient. Patient will be discharged to home.

25-3a.   Admit diagnosis: _____

25-3b.   Discharge disposition: _____

25-3c.   Principal diagnosis: _____

25-3d.   Secondary diagnoses (indicate POA status for secondary diagnoses):

_____

_____

_____

_____

_____

_____

_____

25-3e.   Principal procedure: _____

25-3f.   Secondary procedures: _____

_____

25-3g.   Assign MS-DRG: _____

25-3h.   Relative weight of MS-DRG: _____

25-3i.   Can this MS-DRG be optimized with the addition of a CC? Yes or No
        Can this MS-DRG be optimized with the addition of an MCC? Yes or No

25-3j.   Is there a main guideline pertinent to selection of the principal diagnosis in this case study?

_____

_____

25-3k.   Is there another diagnosis that meets the definition for principal diagnosis? Yes or No

25-3l.   If yes, what is the other diagnosis? _____

25-3m. Is there any opportunity for physician query?

_____

_____

25-3n.   What is the drug tPA used to treat? _____

26 Reimbursement Methodologies

ABBREVIATIONS/ACRONYMS

Without the use of reference materials, define the following abbreviations or acronyms.

1. PEPPER _____

2. RW _____

3. RAC _____

4. ALOS _____

5. CMI _____

6. GMLOS _____

7. IPPS _____

8. QIO _____

9. PPS _____

10. HPR _____

GLOSSARY DEFINITIONS

Match the glossary term to the correct definition.

1. _____ Principal diagnosis

2. _____ Complication

3. _____ Grouper

4. _____ Optimization

5. _____ Comorbidity

6. _____ Encoder

7. _____ Maximization

8. _____ HMO

9. _____ Revenue code

10. _____ Chargemaster

11. _____ Medical necessity

12. _____ National coverage determinations

13. _____ Department number

14. _____ Charge description number

15. _____ Local coverage determinations

A. Coding software used to assign the appropriate MS-DRG

B. Condition established after study as chiefly responsible for occasioning admission of the patient to the hospital for care

C. Condition that arises during a patient's hospitalization which may lead to increased resource use

D. Coding software that is used to assign diagnosis and procedure codes

E. Manipulation of codes to ensure maximum reimbursement without supporting documentation in the health record, or with disregard for coding conventions, guidelines, and UHDDS definitions

F. Preexisting condition that may lead to increased resource use

G. Process of striving to obtain optimal reimbursement or the highest possible payment to which the facility is legally entitled, on the basis of documentation in the health record

H. Type of managed care in which care is provided at a discounted rate

I. Listing of the services, procedures, drugs, and supplies that can be applied to a patient's bill

J. A number that designates a particular service or procedure and is used to generate a charge on a patient bill

K. Ancillary departments such as Radiology, Laboratory, and Emergency Room will have a specific hospital departmental number

L. Local policy that may include certain time frames for testing, that a patient be a certain age, and that a particular diagnosis or condition is present to be considered medically necessary

M. Criteria or guidelines for what is determined to be reasonable and necessary for a particular medical service

N. National policy that may include certain time frames for testing, that a patient be a certain age, and that a particular diagnosis or condition is present to be considered medically necessary

O. A four-digit code that is utilized on the UB-04 to indicate a particular type of service

MULTIPLE CHOICE/SHORT ANSWER

Select the correct answer or fill in the blank for each of the following.

1. If a patient was admitted to the hospital for a kidney problem, which MDC would be assigned?
   A. MDC 10
   B. MDC 11
   C. MDC 12
   D. MDC 13

2. Other factors that may play a role in MS-DRG assignment besides principal and secondary diagnoses and procedures include
   A. The patient's sex
   B. The patient's discharge disposition
   C. The birthweight for neonates
   D. All of the above

3. An electronic report sent to hospitals that contains hospital-specific information for specific MS-DRG target areas is known as
   A. SOW
   B. PEPPER
   C. QIO
   D. None of the above

4. An organization that acts under the direction of CMS and is contracted to monitor the quality of health care and to make sure that Medicare pays only for services that are reasonable and necessary is
   A. SOW
   B. PEPPER
   C. QIO
   D. None of the above

5. Calculate the MS-DRG payment for MS-DRG 055 if the hospital payment rate is $4000.00. _____

6. Describe the purpose of a CDIP. _____

7. During the month of July, the following Medicare patients were discharged from Hospital B. Using the MS-DRG weights, calculate the case mix for the following:
   2 patients   MS-DRG 100
   2 patients   MS-DRG 460
   1 patient   MS-DRG 066
   3 patients   MS-DRG 740
   2 patients   MS-DRG 418
   The CMI for July is _____ .

8. List four commonly missed CCs or MCCs.

   _____

   _____

   _____

   _____

9. Compare and contrast a retrospective payment system (RPS) with a prospective payment system (PPS).

   _____

   _____

   _____

   _____

   _____

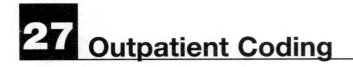

27 Outpatient Coding

ABBREVIATIONS/ACRONYMS

Without the use of reference materials, define the following abbreviations or acronyms.

1. HCPCS _____

2. COPD _____

3. AMA _____

4. ER _____

5. OPPS _____

6. CPT _____

7. PCP _____

8. APC _____

GLOSSARY DEFINITIONS

Match the glossary term to the correct definition.

1. _____ Professional service

2. _____ Encounter

3. _____ Observation unit

4. _____ Ancillary service

5. _____ Uncertain diagnosis

6. _____ Contraindication

A. Service rendered by a physician or a nonphysician practitioner

B. Area outside the Emergency Department where unstable patients are admitted for a stay of less than 48 hours; the patient is being observed for admit to the hospital or discharge home

C. Services provided by a hospital that are additional to a professional service, such as Lab, Radiology, and Pathology

D. Diagnosis that has not been verified by tests

E. Face-to-face visit with a healthcare provider

F. Reason that would make a medical treatment unadvisable

CODING

Using the code book, code the following.

1. Routine prenatal visit at 16 weeks; patient had a miscarriage 1 year ago _____

2. Infant brought to the clinic for evaluation of diaper rash _____

3. Child seen in the ED with impetigo of eyelid _____

4. Patient seen in the ER because of right flank pain Diagnosis: possible kidney stone _____

347

5. Patient had liver function test because of the medication he takes for hypercholesterolemia   _____

6. Patient was seen in clinic by dermatologist for severe acne   _____

7. Patient was evaluated by podiatrist for bunion left big toe   _____

8. Patient seen in clinic with symptoms of polydipsia, polyuria, fatigue, and weight loss in spite of extreme hunger; patient has a family history of DM; patient will need fasting blood work to rule out diabetes mellitus   _____

9. Patient has pain in right heel; physician ordered x-rays   _____ to rule out calcaneal spur; x-ray confirms a calcaneal spur

10. Patient seen in clinic for amenorrhea   _____

11. Patient seen in the ED for swollen left foot and ankle   _____ Diagnosis: cellulitis

12. Patient had a screening mammogram   _____

13. Cerumen both ears; irrigation performed   _____

14. Patient is seen for interrogation of AICD   _____

15. Employment physical   _____

CASE SCENARIOS

Using the code book, code the following cases.

1. Patient is seen for influenza vaccination. Patient has a history of diabetes and asthma. Flu vaccine was administered.

   _____

   _____

2. Preoperative examination. Patient has asthma/COPD and is scheduled for a CABG for three-vessel CAD.

   _____

   _____

3. Patient admitted for outpatient chemotherapy. Patient had a left mastectomy for breast cancer, which has spread to the axillary nodes.

   _____

   _____

4. Patient was seen in the clinic because of fever, sore throat, headache, swollen glands, fatigue, and anorexia. A monospot was done that was positive for mononucleosis. Instructions for rest, pain control, fluids, and activity were given.

_____

_____

5. Female infant was brought to the clinic for fussiness and fever. The infant was nursing well and had wet diapers. Examination of ears showed bilateral otitis media.

_____

_____

6. Patient was seen in the clinic for renewal of birth control pills. She has had no adverse effects. She has no risk factors for taking the pill. She does not smoke.

_____

_____

7. Patient is seen for increasing chest pain on exertion. The pain was relieved with rest. A chest x-ray was negative. A stress test was ordered to rule out angina and will be done next week. Patient will return after undergoing stress test.

_____

_____

8. Patient was seen in the ED following an MVA. Patient was an unbelted driver who ran into a tree. Patient complains of neck and left shoulder pain. X-rays were taken. No fractures were identified.
   Diagnosis: Sprain of neck and injury to shoulder.

_____

_____

9. Patient was seen in the clinic because of dysuria and frequency. UA was taken. Patient was given a prescription for antibiotics.
   Diagnosis: Dysuria due to UTI.

_____

_____

10. Patient was seen in the clinic for evaluation of diabetic right foot ulcer. The ulcer appears to be improving, and diabetes is well controlled. Return in 3 weeks.

_____

_____

349

Additional Practice Exercises

Identify the principal diagnosis in the following cases. Assign and sequence the codes for diagnosis and procedures.

1. The patient was admitted to the hospital after a fall from a snowmobile, sustained while riding in a public park. The patient has a fracture of the skull, a broken right little finger, and a 3-cm laceration of his right thigh. The laceration was sutured in the ER, and he was admitted to the floor for further treatment and care.

   Principal diagnosis: _____

   Code(s): _____

   Main guideline pertinent to selection of principal diagnosis: _____

2. The patient was admitted to the hospital for bowel resection because of adenocarcinoma of the sigmoid colon, which was proven by biopsy. Before incision, the patient developed atrial fibrillation in the OR, and the procedure was canceled. A cardiologist will be consulted before the surgical resection is attempted.

   Principal diagnosis: _____

   Code(s): _____

   Main guideline pertinent to selection of principal diagnosis: _____

3. The patient has been at the beach all day and after falling into a bonfire was admitted to the hospital for treatment of the second-degree burns on his feet, first- and second-degree burns on the back of his hands, and third-degree burns on 50% of his chest. On the fourth hospital day, his third-degree burns were excisionally debrided by the doctor.

   Principal diagnosis: _____

   Code(s): _____

   Main guideline pertinent to selection of principal diagnosis: _____

4. The patient was admitted to the hospital because of inability to eat and drink. Mucous membranes were dry, and skin turgor was poor. The patient was given a bolus of IV fluids 500 mL initially, and it was reduced to 150 mL/hr. The physician has documented that the dehydration is due to her chemotherapy treatments. The patient underwent a right mastectomy 1 month ago for breast cancer.

   Principal diagnosis: _____

   Code(s): _____

   Main guideline pertinent to selection of principal diagnosis: _____

5. The patient was admitted to the hospital with pneumonia and exacerbation of congestive heart failure. IV antibiotics were started after blood cultures were drawn. The physician ordered Lasix 20 mg IV every 12 hours. The patient went home on oral antibiotics and oral Lasix. The patient will return in 1 week for follow-up.

   Principal diagnosis: _____

   Code(s): _____

   Main guideline pertinent to selection of principal diagnosis: _____

6. The patient was admitted with severe abdominal pain. IV analgesics were administered, and the patient was treated with IV Pepcid. A history of gallbladder attack 3 years ago was reported. Upper GI and abdominal ultrasound will be done on an outpatient basis.

   Final diagnosis: Abdominal pain due to peptic ulcer versus cholelithiasis.

   Principal diagnosis: _____

   Code(s): _____

   Main guideline pertinent to selection of principal diagnosis: _____

7. The patient is known to have cancer of the prostate with metastasis to the bones. The patient is in extreme pain and is being admitted to the hospital for better pain control. Measures taken by the home health nurse were unsuccessful in managing this man's pain. He will be treated with IV morphine.

   Principal diagnosis: _____

   Code(s): _____

   Main guideline pertinent to selection of principal diagnosis: _____

8. The patient was admitted to the hospital for treatment of congestive heart failure. Chest x-rays showed evidence of pleural effusion. No procedures were performed.

   Principal diagnosis: _____

   Code(s): _____

   Main guideline pertinent to selection of principal diagnosis: _____

9. The patient was admitted to the hospital with symptomatic angina. After admission to CCU, serial cardiac enzymes and EKGs showed an elevation of CPK, and an anterior wall infarct was suspected on the basis of EKG results.

   Principal diagnosis: _____

   Code(s): _____

   Main guideline pertinent to selection of principal diagnosis: _____

10. The patient was admitted to the hospital with septic shock. Blood cultures were drawn and were positive, with both of the blood cultures growing *Staphylococcus aureus*.

    Final diagnosis: Septic shock due to *Staphylococcus aureus*.

    Principal diagnosis: _____

    Code(s): _____

    Main guideline pertinent to selection of principal diagnosis: _____

11. The patient was admitted to the hospital with external abdominal wound dehiscence. The patient underwent a cholecystectomy and was discharged 3 days ago. The patient had a coughing spell at home and was admitted; the dehiscence was repaired.

    Principal diagnosis: _____

    Code(s): _____

    Main guideline pertinent to selection of principal diagnosis: _____

12. The patient, a known diabetic with peripheral vascular disease and atherosclerosis of the lower extremities, developed diabetic gangrene on the second toe of the left foot. The patient was admitted for aggressive treatment of the gangrene. If this fails, a below-knee amputation may have to be considered.

    Principal diagnosis: _____

    Code(s): _____

    Main guideline pertinent to selection of principal diagnosis: _____

13. The patient was admitted to the hospital with chest pain. Nitroglycerin sublingually relieved the patient's symptoms initially. The patient was monitored in the ICU, and the consulting cardiologist confirmed that the patient's chest pain was due to unstable angina.

   Final diagnosis: Chest pain.

   Principal diagnosis: _____

   Code(s): _____

   Main guideline pertinent to selection of principal diagnosis: _____

14. Patient is admitted through the ER for a fever and hacking cough. IV antibiotics were initiated in the ER. CXR is taken and shows infiltrates. Labwork is done as physician suspects H1N1 pneumonia. The discharge summary lists community acquired pneumonia.

   Principal diagnosis: _____

   Code(s): _____

   Main guideline pertinent to selection of principal diagnosis: _____

15. Patient is admitted through the ER with severe chest pain. Diagnostic and laboratory work reveals severe GERD and a hiatal hernia. The attending physician lists both conditions as the cause of this patient's chest pain.

   Principal diagnosis: _____

   Code(s): _____

   Main guideline pertinent to selection of principal diagnosis: _____

16. The patient was treated in the outpatient surgery area for a senile left cataract by phacoemulsification and aspiration of the cataract with insertion of an intraocular lens. In the post anesthesia care unit the patient developed elevated blood pressure. It was determined that the patient should be admitted as an inpatient to monitor his blood pressure.

   Principal diagnosis: _____

   Code(s): _____

   Main guideline pertinent to selection of principal diagnosis: _____

17. In the discharge summary the attending physician lists the diagnoses as pneumonia, COPD exacerbation, and exacerbation of CHF. The record reveals that the patient had been admitted and discharged 7 days prior to this admit with a diagnosis of pneumonia. At that discharge, the patient was instructed to continue taking antibiotic PO for another three days.

   Principal diagnosis: _____

   Code(s): _____

   Main guideline pertinent to selection of principal diagnosis: _____

CASE STUDIES

Using the code book, assign and sequence the codes for diagnosis and procedures.

18. CASE STUDY

Title of Operation

Closed reduction and percutaneous skeletal fixation

Indications for Surgery

This patient has a type 2 supracondylar fracture with extension and valgus, and wants to reduce and stabilize this.

Preoperative Diagnosis

Supracondylar fracture, right distal humerus.

Postoperative Diagnosis

Supracondylar fracture, right distal humerus.

Anesthesia

General.

Prosthetic Device/Implant

Two 3/32-inch smooth Steinmann pins.

Surgeons Narrative

Procedure in Detail: The patient was taken to the operating room and given general anesthetic. A time-out was held. Right arm was prepped and draped in sterile fashion. It was reduced. It was pinned using two 3/32-inch Steinmann pins, first in the lateral side and then in the medial side. Medial was done with a small incision, carefully palpating the medial epicondyle, visualizing fluoroscopically and holding the elbow in extension. There was bicortical fixation, it was stable, anatomic reduction, the images were saved, the wound was sterilely dressed, and it was placed in a long-arm splint. No complications. No blood loss.

Principal diagnosis code(s):

_____

Procedure code(s):

_____

19. CASE STUDY

Title of Operation

Right carotid endarterectomy and Hemashield Dacron patch angioplasty using intra-luminal shunt.

Indications for Surgery

This 64-year-old woman recently underwent a screening carotid duplex scan, which suggested a significant right carotid stenosis. She was referred here for a formal vascular surgical consultation and repeat duplex scan at this institution, which confirmed a high-grade, 70-99%, right internal carotid stenosis. In view of this significant right carotid lesion and a family history of stroke, as well as her otherwise apparent good medical risk, the patient elected to proceed at this time with right carotid endarterectomy.

Preoperative Diagnosis

Severe right internal carotid stenosis.

Postoperative Diagnosis

Severe right internal carotid stenosis.

Additional Practice Exercises

General.

Hemashield Dacron patch.

Procedure: With the patient in the supine position and the head extended and turned to the left, the right neck and chest regions were prepped and draped in the usual fashion. A longitudinal incision was made along the anterior border of the sternocleidomastoid muscle and deepened through the subcutaneous tissues and platysma. The sternocleidomastoid muscle was sharply dissected posteriorly. The internal jugular vein was identified, medial branches were ligated with 2-0 silk sutures and divided, and the internal jugular vein was mobilized posteriorly. Using sharp and blunt dissection, the common carotid artery was identified, it was sharply freed from its surrounding tissues, and controlled well proximal to the bifurcation with an umbilical tape. The dissection was carried distally and using sharp and blunt dissection, individual control was obtained of the internal carotid artery several centimeters beyond the bifurcation where it appeared to be disease-free, and the external carotid artery just beyond bifurcation, with vessel loops. An unusual branch of the common carotid artery posteriorly was identified and controlled with a 2-0 silk suture. The hypoglossal nerve was identified at the apex of the incision and the vagus nerve deep to the artery, and both the nerves were carefully protected throughout the course of the procedure. There appeared to be a calcified plaque at the carotid bifurcation with extension into the proximal internal carotid artery.

The patient was given 5000 units of heparin intravenously. After 3 minutes, the internal, common, and external carotid arteries were clamped. A longitudinal ateriotomy was made in the common carotid artery and carried through a dense and eccentric arthrosclerotic plaque at the carotid bifurcation for approximately 2 cm up the internal carotid artery to where the intima normalized in appearance. A #10 shunt was then placed into the internal carotid artery and while back-bleeding was placed into the common carotid artery and a pump tourniquet was cinched down. Total ischemic time prior to shunt placement was less than 1 minute.

A good endarterectomy plane was begun in the common carotid artery and completed circumferentially. The plaque feathered to a good endpoint proximally. The endarterectomy was then carried distally and a short plug of atheromatous plaque was everted out of the origin of the external carotid artery. The endarterectomy was then carried distally and the plaque feathered to an excellent endpoint in the proximal internal carotid artery. Free fronds of intima were removed. The vessel was then vigorously irrigated with heparinized saline solution, and no free intimal edges were identified proximally or distally.

The arteriotomy was then closed with a Hemashield Dacron patch using running 6-0 Surgipro suture material. Prior to completing the patch closure, the shunt was removed, the common carotid artery was flushed, the internal and external carotid arteries were back-bled. The vessel was again vigorously irrigated with heparinized saline solution, and then patch closure was completed. The internal carotid clamp was then released and the vessel was occluded at its origin, and flow was initially established up to the external carotid artery. After several beats, the internal carotid clamp was released. There were now strongly palpable pulses noted in both the internal and external carotid arteries, confirmed with physiologic Doppler signals.

The wound was irrigated with copious amounts of warm bibiotic solution. A meticulous search for hemostasis was carried out. Once the hemostasis has been achieved, a round 3/16 inch Davol drain was placed and secured with a 3-0 nylon suture. The incision was then closed with running 2-0 Prolene to the platysma and running 4-0 Polysorb to the subcuticular layer, with Ster-Strips applied to the skin. A dry sterile pressure dressing was applied. The sponge, needle, and instrument counts were correct x2. The patient tolerated the procedure well; she immediately awakened to the stable neurologic condition in the Operating Room, was extubated, and transferred to SICU in stable condition for post-operative monitoring.

Principal diagnosis code(s):

_____

Procedure code(s):

_____

20. CASE STUDY

Title of Operation

Right craniotomy for resection of tumor using frameless stereotaxy and placement of Gliadel wafer.

Indications for Surgery

The patient with an enlarging and enhancing mass, who is having surgery for diagnosis and potential therapy with Gliadel.

Preoperative Diagnosis

Recurrent malignant brain tumor.

Postoperative Diagnosis

Recurrent malignant brain tumor.

Surgeon's Narrative

Procedure: The patient was brought to the Operating Room and general anesthesia was induced in the usual fashion. After appropriate lines were placed, the patient was placed in Mayfield two-point head fixation, and the right side of the head was exposed. The timeout was held with nursing and anesthesia. Intraoperative navigation was registered to the patient. The area of the old incision was shaved. In this area, the head was prepped and draped in the usual fashion. The incision was made, and Raney clips were placed on the skin. The temporalis muscle was taken back with the skin to expose the old craniotomy. Using intraoperative navigation, this craniotomy did not cover the area of the enhancement. For this reason, a new craniotomy needed to be turned, and this was carried out with a craniotome after dissecting the dura from the inner table. Using intraoperative navigation, the dura was then opened over the enhancing area. The surface of the brain was very abnormal. This mapped out to the findings on the intraoperative navigation, and the cortex of this area was bipolared and opening in a circumferential fashion.

Specimen was sent to pathology, which came back as recurrent tumor. This tumor was very distinct compared to normal brain. Specimen was removed with suction and bipolar as well as a Cavitron. It was taken back to normal-appearing white matter. Intraoperative navigation was used constantly to gauge the degree of the resection. At the end of the resection, there was no grossly abnormal tissue remaining, and all walls were normal white gliotic brain. Hemostasis was then achieved with thrombin-soaked Avitene. This was washed out, and the 8 Gliadel wafers were placed. Surgicel was laid over the Gliadel wafers. The dura was closed in a watertight fashion with multiple interrupted 4-0 Nurolons. Hemashield was used to seal this. Two central tacking stitches were placed, and Gelfoam was laid over the dura. The bone flap was reattached with Leibinger plates. A subgaleal drain was left in place. The 0 Vicryls were used to close the temporalis muscle fascia, 3-0 Vicryls in the galea, and staples on the skin.

356

The patient tolerated the procedure well, was taken to the ICU in stable condition.

Principal diagnosis code(s):

_____

Procedure code(s):

_____

21. CASE STUDY

Title of Operation

Nesbit procedure.

Indications for Surgery

The patient had developed a penile deformity following radical prostatectomy. He was counseled regarding management options and elected to undergo surgical correction. Consent was obtained for surgery.

Preoperative Diagnosis

Peyronie's disease.

Postoperative Diagnosis

Peyronie's disease.

Anesthesia

General.

Specimen (Bacteriologic, Pathologic, or Other)

None.

Surgeon's Narrative

The patient was brought in to the Operating Room, whereupon general anesthesia was performed. He was maintained supine on the Operating Room table. He received antibiotic prophylaxis. There was standard prep and drape over the lower abdomen and genitalia. Initially, an artificial erection was induced using a 21-gauge butterfly needle, passed through the glans into the left corpus cavernosum. A Penrose tourniquet was placed at the base of penis. An injection of saline was then done through the needle, showing that there was a significant dorsal curvature of about 60 degrees. The artificial erection was released. Based on this evaluation, it was felt that the approach for the Nesbit procedure would be a midline ventral incision at the area of the penile shaft raphe with access gained to the ventral aspect for plications. The incision was then made over a distance of about 5 cm in length. The dissection was carried out to the skin, dartos fascia, and then through Buck fascia where appropriate on both the corporal bodies ventrally. It was felt that two separate plication locations would be best performed. One was done toward the proximal third of the penile shaft and the second one toward the distal third of the penile shaft. Buck fascia was dissected, exposing the tunica albuginea at each of these locations. Small elliptical incisions were made involving only the longitudinal fibers of the tunica albuginea. Thereafter, the plication was carried out with running 3-0 Maxon suture in a hemostatic fashion. Repeat artificial erections were induced in stages and there was confirmation of penile straightening at end of the case. Buck fascia was reapproximated with running 4-0 Vicryl suture. Additional closure involved running 3-0

Vicryl suture at the dartos fascial level and interrupted 4-0 chromic suture at the skin level. Bacitracin ointment was applied over the wound site, followed by fluff dressing and an athletic supporter. Straight catheterization was performed at the end of the case to evacuate urine from the bladder. The patient was awakened from anesthesia, transferred to a stretcher, and then taken away to the recovery room in satisfactory condition. Blood loss associated with the case was negligible.

Principal diagnosis code(s):

_____

Procedure code(s):

_____

22. CASE STUDY

Title of Operation

Laparoscopic converted to open cholecystectomy.

Indications for Surgery

This is a 71-year-old gentleman who was referred to me for elected cholecystectomy. Unfortunately, one day prior to his scheduled cholecystectomy, he was admitted to the hospital with acute cholangitis. He underwent successful ERCP and biliary sphincterotomy and was discharged home after a mild case of post ERCP pancreatitis. He returned today for elective cholecystectomy.

Preoperative Diagnosis

Acute cholecystitis.

Postoperative Diagnosis

Necrotic gangrenous cholecystitis.

Anesthesia

GETA

Specimen (Bacteriologic, Pathologic, or Other)

Gallbladder

Surgeon's Narrative

The patient was brought into the Operating Room and placed supine on the Operating Room table. General endotracheal anesthesia was established and intravenous antibiotics were administered. Bilateral sequential compression devices were placed on both lower extremities and a Foley catheter was placed sterilely. The patient's abdomen was now prepped and draped in the usual sterile fashion. A supraumbilical incision was made and Hasson technique was used to place a trocar into the abdominal cavity. The abdomen was insufflated to 15 mm Hg pressure and a camera was inserted into the abdomen and revealed no evidence of injury from the trocar placement. Under direct visualization, two 5-mm trocars were placed in the right upper quadrant and an additional 5-mm trocar was placed in through the epigastrium. The patient was placed in reverse Trendelenburn position and immediately we noted that there were dense adhesions of the hepatic flexure of the colon to the liver edge, making

358

visualization of the gallbladder impossible. Using a harmonic scalpel, we carefully started taking the adhesions down from the liver edge, taking care to avoid injury to the colon itself. Eventually, we were able to identify the dome of the gallbladder, which was completely intrahepatic and was obviously necrotic. Attempt to grasp the dome of the gallbladder revealed that there was gross purulence within the lumen of the gallbladder. We dissected for an additional 30 minutes using the combination of sharp dissection and harmonic scalpel, eventually clearing most of the adhesions away from the gallbladder; however, we were unable to identify any anatomy whatsoever in the infundibulum and the gallbladder. Due to the dense adhesions and the inability to visualize the critical structures, we elected at this point to convert to an open cholecystectomy. In order to do that we removed all three 5-mm trocars and made an incision connecting all three of them by making a right subcostal incision. The electrocautery was now used to divide the muscle and to enter the intraabdominal cavity. A Bookwalter retractor was now placed to gain adequate intraabdominal visualization. We carefully grasped the gallbladder fundus and started working from the fundus down toward the infundibulum. Of note, the gallbladder was frankly necrotic with pus within the lumen of the gallbladder; in addition it was very contracted and intrahepatic, making dissection of the back wall of the gallbladder out of the liver bed very difficult and in some portions of the gallbladder not possible. We eventually cleared approximately 3/4 of the gallbladder from the liver bed using a combination of electrocautery and argon beam coagulation and started working carefully down at the infundibulum. We were able to clear and also dissect tissue away in order to clearly identify the common bile duct; however, we cannot definitively identify the cystic duct and we were able to identify that the infundibulum of the gallbladder was fused/fistulized to the common bile duct in a Mirizzi syndrome type stricture. I knew that we would be unable to safely separate the infundibulum from the common bile duct and therefore we elected to perform a subtotal cholecystectomy. In order to do that we transected the majority of the gallbladder using electrocautery and passed that off the field as a specimen. We do not definitively identify a cystic artery. At this point, we have oversewn the infundibulum at the gallbladder with a running 2-0 Prolene suture. Of note, we had noted that there was no back spillage of bile from the nectrotic gallbladder remnant. We were confident, however, that we had not entered the common bile duct, as we could visualize it in its entirety, and as mentioned, the cystic duct was not clearly identified. At this point, we turned our attention to the liver bed. There were areas that required an argon-beam coagulation for hemostasis and the entire liver bed was carefully argon-beam coagulated, making sure that any remnants of gallbladder mucosa were completely obliterated. At this point, we now placed a 3/16 round JP drain in the liver bed and brought it out through a separate stab incision in the right quadrant. We irrigated the entire right upper quadrant with normal saline with clear effluent noted. We re-inspected the hepatic flexure of the colon and noted no inadvertent enterotomies. The duodenum was visualized in its entirety as well as the stomach. These, too, were free of injury. At this point, we now closed the subcostal incision with 2 running #1 Maxon sutures. The skin was closed with skin staples after irrigating with normal saline and bibiotic solution. The Hasson trocar from the umbilicus was removed and the fascial defect at the umbilicus was closed with a figure-of-eight Vicryl suture and the skin was closed with Biosyn. Sterile dressings were now placed. The patient tolerated this procedure hemodynamically well. He was extubated at the end of the case, transferred to a stretcher, and brought to the recovery room in good condition.

Principal diagnosis code(s):

_____

Procedure code(s):

_____

Title of Operation

Lumbar laminectomy; inferior half of the L2, all of the L3, all of L4, all of L5, superior half of S1 with bilateral laminoforaminotomies L2-L3, L3-L4, L4-L5, and L5-S1.

Indications for Surgery

The patient is a 78-year-old gentleman with buttock, posterior thigh, and lateral thigh pain with standing and walking, limiting standing and walking. The patient was unresponsive to nonoperative measures. This was interfering with his activities of daily living. CT monogram demonstrated lumbar spinal stenosis primarily from facet hypertrophy at the L3-L4 and L4-L5 as well as the L5-S1 levels. His alignment was normal. His disc spaces were collapsed, but there was no spondylolisthesis or instability or lateral flexion extension views. After discussion of the risks, benefits, nature, alternatives, and complications of the procedure, the patient signed the informed consent and was taken to the Operating Room.

Preoperative Diagnosis

Lumbar spinal stenosis.

Lumbar spondylosis without myelopathy.

Postoperative Diagnosis

Same

Anesthesia

GET

Specimen (Bacteriologic, Pathologic, or Other)

None

Prosthetic Device/Implant

None

Pathology

None

Cultures

None

Drain

1/8-inch Hemovac drain beneath lumbar fascia exiting through a separate stab wound.

Surgeon's Narrative

Description of Procedure: The patient was identified and the surgical site was marked in the preoperative area. He was then brought to the Operating Room and placed under general endotracheal anesthesia by the anesthesiologist. Prior to being brought to the Operating Room, his pacemaker was turned off and he had a patch placed for extra pacing as necessary. A time-out was performed and prophylactic intravenous antibiotics were given. The patient was then placed prone on a Wilson frame. All pressure points were protected and the eyes were left free. Back was then prepped and draped in the usual fashion. A vertical skin incision was made in the posterior midline and carried down to the fascia. Subperiosteal dissection was performed in the inferior half of the L2 to the sacrum. The pars were identified throughout the surgical site as well as the facet joints. The facet joint capsules were not violated. Lateral radiographs showed Kocher clamps placed on the L4 spinous process. Next, a Horsley Bone Cutter was used to remove the spinous process of L3, L4, and L5 inferior through L2. Leksell rongeur and Kerrison punches were then used to perform laminectomy on all of L5, all of L4, all of L3, inferior half of the L2, and superior portion of S1, with bilateral laminoforaminotomies at the L2-L3, L3-L4, L4-L5, and L5-S1 levels.

There was good decompression of the nerve roots and foramen in all of these levels. There was a significant amount of facet hypertrophy noted at all of the levels; however, it was particularly severe on the left at the L3-L4 level. Next, the wound was irrigated with Bibiotic solution. Bone wax was placed into the interstices of the bleeding cancellous bone along with the laminectomy site. An 1/8-inch Hemovac drain was placed beneath the fascia exiting through stab wounds. The fascia was then closed with #1 Vicryl in figure-of-eight sutures. Subcutaneous tissue was closed with 0-Vicryl interrupted simple sutures. Skin was closed with staples. The wound was sterilely dressed and the drain was placed through a standard collection drainage system. The patient was then awoken from general endotracheal anesthesia, found to be neurologically unchanged from preoperative examination, and taken to the surgical intensive care unit in good condition. He was taken to the surgical intensive care unit because of his prior cardiac history.

Principal diagnosis code(s):

_____

Procedure code(s):

_____

24. CASE STUDY

Title of Operation

Left hip uncemented hemiarthroplasty.

Indications for Surgery

The patient is a very pleasant 92-year-old woman who fell and sustained a left femoral neck fracture. When she was cleared by medicine, she was taken for surgery. Informed consent was obtained. Risks include pain, bleeding, infection, damage to blood vessels and nerves, dislocations, leg length discrepancy, among others.

Preoperative Diagnosis

Left femoral neck fracture.

Postoperative Diagnosis

Left femoral neck fracture.

Anesthesia

General endotracheal anesthetic.

Her femoral neck was sent.

Prosthetic Device/Implant

Uncemented Stryker Howmedica Accolade Bipolar system, using a size-3 femoral neck and 41 head.

Surgeon's Narrative

The patient was brought back to the operating theater, where she was given general endotracheal anesthetic. She was placed in the right lateral decubitus position with her left hip up. The patient was prepped and draped in the usual sterile fashion. Incision was carried down to the posterior hip; this was carried down through the gluteus maximus to the posterior capsule of the hip. We used a cobra to retract the gluteus medius out of the way. We then incised the hip capsule, piriformis, and short external rotators all in one. This was tied with a tagging stitch. The femoral neck was then taken out using the Christmas tree. We used the cookie cutter to lateralize the femur. We then broached up to a size 3. This fit well. We then measured the head, measured at 38. The smallest size Accolade head was a 41; therefore we trialed a 41 and this did well. It was somewhat tight, but it did stay.

We decided therefore to go with the 3 and a size 41 head. We thoroughly irrigated the hip capsule and debrided soft tissues away. The real implant was placed and reduced, it fit well, it was stable to full flexion and extension, and the leg lengths were compatible. The wound was then thoroughly irrigated. The rotators were attached using 0 Vicryl, closing the remaining soft tissue. The fascia was closed using #1. We then closed the skin with 2-0 and skin staples. Overall, it went well and the patient was extubated and brought to PACU.

Principal diagnosis code(s):

_____

Procedure code(s):

_____

25. CASE STUDY

Title of Operation

Removal of MediPort and loop ileostomy reversal.

Indications for Surgery

The patient is a very pleasant gentleman who is 34 years old and who I saw for rectal cancer and operated on, and things looked great, so we went ahead and scheduled him for a takedown. He did request his MediPort be removed, so we did it at the same time.

Preoperative Diagnosis

Rectal cancer status post neoadjuvant therapy and low anterior resection with diverting loop ileostomy for takedown with stoma.

Postoperative Diagnosis

Rectal cancer status post neoadjuvant therapy and low anterior resection with diverting loop ileostomy for takedown with stoma.

Procedure: The patient was taken to the OR and placed in the supine position with general endotracheal anesthesia administered. The chest and abdomen were prepped in the usual sterile fashion. We began with previous incision for the MediPort. This was carefully opened up and then cauterized down to the MediPort. The MediPort was dissected out. Stitches were removed. The MediPort was brought out, and the edges of the MediPort around the fascial area were freed up and removed. Hemostasis was obtained. The head was lifted up a little bit to lower the central venous pressure. The MediPort opening was stitched closed, and the subcutaneous tissue was reapproximated. Indermil was placed on the skin, and dry, sterile dressing was placed. We then turned our attention toward ileostomy and created a circumferential incision around the ileostomy site and then carefully dissected down around the edges. This was really stuck this time, so we had to spend some time trying to free up the edges. I did make about three serosal entries but no full-thickness, but we finally did get the ostomy to come up. We repaired the serosal defects, but it was pretty adherent, so we thought it best to divide this and do a staples anastomosis. The two ends were divided using a GIA stapler. The ends were brought together. Staple line was partially removed, and a midline anastomosis was made between the two loops of proximal distal bowel. Hemostasis was checked. The final bit of opening was closed with a TA90. The corners were oversewn, and a stitch was placed at the apex of the anastomosis to hold those staples together. The wound was irrigated. The bowel was returned to the abdomen. The abdomen was irrigated. The fascia was freed up and closed with interrupted Maxon in figure-of-eight fashion.

The subcutaneous tissue had a drain placed with 3/16 in size. It was stitched in with 3-0 nylon. The skin was brought together with interrupted 3-0 Vicryl, and then 4-0 Biosyn was used to close the skin. Indermil and a dry, sterile dressing was applied.

Principal diagnosis code(s):

_____

Procedure code(s):

_____

26. CASE STUDY

Title of Operation

Exploratory laparotomy repair of multiple small bowel injuries, ligation of mesenteric bleeders, right retroperitoneal exploration.

Indications for Surgery

The patient is a 24-year-old male who sustained a single gunshot wound to the xiphoid region and was taken emergently to the Operating Room on the basis of peritonitis. Preoperative critical care intervention included type and cross matching, IV fluid resuscitation, IV antibiotics, NG tube, and Foley catheter. The patient was taken to preop.

Preoperative Diagnosis

Gunshot wound to abdomen with peritonitis.

Postoperative Diagnosis

Gunshot wound to abdomen with peritonitis and multiple small bowel injuries as well as injuries to small bowel mesenteric and right psoas muscles and hemoperitoneum.

363

The patient was taken to the Operating Room and placed supine on the table. The chest and abdomen were prepped and draped in a sterile fashion. The abdomen was entered through a midline incision. It was found to have approximately 500 cubic centimeters of hemoperitoneum. The track of the bullet could be seen through the anterior abdominal wall into the abdomen in the upper third and enters through the omentum and multiple loops of small bowel. He had approximately 8 holes in the small bowel and over 1 foot segment of the jejunum with 2 associated injuries to the mesentery. Mesenteric injuries were clamped and electrocoagulated. There was a second segment of midjejunum that had 2 holes with tissue necrosis. These injuries were incorporated with 2 segmental resections. These resections were performed with the GIA stapler to isolate and divide bowel as well as to perform a small bowel to small bowel anastomosis and a TA60 staple with the third arm of the anastomosis on 2 cases; thus 2 small bowel anastomoses were created and the mesenteric defects associated with those were closed with figure-of-eight silk sutures. Hemostasis about the anastomosis was assessed to be adequate, as well as patency about the anastomosis. A seromuscular soak was placed on the bowel walls to ensure the anastomosis is tension free. Attention was then paid to the rest of the abdomen. The patient was found to be free of injury in the retroperitoneum, and the mid aspect of the abdomen was similarly uninjured. The liver and spleen, stomach, lesser sac, and pancreas were all looked at individually, and the right retroperitoneum over the area of the inferior vena cava and the common iliac vein and artery were identified to be normal. Upon completion of the exploration, the track could be seen to have gone through the small bowel and ended up in the right iliopsoas muscle lateral to the retroperitoneal structures. Thus the patient did have some muscle bleeding to explain his right retroperitoneal hematoma. Hemostasis again about the abdomen was assessed to be adequate. The peritoneal cavity was irrigated with saline solution and the fascia was closed with a running #1 looped Maxon suture. The subcutaneous tissues were irrigated and the skin was closed with staples. The patient tolerated the procedure well, was extubated, and was taken to the postop recovery room in guarded condition.

Principal diagnosis code(s):

_____

Procedure code(s):

_____

27. CASE STUDY

Resection of right pelvis osteochondroma.

The patient is a 21-year-old male with a history of a symptomatic right pelvis osteochondroma. Risks, benefits, and alternatives to resection versus observation were discussed with him and he desired to undergo elected resection for pain relief. He is a football player. He has finished his season. Informed consent was obtained.

Right iliac crest osteochondroma.

Right iliac crest osteochondroma.

General with an epidural.

Osteochondroma

None

Operative Findings: Large osteochondroma coming off the lateral aspect of the iliac crest.

Operative Technique: The patient was taken to the Operating Room and placed in the supine position. Once anesthesia had been obtained, he was changed to lateral decubitus position with the right side up. Attention was turned to the right iliac crest. A 15-cm incision was then marked out transversely in line with the iliac crest, directly over the osteochondroma. After the time-out was performed, an incision was made through skin using a scalpel. Subcutaneous tissues were then incised using Bovie electrocautery. Hemostasis was achieved using Bovie electrocautery. The capsule of the osteochondroma was identified and was incised using Bovie electrocautery in line with the incision. Using blunt dissection, the remaining adhesions and capsule were peeled off the osteochondroma, revealing a multilobulated mass. The abductors were peeled off the capsular adhesions using blunt dissection distally and the abdominal muscle-tendinous insertions were also peeled off using blunt dissection proximally. There were no direct muscle attachments into the osteochondroma. Once the muscle and any capsular adhesions had been cleaned off, the osteochondroma was then removed using a large osteotome. Using C-arm fluoroscopy, a large bulk of the osteochondroma was removed in 1 piece; however, there was residual osteochondroma seen on the x-rays and also certain areas of stalks were able to be palpated. The remainder of these were removed using osteotomes. Again, using C-arm fluoroscopy, it was verified that the osteochondroma was removed. The sessile stalk area was smoothed out using a rasp. There was no osteochondroma remaining once this was performed. The wound was then copiously irrigated using about a liter of pulsatile lavage, normal saline. Hemostasis was achieved using Bovie electrocautery. There was no active bleeding. There were no hernias detected. The fascial insertions of the abdominal muscles and the abductors on the remaining iliac crest were intact. Deep tissues were then closed with interrupted 0 absorbable suture. Subcutaneous closures were closed using buried interrupted 2-0 absorbable sutures. Skin was reapproximated using interrupted 2-0 nylon sutures. Sterile dressing was applied. The patient tolerated the procedure and was extubated. He was transferred to the recovery room in stable condition. There were no immediate complications.

Drain: A one-eighth-inch Hemovac drain coming out proximally in line with the incision, which was left in the deep tissues.

Principal diagnosis code(s):

_____

Procedure code(s):

_____

Title of Operation

Radical retropubic prostatectomy.

Pelvic lymph node dissection.

Preoperative Diagnosis

Carcinoma of the prostate.

Postoperative Diagnosis

Stage T1c adenocarcinoma of the prostate.

Anesthesia

Spinal.

Surgeon's Narrative

While the patient was in the supine position under anesthesia, the skin was prepared and draped in the usual way. A midline lower abdominal incision was made, and a bilateral pelvic lymph node dissection was performed. Gross inspections of the specimens were negative for tumor. The endopelvic fascia was opened, the puboprostatic ligaments were divided, and the dorsal vein was divided and oversewn with 3-0 Monocryl. The urethra was partially transected and five 3-0 Monocryl sutures were placed through the edges of the smooth muscle and mucosa at 7, 11, 12, 1, and 5 o'clock. During transaction of the posterior urethra and posterior portion of the striated sphincter, the 6 o'clock suture was placed. At this point in the operation there was excellent hemostasis.

The lateral pelvic fascia was released and both neurovascular bundles were preserved. The lateral pedicles were divided without ligation using hemoclips to secure arterial and venous bleeders.

The bladder neck was divided, and the prostate, seminal vesicles and vasa deferentia were removed. The bladder neck was reconstructed with interrupted 2-0 Caprosyn and 4-0 Caprosyn to exteriorize the mucosa. Maxon 2-0 was used next to intussuscept the bladder neck, and the anastomosis was completed with six interrupted 3-0 Monocryl sutures. A #16 Foley catheter with 15 cc in the balloon was used to stent the anastomosis.

Davol catheters were placed, and the incision was closed with a running #2 nylon and skin clips. The patient tolerated the procedure very well and was returned to the recovery room in good condition.

Principal diagnosis code(s):

_____

Procedure code(s):

_____

Title of Operation

Minimally invasive mitral valve repair.

Indications for Surgery

The patient is a 69-year-old woman presenting with severe mitral regurgitation due to severe bileaflet mitral prolapse. She has become increasingly symptomatic over the last several months and has been referred for a minimally invasive mitral valve repair. She has relatively well-preserved left ventricular function and no flow-limiting coronary artery disease. All risks with respect to the operation include bleeding, infection, stroke, heart failure, and mortality were carefully explained to the patient and she wished to proceed.

Preoperative Diagnosis

Mitral insufficiency.

Postoperative Diagnosis

Mitral insufficiency.

Anesthesia

General endotracheal anesthesia.

Prosthetic Device/Implant

Mitral Annuloplasty Band Data: Edwards-Cosgrove 32-mm annuloplasty band, model 4600.

Surgeon's Narrative

Operative Findings: The patient's aorta was soft, nonaneurysmal, without significant calcifications. The patient's biventricular function was within normal limits. The patient had a markedly dilated left atrium with severe bileaflet mitral prolapse due to myxomatous changes. She has a moderately dilated mitral annulus as well. Completion transesophageal echocardiography revealed no residual mitral regurgitation after the repair.

Operative Summary: After the patient was successfully induced with general endotracheal anesthesia, she underwent placement of a right internal jugular 15-French Bio-Medicus venous cannula, a right radial arterial line, double-lumen endotracheal tube, and right internal jugular introducer. The patient was then placed in a modified left lateral decubitus position and her chest, abdomen, and groins were prepped and draped in the usual sterile fashion. A 3-inch right submammary incision was made with dissection up the chest wall behind the right breast. Entry into the fourth intercostal space under single lung isolation was performed easily. After placing a medium CardioVations soft tissue retractor, an Estech rib spreader was placed. The pericardium was then divided transversely 2 cm anterior to the course of the right phrenic nerve, which was carefully visualized and preserved throughout its course.

Appropriate diaphragmatic and pericardial retraction sutures were placed. Transpleural CO_2 and spring vent lines were placed.

Our attention was then turned to the right common femoral vessels, which were isolated through a right lung inguinal crease incision. After systemic heparinization was delivered, 4-0 Prolene pursestring sutures were placed on the anterior surfaces of these vessels. A 21-French Bio-Medicus venous cannula was directed up the right common femoral vein and a 19-French Bio-Medicus arterial cannula was placed up the right common femoral artery. Cardiopulmonary bypass was then initiated with placement of an aortic root vent. A Chitwood transthoracic cross-clamp was placed across the aorta via the transverse sinus. It was applied and 800 cubic centimeters of cold blood cardioplegia was delivered down the aortic root, achieving a clean diastolic arrest of the heart. Systemic cooling to 26 degrees Celsius was commenced.

After developing Sondergaard's groove with electrocautery, a transverse left atriotomy was performed. An Estech atrial lift system was used to achieve reasonable exposure of the mitral valve. It was clearly myxomatous with severe bileaflet prolapsed from redundant tissue. The mitral annulus was also moderately dilated and the left atrium was markedly dilated. A series of 11 nonpledgeted 2-0 Ti-Cron horizontal mattress sutures were placed from right to left fibrous trigone across the posterior mitral annulus. The P2 and A2 scallops were then reapproximated with a running double layer 4-0 Prolene suture in an Alfieri pattern. A 32-mm Edwards-Cosgrove annuloplasty band was then selected and sutures were passed through this band. The band was lowered into position and the sutures were tied and cut. Insufflation of the left ventricle revealed the mitral valve to be fully competent. The left atriotomy was then closed with a running 3-0 Prolene suture.

The patient was then placed in a steep Trendelburg position and the aortic cross-clamp was removed. The heart was then resuscitated, de-aired, and rewarmed. After spontaneous biventricular function was regained, tranesophageal echocardiography revealed excellent biventricular function, no intracardiac air, and no residual mitral insufficiency. At this point, the aortic root vent was removed and its site was oversewn with two pledgeted 4-0 Prolene horizontal mattress sutures. Temporary ventricular pacing wires were placed on the right ventricle. Cardiopulmonary bypass was then carefully weaned off with sequential removal of the venous and arterial cannula. The cannulation sites were reinforced with 5-0 Prolene horizontal mattress sutures. The right inguinal crease incision was closed in the usual fashion.

A 28-French right thoracostomy tube was placed followed by a 24-French posteriorly placed Black drain. The right mini thoracotomy incision was then closed in the usual fashion. All sponge and needle counts were found to be correct. The patient tolerated the procedure well. The patient was transported to the cardiac surgical intensive care unit in stable condition.

Cardiopulmonary Bypass Data: Cardiopulmonary bypass time 132 minutes, aortic cross-clamp time 85 minutes, and lowest temperature achieved 24.7° Celsius.

Principal diagnosis code(s):

_____

Procedure code(s):

_____

Title of Operation

Percutaneous liver biopsy with ultrasound guidance.

Indications for Surgery

The patient is a 2-month-old girl with direct hyperbilirubinemia and acholic stools concerning for biliary atresia.

Preoperative Diagnosis

Direct hyperbilirubinemia.

Postoperative Diagnosis

Direct hyperbilirubinemia.

Anesthesia

General with LMA.

Specimen (Bacteriologic, Pathologic, and Other)

Liver biopsy.

Prosthetic Device/Implant

Bard 0.7 cm notch.

Surgeon's Narrative

Description of the Procedure: The patient's mother was informed of the risks, benefits, and alternatives of the procedure and all questions were answered. Informed consent was obtained and documented in the patient's room. The platelets and coagulation times were reviewed: Platelets 529, PT 10.1, INR 1.0, PTT 25.1. The patient was moved to the Operating Room where a time-out was performed with the attending gastroenterologist in the room. General anesthesia was induced. Ultrasound was present in the Operating Room and identified the site for biopsy at the ninth intercostal space. The area was marked. The patient was prepped and draped in sterile fashion and sterile technique was used throughout the procedure. 0.1 cc of 1% lidocaine was used for local anesthetic. A 2-mm incision was made at the marked site with an 11-blade. The biopsy needle was inserted 3 mm through the incision and fired one time. A biopsy was obtained that was approximately 2 mm in length. Therefore, the biopsy needle was inserted a second time through the incision and fired again. The second biopsy was approximately 5 mm in length. There was minimal bleeding at the site. Ultrasound was performed immediately post biopsy and there was no visible hematoma or apparent perforation of the surrounding organs. The area was dressed. The patient was extubated without incident and transferred to the recovery room in stable condition. The liver biopsy was sent for a rush processing. The attending was present during the entire procedure.

Complications: None.

Condition: Stable.

Principal diagnosis code(s):

_____

Procedure code(s):

_____

Title of Operation

Left deep inferior epigastric perforator flap with partial rib resection, tissue expander removal, and pectoralis major muscle advancement flap.

Indications for Surgery

The patient had previously been followed and found to be a candidate for exchange of the tissue expander for autologous tissue from the abdomen. The operative plan was confirmed. Informed consent was obtained. The patient expressed understanding of the risks and benefits of the procedure and has desired to continue. Please see the informed consent document for details. History and physical examination were reviewed and updated on the preoperative data sheet. The patient's markings were placed with her in a standing position along with the planned superior and inferior transverse abdominal incisions as well as the midline in the inframammary fold bilaterally.

Preoperative Diagnosis

Left mastectomy defect with tissue expander.

Postoperative Diagnosis

Left mastectomy defect with tissue expander.

Anesthesia

General.

Specimen (Bacteriologic, Pathologic, or Other)

Left mastectomy scar, left breast tissue expander.

Surgeon's Narrative

Estimated Blood Loss: 300 cubic centimeters.

Urine Output: 450 cubic centimeters.

Intravenous Fluids: 4.6 liters of crystalloid.

Drains: One in the left breast, 2 in the abdomen.

Complications: None.

Operative Findings: The patient was taken to the Operating Room and placed supine on the Operating Room table. TEDs and SCDs were placed. The arms were padded, the left was tucked, and the right was placed on an arm board and abducted to slightly less than 90 degrees. General anesthesia was induced. The patient was intubated. The chest and abdomen were exposed, prepped sterilely with ChloraPrep, and draped in a sterile fashion. A knife was used to excise the mastectomy scar and electrocautery was used to dissect the skin and subcutaneous tissue off the pectoralis major muscle, and access capsulotomy was made at the inferior border of the pectoralis major muscle. The pectoralis major muscle was then advanced over a width of 12 cm and a length of 4 cm to the inframammary fold and sutured in place with 3-0 Vicryl sutures. The superior pectoralis was split in the direction its fibers ran and a medial costal cartilage was excised. The internal mammary artery and vein were identified. A knife was used to incise around the umbilical stalk and curved Mayo scissors were used to dissect the umbilical stalk. A knife was used to incise the superior and inferior transverse abdominal incisions and electrocautery was used to dissect through the subcutaneous fat to the fascia of the abdominal wall. The flap was then elevated from lateral to medial bilaterally identifying a large periumbilical perforator medially on each side. A lower lateral row perforator was also found to and preserved on each side bilaterally. It was determined that the hemi-flap was larger than the breast reconstruction needed, therefore the flap was divided in the midline and the left side was preserved as a back up. The lateral row perforator was ligated and divided. There appeared to be good arterial inflow and venous outflow through the remaining perforator based on Doppler signal and physical examination of the skin color, temperature, turgor, and dermal bleeding. A fascial button was incised and the flap was dissected as it wrapped medially around the rectus muscle and then traveled on the posterior aspect of the rectus muscle toward its origin in the groin. Then 3000 units of intravenous heparin were administered. The pedicle was ligated and divided in the groin. A flap was weighed in approximation to the chest. Microscope was used to clean the internal mammary artery and vein as well as the pedicle artery and vein, and a 3.0-mm coupler was used to anastomose the internal mammary vein to the pedicle vein after clipping the internal mammary vein distally, placing a single-vessel clamp proximally and dividing the vessel. Following this, there appeared to be good venous backflow through the anastomosis. A clip was placed on the distal internal mammary artery. A double-opposing Acland clamp was placed proximally. The vessel was divided. The pedicle artery was placed in the second clamp and 9-0 nylon simple interrupted sutures were used to anastomose the artery. At the completion of this, there appeared to be good arterial inflow and venous outflow based on inspection of the pedicle, Doppler signal of the pedicle, and the skin paddle as well as skin color, temperature, turgor, and dermal bleeding. Additional tissue was resected from the flap for a total flap weight of 599 grams and this was inset into the left breast. De-epithelialization was performed around the skin paddle. The breast incision was closed with 3.0 vicryl dermal sutures and skin glue. The drain was placed in the subcutaneous space and held in place with a nylon drain suture through a separate stab incision in the anteroinferior axilla. Ischemia time was one hour and 56 minutes. The skin and subcutaneous tissue were dissected off the abdomen toward the costal margin. The patient was placed in a flexed position. Drains were exited through the lateral aspect of the incision in the abdomen bilaterally and held in place with nylon drain sutures. Then 2-0 Vicryl sutures were placed in Scarpas fascia, 3-0 Vicryl dermal sutures were placed, and 4-0 Biosyn subcuticular stitch was placed. The umbilicus was delivered through a V-shaped incision in the midline and held in place with 3-0 Vicryl dermal sutures. Skin glue was applied to all incisions. The patient was awakened, extubated, and transferred to the bed in the recovery room with the patient in flexed position; the flap was viable at the completion of this.

Principal diagnosis code(s):

_____

Procedure code(s):

_____

32. CASE STUDY

Title of Operation

Exploratory laparotomy and lysis of adhesions.

Resection of hernia sac and ventral hernia repair with biologic AlloDerm mesh.

Preoperative Diagnosis

Small bowel obstruction.

Postoperative Diagnosis

Small bowel obstruction.

Procedure: The patient was taken to the Operating Room, where he was prepped and draped in a standard surgical fashion in the supine position.

We entered the abdomen and there were numerous loose filmy adhesions of the small bowel, although the abdomen was not difficult to access or difficult to dissect, because the adhesions were so loose and filmy. There were marked adhesions, which were causing torsion of the proximal small bowel. There was a segment of approximately 20 to 30 centimeters of jejunum, which was torsed on itself around numerous filmy adhesions. We divided the adhesions around the torsed area of small bowel. It took approximately one hour. We then noted a large defect, approximately 12-cm long on the side and 16-cm long at the upper abdomen, skewed toward the left side. The defect had a large hernia sac, which was excised, and the defect closed in a tension-free manner with an AlloDerm underlay placed in uninterrupted U stitches using 0 Prolene. We had excellent coverage of the defect. The sponge and needle counts were correct. We placed a Jackson-Pratt drain in the subcutaneous space and closed the Scarpa layer with three interrupted 3-0 Vicryl stitches. The skin was closed with staples. The patient tolerated the procedure well and was extubated in stable condition.

Principal diagnosis code(s):

_____

Procedure code(s):

_____

33. CASE STUDY

Title of Operation

Urgent primary low-segment transverse cesarean section after vaginal delivery, twin gestation.

Indications for Surgery

The patient is a 38-year-old para 0 at 39 and 0/7 weeks, who was admitted for induction of labor secondary to preeclampsia. She was started on Pitocin and magnesium sulfate for seizure prophylaxis. She reached full dilation, had a full-term vaginal delivery of twin A and cord prolapsed prior to the delivery of twin B, therefore we proceeded with an urgent low-segment transverse C-section.

Preoperative Diagnosis

Intrauterine pregnancy at 39 and 0/7 weeks, cord prolapse.

Postoperative Diagnosis

Intrauterine pregnancy at 39 and 0/7 weeks, cord prolapse, delivered.

Anesthesia

Epidural.

Specimen (Bacteriologic, Pathologic, or Other)

Placenta and arterial cord gas ×2.

Surgeon's Narrative

Estimated blood loss for the cesarean section was 1500 cubic centimeters for total of 1800 cubic centimeters.

Intravenous Fluids: 6000 cubic centimeters.

Urine Output: 200 cubic centimeters, clear.

Findings: Twin A was a female infant, birth weight 2309 grams, Apgars were 8 at 1 minutes and 9 at 5 minutes. Arterial cord gas pH was 7.24, base excess of -5. Twin B was a female infant, birth weight 3220 grams, Apgars were 2 at 1 minute, 3 at 5 minutes, and 3 at 10 minutes. Arterial cord gas pH was 7.25, base excess of -6. Normal tubes and ovaries bilaterally. Normal postpartum uterus with moderate amount of uterine atony, improved after uterotonic agents.

Complications: Extension of the lower uterine segment.

Procedure: The patient had undergone an induction of labor for preeclampsia with Pitocin and was started on magnesium sulfate for seizure prophylaxis. The presentation on sonogram, dichorionic diamniotic twins with vertex to vertex. She progressed well, was fully dilated and was taken to the Operating Room for double setup. She pushed and had a full-term spontaneous vaginal delivery of twin A. An ultrasound confirmed that baby B was still vertex and membranes were intact, the head was engaged, and the membranes were ruptured. After rupture, there was a cord prolapse diagnosed and the head was elevated with a vaginal hand. Therefore, we proceeded with an urgent low-segment transverse C-section for baby B. The patient had been placed in the dorsal lithotomy position with stirrups, and she was prepped with ChloraPrep and draped.

A Pfannenstiel skin incision was made with a scalpel. The incision was carried down to the fascia using a second scalpel. The fascia was grasped with a Kocher clamp and dissected off, and the rectus muscles were dissected off bluntly and sharply with a scalpel. The same was done in the inferior aspect of the fascia. The rectus muscles were spread in midline bluntly. No adhesions were noted. The bladder blade was inserted. The vesicouterine peritoneum was entered sharply and extended laterally using Metzenbaum scissors. The bladder flap was created digitally and the bladder blade was reinserted.

A transverse incision was made in the lower uterine segment with a scalpel and extended laterally using blunt traction and bandage scissors. The fetal head had been elevated by the vaginal hand and was brought to the incision and delivered with the assistance of vacuum. The body and extremities followed. The cord was clamped and cut ×2 and the infant was handed to the awaiting pediatricians. Arterial cord gas was obtained and sent.

The placenta was delivered with intact membranes manually. The uterus was exteriorized and manually cleared of clots. There was a 3-cm extension noted on the inferior aspect of the hysterotomy in the midline extended toward the vagina. It was repaired separately using 3-0 Polysorb in a running locked fashion. The uterus was closed in a single layer using #0 Vicryl in a running locked fashion. Several figure-of-eight sutures were placed for additional hemostasis. The uterus was returned to the abdomen and the gutters and hysterotomy were copiously irrigated. Good hemostasis was noted. Surgicel was placed below the hysterotomy at the side of the bladder flap for additional hemostasis. Rectus muscles and fascia were inspected and left rectus muscle was cauterized. A JP drain was placed below the fascia and the fascia was closed in running fashion using #1 Vicryl. The subcutaneous tissue was irrigated and reapproximated using 3-0 Vicryl in an interrupted fashion. The skin was closed using staples. The patient tolerated the procedure well. An x-ray was performed at the conclusion of the case because the count was incomplete prior to beginning the procedure. There were no foreign bodies identified by Radiology. The patient was taken to the recovery room in stable condition.

Principal diagnosis code(s):

_____

Procedure code(s):

_____

Title of Operation

Diagnostic laparoscopy and right salpingo-oophorectomy.

Indications for Surgery

The patient is a 10-year-old female, gravid 0, para 0 with a history of a right adnexal mass. She reports the history of right lower quadrant pain for approximately 24 hours. She was evaluated in an outside hospital. CT scan and abdominal ultrasound demonstrated a right adnexal mass. She was transferred for further evaluation. Ultrasound was performed. The study demonstrated an enlarged right adnexal mass consistent with torsion of the right ovary. Although there had been flow detected in the mass on the outside studies, flow is no longer seen. An area is noted consistent with the fallopian tube. The uterus and left ovary are normal. Given the findings, her mother consented for us to perform a diagnostic laparoscopy, possible right ovarian cystectomy, possible right salpingo-oophorectomy, possible staging, and possible open procedure. The risks, benefits, indications of the procedure were reviewed. Questions were answered. Options were discussed. Her mother consented for us to proceed.

Preoperative Diagnosis

Right lower quadrant pain, probably torsed right ovary.

Postoperative Diagnosis

Torsion of right tube and ovary with evidence of necrosis.

Anesthesia

General endotracheal.

Specimen (Bacteriologic, Pathologic, or Other)

Right tube and ovary.

Surgeon's Narrative

Estimated Blood Loss: Minimal.

Complications: None.

Drains: Foley catheter.

Procedure in Detail: The patient was brought to the Operating Room, and after the induction of adequate anesthesia, was placed in the dorsal lithotomy position in Yellowfin stirrups. Rectal examination revealed approximately 5-cm mass posterior to the uterus. The mass extended to the right. She was prepped and draped in the usual sterile fashion. A Foley catheter had been placed in the Emergency Room.

Initially, performed a diagnostic laparoscopy. A 5-mm infraumbilical incision was made. A Veress needle was placed. A pneumoperitoneum was achieved. A 5-mm trocar was placed and positioned within the peritoneal cavity, confirmed with laparoscope. The umbilical trocar was ultimately upsized to 10 mm. Then 5-mm trocars were placed in the right and left lower quadrants under direct visualization. The liver and diaphragm surfaces were without lesion. The gallbladder was without lesion. The stomach and omentum were without lesion. The appendix appears to be retrocecal. The left tube and ovary were within normal limits. The uterus was within normal limits. An approximately 6-cm mass was noted on the right. The right tube and ovary were

374

torsed. The right ovary and distal portion of the right tube appeared necrotic. The right tube and ovary were detorsed. After approximately 5 minutes, there was no evidence of improvement in the appearance of the right tube and ovary. The decision was made to proceed with the right salpingo-oophorectomy.

The broad ligament was opened. Retroperitoneal space was developed. The ureter was identified and traced throughout the course of the pelvis. The right infundibulopelvic vessels were ligated and cut with LigaSure. The right adnexa was mobilized. The right fallopian tube and right uteroovarian ligaments were ligated and cut with LigaSure. The right tube and ovary were placed in an EndoCatch bag and the specimens were removed through the umbilical incision. The intraoperative pathology demonstrated no evidence of malignancy.

The abdomen and pelvis were irrigated with copious amounts of warm saline. Hemostasis remained adequate. The pneumoperitoneum was released. Hemostasis remained adequate. All instruments were removed on direct visualization. The fascia of the umbilical site was closed with interrupted stitches of 2-0 Vicryl. The subcutaneous tissue was reapproximated with 4-0 Vicryl. The skin was reapproximated with subcuticular stitch of 4-0 Biosyn. Dressings were applied. All sponge, needle, and instrument counts were correct ×2. The patient was taken in stable condition to the recovery room.

Principal diagnosis code(s):

_____

Procedure code(s):

_____

35. CASE STUDY

Title of Operation

Total thyroidectomy for a substernal goiter.

Autotransplantation of left upper parathyroid gland.

Intraoperative nerve monitoring.

Indications for Surgery

Clinical Note: This patient had been diagnosed with a multinodular goiter with compressive symptoms. Needle aspiration biopsies were most consistent with adenomatoid nodules and lymphocytic thyroiditis. Due to the interval growth of her goiter and compressive symptoms, thyroidectomy was recommended, and the patient was accepting of this recommendation. The risks of the procedure, including bleeding, infection, nerve injury, hypoparathyroidism, voice change, and the requirement for a cervical skin incision, were explained to the patient, and she wished to proceed.

Preoperative Diagnosis

Multinodular goiter with compressive symptoms.

Postoperative Diagnosis

Multinodular goiter with compressive symptoms.

Anesthesia

GETA

Total thyroidectomy

Operative Findings: A total thyroidectomy was performed in standard fashion without complication. Both recurrent laryngeal nerves were identified with the aid of the nerve stimulator and stimulated normally at the completion of the procedure. The left upper parathyroid gland was in a subcapsular anterior position and could not be preserved in its blood supply. Thus, a small portion of it was sent for confirmatory biopsy, and it was subsequently autotransplanted into the sternocleidomastoid muscle.

Details of the Procedure: With the patient in the supine position and the neck extended, the skin was prepped and draped in standard fashion. A cervical skin incision was fashioned and superior and inferior skin flaps raised. The superficial layer of the deep cervical fascia was incised in the midline and the strap muscles dissected off the left lobe of the thyroid. The lobe was markedly enlarged and nodular. The lobe was retracted medially. The middle thyroid vein was ligated and divided between 3-0 silk ties. The left recurrent laryngeal nerve was identified in the tracheoesophageal groove with the aid of the nerve stimulator and carefully preserved. The left lower parathyroid gland was dissected laterally off the thyroid. The superior pole vessels on the left side were then ligated and divided between 0 silk ties with dissection proceeding lateral to the cricothyroid muscle directly on the upper pole of the thyroid to preserve the external branch of the superior laryngeal nerve. The lobe was then retracted further medially, and the left upper parathyroid was noted to be in a subcapsular position and very anterior, and it was clear that it could not be preserved laterally on its blood supply. Thus, this gland was resected, a small piece sent for confirmatory frozen section, and the remainder stored on iced saline for subsequent autotransplantation.

Following this, the recurrent laryngeal nerve was then re-identified and traced to its distal insertion, carefully preserved with secondary branches of the inferior thyroid artery, and ligated and divided between 3-0 silk ties, as were several small inferior thyroid veins. With the nerve in clear view, the ligament of Berry was divided using bipolar electrocautery, and dissection was continued beneath the left lobe of the thyroid and the isthmus. We next mobilize the strap muscles off of the right lobe of the thyroid. The lobe was retracted medially. The middle thyroid vein was ligated and divided between 3-0 silk ties. The right recurrent laryngeal nerve was identified deep in the neck with the aid of the nerve stimulator and carefully preserved. A capsular dissection technique was then used to dissect the right lower parathyroid laterally off the thyroid. The superior pole vessels on the right side were then ligated and divided between 0 silk ties with dissection proceeding lateral to the cricothyroid muscle directly on the upper pole of the thyroid to preserve the external branch of the superior laryngeal nerve. The lobe was then retracted further medially and the right upper parathyroid gland dissected laterally off the thyroid. The recurrent nerve was then re-identified and traced to is distal insertion, carefully preserved with the secondary branches of the inferior thyroid artery, and ligated and divided between 3-0 silk ties, as were several small inferior thyroid veins. With the nerve in the clear view, the ligament of Berry was divided using bipolar electrocautery, and dissection was continued beneath the right lobe and isthmus until the total thyroidectomy specimen was now free and handed off for pathologic evaluation.

Meticulous hemostasis was then assured in the left and right neck and both recurrent laryngeal nerves re-stimulated with a nerve stimulator and found to stimulate normally. Following this, the strap muscles were closed with a running 3-0 Biosyn suture. A small pocket was then created in the left sternocleidomastoid muscle, and the parathyroid tissue, which had been stored in iced saline, was finally minced and deposited into this pocket, which was closed with a 3-0 Prolene suture and marked with a clip. Following this, the platysma muscle was closed with interrupted 3-0 Biosyn sutures, and the skin was closed with a running 4-0 subcuticular Biosyn suture and Steri-Strips applied.

Estimated blood loss during the procedure was minimal. There were no complications. Sponge, needle, and instrument counts were correct, and the patient was transported to the recovery room in stable condition.

Principal diagnosis code(s):

_____

Procedure code(s):

_____

36. CASE STUDY

Title of Operation

Right frontal burr hole, endoscopic third ventriculostomy.

Indications for Surgery

The patient is a 6-year-old with a history of aqueductal stenosis. She recently has had episodes concerning for a seizure activity. Her EEG was confirmatory. She was recently placed on antiepileptic medications. The MRI evaluation revealed evidence of hydrocephalus from aqueductal stenosis. She is therefore being brought to the Operating Room for an endoscopic third ventriculostomy. The risks and indications of the procedure were discussed with legal guardians prior to the surgery and informed consent was obtained.

Preoperative Diagnosis

Obstructive hydrocephalus.

Postoperative Diagnosis

Obstructive hydrocephalus.

Anesthesia

General.

Specimen (Bacteriologic, Pathologic, or Other)

None.

Prosthetic Device/Implant

None.

Surgeon's Narrative

Estimated Blood Loss: 10 cubic centimeters.

Operative Findings: Stenosis of the aqueduct visualized. We created a ventriculostomy on the floor of the third ventricle and opening in Liliequist's membrane for visualization of the prepontine cistern.

Description of the Procedure: The patient was brought to the Operating Room and general endotracheal anesthesia was induced. She was then placed in the supine position with the head on a horseshoe head rest and in the flexed position. We then prepared for a right frontal burr hole, which was about 1 cm in front of the coronal suture in the midpupillary line. We shaved the hair and prepared for a linear incision. We then prepped and draped the skin in the sterile fashion. We injected local anesthesia. With a 15-blade knife, we made an incision in the skin. Then we used Bovie cautery to dissect down to the pericranium. We reflected the pericranium and placed a self-retaining retractor. We then used an acorn bit on the Anspach drill. We created a burr hole without incident. We then used a curette and Kerrison punches to widen the burr hole. We used bipolar cautery and coagulated the surface of the dura. Then, we used a knife and opened the dura in a cruciate fashion. We did have some dural bleeding from the left edge. In the end, we extended the opening of the burr hole to the left and controlled this bleeding successfully using bipolar cautery. We then coagulated the surface cortical vein. Then, we made a small opening in the cortex using bipolar cautery. We then inserted 14-French peel-away sheath with a trocar and placed it through the cortex toward the ventricle. We then peeled away the plastic and stapled it down to the drapes. We had brisk outflow of CSF. Then, we introduced our endoscope. Through the scope, we visualized the widened foramen of Monro. We then advanced through the foramen and visualized the floor of the third ventricle. In the posterior direction, we also visualized the posterior commissure and the stenotic aqueduct of Sylvius. We then found a thinned membrane in the front of the mamillary bodies. We advanced our endoscope and inserted a biopsy forceps through the membrane and opened the jaws of the forceps to widen the opening. Beyond the opening, we did visualize an arachnoid membrane consistent with Liliequists's membrane. We did visualize some pulsations on the floor of the third ventricle. With this maneuver, we had then made an opening in the Liliequist's membrane. Past the membrane, we advanced the endoscope and visualized the prepontine cistern along with pontine perforators and the basilar artery. We then withdrew the endoscope into the third ventricle and visualized bounding pulsations on the floor of the third ventricle and we were comfortable with our opening. We withdrew our endoscope into the lateral ventricle and did not visualize any spontaneous bleeding. We withdrew our endoscope completely. Then, down the peel-away sheath, we placed a rolled up piece of Gelfoam. We removed the sheath with the Gelfoam in place. We irrigated the wound with copious amounts of saline. Next, we placed a piece of Gelform in the burr hole. We then closed the incision with an interrupted 3-0 Vicryl sewn in an inverted fashion in the galea. Then, we closed the skin with a running Caprosyn suture. The incision was sealed with Histoacryl. Then, the drapes were removed and the patient was extubated and transported into the recovery room in stable condition.

Principal diagnosis code(s):

_____

Procedure code(s):

_____

Electrophysiology Procedure Report

Procedure Performed

- Upper extremity venogram
- Vascular access
- PPM/ICD system revision

History

The patient is a 75-year-old man with ischemic cardiomyopathy (EF 15%), history of PCI and monomorphic ventricular tachycardia who underwent BiV ICD implantation in May 2005. Routine device interrogation noted 8 episodes of ATP for NSVT. Examination of electrograms revealed a high frequency signal in the right ventricular sensing channel. EP study demonstrated an abnormal RV pacing/defibrillating lead; however, new lead insertion was unsuccessful given significant left subclavian vein stenosis. The patient is referred for repeat attempt of RV pacing/defibrillating lead implantation with possible extraction of the abnormally functioning RV lead.

Procedure Description

After the usual sterile prep and drape, the site was locally anesthetized and vascular sheath(s) were inserted as described below.

After written, informed consent was obtained, the patient was brought to the Electrophysiology Laboratory. An intravenous infusion of prophylactic antibiotic was begun. The device site was extensively prepped with an antibiotic soap and disinfectant, and draped appropriately. Following infiltration with 1% lidocaine, an incision was made immediately superior to the upper margin of the old generator, taking care to avoid the leads. Using blunt and sharp dissection, the incision was extended down to the generator and the generator and leads were dissected free of adhesions. Lead and device testing and revision were performed as described below. Any new or revised leads advanced into the cardiac chambers under fluoroscopy and secure locations were found. Such leads were sutured to the underlying pectoral muscle with interrupted 2-0 silk sutures over a plastic collar. After, revision lead thresholds were found to be satisfactory. A generator was connected to the leads and found to perform appropriately. After irrigation with antibiotic solution, the pocket was inspected and no bleeding was seen. The generator was inserted into the pocket and the wound was closed with subcutaneous sutures. A pressure dressing was applied.

The attending physician performed the procedure and interpreted the results.

Impressions:
1. Biventricular pacing at baseline.
2. Excellent parameters on all leads.
3. Venogram showed tight stenosis at left subclavian vein.
4. Access to lateral left subclavian vein was achieved without difficulty.
5. With great difficulty, a 0.035 glide wire passed through LSCV and innominate vein steonsis.
6. Van Andel straight diagnostic catheter was placed over the glide wire and past the stenosis.
7. The wire was then upgraded to an Amplatz Super Stiff wire.
8. Serial dilation to 12F dilator was performed (long).
9. 9F peel away long sheath successfully inserted.

10. New active fixation RV lead (defib) placed to RV apical septum with moderate difficulty.
11. DFT = 17J
12. All lead parameters stable.

Recommendations:
1. Maintain head of bed to 60 degrees.
2. CXR and device interrogation in the morning.
3. Continue prophylactic antibiotics with cefazolin and vancomycin for 24 hours. Tomorrow afternoon, change antibiotics to keflex 500 mg po qid × 3 days.
4. Maintain pressure dressing. Site should remain dry for 3 days.
5. Resume all other oral medications. Avoid heparin or lovenox.
6. Please page with any questions.

Complications

No immediate complications were appreciated.

Procedure Data

CASE MEDICATIONS

Cefazolin	1 g	iv
Fentanyl	500 mcg	iv
Midazolam	23 mg	iv
Vancomycin	1 g	iv

CONTRAST

Visipaque: 45.0 cc, Vascular

VITAL SIGNS

	Pre-case	Post-case
Pulse beats/min	68	72
SBP (auto cuff) mm Hg	118	128
DBP (auto cuff) mm Hg	80	63
Respiration rate	18	16
Arterial O$_2$ sat %	97	96

Devices

GENERATOR

	Implanted	Explanted
Manufacturer	Guidant	Guidant
Model	H210	H170
Serial #	309063	400151
Implanted By	_____	_____
Type	Bi-ventricular ICD	Bi-ventricular ICD

Lead

	Implanted	Pre-existing Acti	Pre-existing Acti	Deactivated
Manufacturer	Guidant	Guidant	Guidant	Guidant
Model	0158	1688	4537	1581
Serial #	160098	DN288694	154017	RH28177
Implanted By	_____	_____	_____	_____
Implant Date	2007-05-01 14:00:00.0	2004-05-24 00:00:00.0	2004-05-24 00:00:00.0	2004-05-24 00:00:00:.0
Type	Pace + defibrillating	Pacing	Pacing	Pacing + defibrillating
Location	Right ventricle	Right atrium	Coronary sinus	Right ventricle

Upper Extremity Venogram

Tight stenoses of left subclavian vein and innominate vein were visualized, with extensive collaterialization.

Vascular Access

Vessel: Vein-subclavian
Access Type: Pocket puncture
Sheath Count: 1

Vessel Side: Left
Sheath Size: 9.0
Vascular Closure: Manual compression

Guidance Methods, Needles, and Wires

Guidance method: Angiography/venography - successful.

PPM/ICD System Revision

Indication(s)

Primary Indication: Complication/failure of ICD or lead

Summary Findings

	Observation
Qualifiers	Implanted bi-ventricular ICD generator, explanted bi-ventricular ICD generator, implanted right ventricle pace + debfibrillating lead, preexisting active right atrium pacing lead, preexisting active coronary sinus pacing lead, deactivated right ventricle pace + defibrillating lead
Main reason for revision	Other (see history)
Primary finding/diagnosis	Sensing unacceptable
Primary treatment	Lead replaced
Old generator type	BiV dual-chamber ICD
Original generator location	Left infraclavicular
Old vs. new generator implant	New-EOL/ERI replacement
New generator type	BiV dual-chamber ICD
Final generator location	Left infraclavicular
Culprit lead	Ventricular
Venogram?	Yes
Intra-procedural antibiotic	Vancomycin

Revision Procedures (in order)

	Obs #1	Obs #2	Obs #3	Obs #4
Qualifiers	Explanted bi-ventricular ICD generator	Implanted right ventricle pace + defibrillating lead	Deactivated right ventricle pace + defibrillating lead	
Procedure	Generator explanted	New lead(s) implanted	Lead(s) capped	Generator implanted
Procedure successful?	Yes	Yes	Yes	Yes

Generator Pacing Parameters

	Observation
Qualifiers	Implanted bi-ventricular ICD generator
Pacing mode	DDDR
Lower rate limit bpm	70
Upper rate limit bpm	130
Mode switching	On

Leads

	Obs #1	Obs #2	Obs #3
Qualifiers	Preexisting active right atrium pacing lead	Preexisting active coronary sinus pacing lead	Implanted right ventricle pace + defibrillating lead
Lead type	Old	Old	New implant
Lead status	Active	Active	Active
Insertion site	Left axillary	Left axillary	Left axillary
Tunneled?	No	No	No
Vascular access method			Puncture
Number of access attempts			4
Fixation method			Active
Number of fixation attempts			1
P/R wave amplitude mV	1.20	13.00	11.00
Threshold at 0.5 msec V	0.8	0.4	1.0
Impedance ohms	398	612	550
Polarity	Bipolar	Bipolar	Bipolar
Output V	2.40	2.40	3.50
Pulse width (msec)	0.50	0.50	0.50
Sensitivity (mV)	0.75	2.50	2.50

	Obs #1	Obs #2
Qualifiers	Implanted bi-ventricular ICD generator	Implanted bi-ventricular ICD generator
Induction method	Shock on T wave	Shock on T wave
Rhythm induced	Ventricular fibrillation	Ventricular fibrillation
Shock polarity	Standard	Standard
Anode	RV	RV

Cathode	SVC/Can	SVC/Can
Energy delivered J	17.0	11.0
Shock impedance ohms	38	37
Resulting rhythm	Sinus	VF
Rescue mode		Internal ICD shock
Rescue energy J		21

FINAL DEFIBRILLATION THRESHOLD

Observation

Qualifiers	Implanted bi-ventricular ICD generator, implanted right ventricle pace + defibrillating lead
Defibrillation threshold J	17.0
DFT adequacy	Adequate
Shock impedance ohms	38
Lead configuration	RV to SVC/Can

FINAL ZONE SETTINGS

	Obs #1	**Obs #2**
Qualifiers	Implanted bi-ventricular ICD generator, implanted right ventricle pace + defibrillating lead	Implanted bi-ventricular ICD generator, implanted right ventricle pace + defibrillating lead
Zone	1	2
Rate cutoff bpm	150	185
Tier 1 therapy	ATP	27 J
Tier 2 therapy	27 J	31 J
Tier ≥3 therapy	31 J × 3	31 J × 3

Principal diagnosis code(s):

_____

Procedure code(s):

_____